Mammalian Sexuality

The Act of Mating and the Evolution of Reproduction

There are more than 6000 species belonging to 27 orders in the Class Mammalia. Comparative studies of this diverse and magnificent array of extant species provide valuable opportunities to formulate and test hypotheses concerning the evolution of reproduction. This is the first book to explore, in depth and breadth, the complex interrelationships that exist between patterns of mating behaviour and the evolution of mammalian reproductive anatomy and physiology. It focuses upon the role that copulatory and post-copulatory sexual selection have played during the evolution of the monotremes, marsupials and placental mammals, and examines the effects of sperm competition and cryptic female choice upon coevolution of the genitalia in the two sexes. In addition, due weight is also given to discussions of the modes of life of mammals, and to the roles played by natural selection and phylogeny in determining their reproductive traits.

Alan F. Dixson is a Professor in the School of Biological Sciences at Victoria University of Wellington, New Zealand. His research has involved comparative studies of reproductive biology and the evolution of sexuality in primates and other mammals. During a distinguished career, he has held posts at the Zoological Society of London (1976–1983), Medical Research Council UK (1983–1999), International Medical Research Centre in Gabon (1989–1992), Sub-Department of Animal Behaviour, University of Cambridge (1993–1998) and was Director of Conservation and Science at the Zoological Society of San Diego in the USA (1999–2005). He has authored, or co-authored, more than 160 papers and books, including *The Mandrill: A Case of Extreme Sexual Selection* (Cambridge, 2015).

Mammalian Sexuality

The Act of Mating and the Evolution of Reproduction

ALAN F. DIXSON DSc
School of Biological Sciences
Victoria University of Wellington
New Zealand

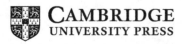

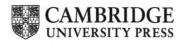

Shaftesbury Road, Cambridge CB2 8EA, United Kingdom

One Liberty Plaza, 20th Floor, New York, NY 10006, USA

477 Williamstown Road, Port Melbourne, VIC 3207, Australia

314–321, 3rd Floor, Plot 3, Splendor Forum, Jasola District Centre, New Delhi – 110025, India

103 Penang Road, #05–06/07, Visioncrest Commercial, Singapore 238467

Cambridge University Press is part of Cambridge University Press & Assessment, a department of the University of Cambridge.

We share the University's mission to contribute to society through the pursuit of education, learning and research at the highest international levels of excellence.

www.cambridge.org
Information on this title: www.cambridge.org/9781108426183

DOI: 10.1017/9781108550758

First published 2021

A catalogue record for this publication is available from the British Library

ISBN   978-1-108-42618-3   Hardback

To Amanda

In your heart my thoughts are born,
In your spirit the source of my words is found.
(Translated from *The Letters of Michelangelo*)

Contents

Preface

This is the first book about mammals that explores, in depth and breadth, the complex interrelationships that exist between their patterns of mating behaviour and the evolution of reproductive anatomy and physiology. It deals with the role played by copulatory and post-copulatory sexual selection, during the evolution of the monotremes, marsupials and placental mammals. Due weight is also given to discussions of the modes of life of mammals, and to the effects of natural selection and phylogeny in determining their reproductive traits.

There are more than 6000 extant species representing 27 orders of mammals. Comparative studies of this diverse and magnificent array of species provide biologists with valuable opportunities to formulate and test hypotheses concerning the evolution of mammalian reproduction. However, to make the most of such opportunities, a broad approach is required, one that gives proper weight to insights derived from research on copulatory behaviour and mating systems, as well as reproductive biology and evolution.

I count myself fortunate, because the seeds of this multidisciplinary approach have indeed germinated, and flowered, during the course of my own career as a zoologist. This process began in 1970 with the publication of Geoffrey Parker's ground-breaking insights concerning sperm competition. Gradually this new field of enquiry expanded and it is now well established that competition between the gametes of rival males for access to a given set of ova has been crucial to the evolution of reproduction in many groups of animals. Moreover, recognition of the phenomenon of cryptic female choice, initially by Thornhill and subsequently by Eberhard in the 1980s, has focused attention upon the potential for the female's behaviour, reproductive anatomy and physiology to influence which male's gametes are most likely to gain access to ova.

Much of the research on post-copulatory sexual selection has involved arthropods and other invertebrates, but there has been a steady increase in the number of studies devoted to vertebrate taxa. The results of work on mammals are still largely confined to specialist journals, however. In addition to these publications, there is a widely scattered literature dealing with mammalian copulatory behaviour, and a huge fund of knowledge concerning the reproductive anatomy and physiology of monotremes, marsupials and placental mammals. My goal has been to create a synthesis of this material, thus making it readily accessible to research workers and to students. If the book achieves this goal, then the four years it took to write will have been time well spent.

Acknowledgements

I am most grateful to the organizations and individuals listed below, for permission to reproduce figures, tables and photographs, either in their original form or as redrawn and modified versions.

Acta Zoologica Sinica: Figure 5.20 upper; *American Psychological Association*: Figure 3.2; *John Anderton*: Figure 2.21; *Cambridge University Press*: Figures 3.7, 3.8A,C, 6.9, 7.5, 8.2B, 8.8 upper, 8.11, 8.18 upper and Table 8.1; *CSIRO Publishing*: Figures 2.5, 5.15, 8.3 and 8.17; *Professor Charles Daugherty*: Figure 2.11D; *De Gruyter*: Figure 5.6; *Dr Jim Dines*: Figure 5.5; *Amanda Dixson*: Figures 2.6A,C,D,E, 2.9, 2.13D and 2.22C; *Edinburgh University Press*: Figure 2.21; *Elsevier Ltd*: Figures 3.3, 5.22B, 5.23, 5.24B, 6.10A,D, 6.16, 7.2C, 7.3 upper, 7.9, 7.10B, 8.2A, 8.4, 8.10, 8.15, 8.16 and 9.3 upper; *Entomological Society of America*: Figure 8.12A; *Fieldiana Zoology*: Figure 5.8; *Gustav Fischer Verlag*: Figures 5.1B and 5.14; *Johns Hopkins University Press*: Figures 2.10 and 2.25; *Karger Publishers*: Figures 2.20, 5.20 lower, 5.24D, 7.6, 7.8 and Table 6.4; *Dr William Keener*: Figure 5.6; *Landsdowne Press*: Figure 2.3; *Dr Elizabeth Miller and colleagues*: Figure 8.13; *Museums and Art Galleries of the Northern Territory*: Figure 5.3B; *Oxford University Press*: Figures 3.1B, 3.9B, 4.1, 4.2, 5.1D,E, 5.4, 5.17, 5.24C, 6.3, 6.7, 7.2A,B, 7.3 lower, 7.7, 7.10D,E, 8.1, 8.2C, 10.1 and Tables 4.3 and 7.1; *Pesquiza Veterinária Brasileira*: Figure 5.16; *PLoS*: Figures 5.1C, 6.15 and 6.17; *Princeton University Press*: Figure 7.10C; *Royal Society Publishing*: Figures 5.2, 5.7, 5.13 and 6.5; *Shutterstock*: Figures 2.2, 2.6B, 2.7, 2.8, 2.11A,B,C,E,F, 2.12, 2.13A,B,C, 2.14, 2.15, 2.16, 2.17, 2.18, 2.19, 2.22A,B,D and 2.24; *Society for Reproduction and Fertility*: Figures 6.6A, 6.10B, 6.14, 7.4, 8.20 lower and 8.22; *Society for the Study of Reproduction*: Figures 5.12 lower, 5.25 and 9.3 lower; *Springer*: Figures 4.5, 8.6 and 8.8; *Springer Nature*: Figures 2.23, 2.26 and 7.11; *Georg Thieme*: Figure 6.8; *University of Chicago Press*: Figures 2.25, 3.1A, 5.15A, 6.1 and 8.14; *University of Utah*: Figure 5.3A; *Professor Frans de Waal*: Figure 3.9C; *Jenny Wardrip*: Figure 3.9A; *Wiley*: Figures 3.8D, 4.4, 5.1G, 5.10, 5.11, 5.21, 5.24A, 5.26 upper, 6.2, 6.4, 6.6B,E, 6.11, 6.13, 8.9A, 8.18 and Table 6.1; *Williams and Wilkins Co.*: Figure 7.1; *Dr Pat Woolley and the Royal Society of New South Wales*: Figure 5.9; *Zoological Society of London*: Figures 5.1F, 6.10C, 6.12, 7.10A, 8.9B, 8.19 lower and 9.2.

Part I

Carnival of the Animals

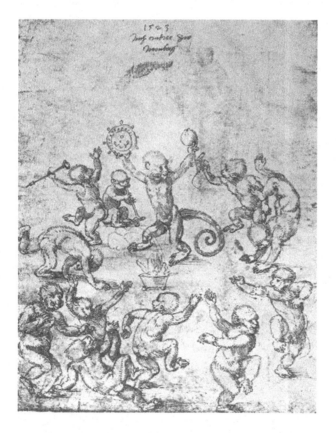

The Monkey Dance
Albrecht Durer, 1523

1 Quo Vadis?

One of the great joys of biology is the realization that there is no end of wonders to discover, to describe, and to attempt to understand.

Janet Leonard (2010)

Representatives of the Class Mammalia are to be found on every continent, and in every ocean of the world. They comprise a handful of extraordinary egg-laying species (the monotremes), as well as 7 orders of marsupials and 19 orders of placental mammals. Phylogeny, and modes of life, as well as sexual selection (via sperm competition and cryptic female choice) have all profoundly influenced mammalian reproductive biology. The reproductive adaptations of these animals have been forged over vast spans of time, beginning some 297–252 million years ago, during the Permian Period, when one branch of the synapsid reptiles (the Therapsida) gave rise to the furry, warm-blooded forerunners of the Class Mammalia (Kemp, 2005). Some therapsids survived a major extinction event that occurred at the close of the Permian; their modern descendants include the echidnas, kangaroos and possums, elephants, whales, rodents, bats and primates, as well as a host of other taxa.

Post-copulatory sexual selection is a relatively new addition to the field of evolutionary biology. This type of selection was unknown to Charles Darwin when he wrote *The Origin of Species* (1859) and *Sexual Selection and the Descent of Man* (1871). At that time, and for almost a century after his death, sexual selection was thought to operate solely with respect to events that take place before the act of mating. Inter-male competition for access to females, and female mate choices for the most attractive males, were viewed as the major drivers by which sexual selection influences individual reproductive success. All this began to change, however, once Geoffrey Parker (1970) had identified the phenomenon of sperm competition, and William Eberhard (1985, 1996) expanded discussions of post-copulatory sexual selection to embrace the concept of cryptic female choice.

The potential for sperm competition arises when a fertile female mates with two or more males. In mammals, sperm competition is usually limited to the 'fertile phase' of the ovarian cycle, during which ovulation occurs and ova are transported to the oviducts prior to fertilization. In some mammals, copulation itself induces ovulation to occur, but sperm competition is still possible if more than one male succeeds in mating with the same partner during the critical phase when fertilization is possible.

However, multiple-partner matings during non-ovulatory periods are not conducive to sperm competition, except in unusual circumstances (e.g. when females store sperm from multiple males, and fertilization is delayed, as happens in some species of bats). These examples serve as indicators that it is the female's reproductive tract and her physiological responses that determine the conditions under which sperm competition and fertilization take place. In mammals, as in other amniotes, spermatozoa must traverse multiple anatomical and physiological sieves and barriers within the female's reproductive system before gaining access to her ova. Therefore, the female's anatomy and physiology might also influence the fate of gametes from rival males in different ways. It is this hidden potential that constitutes cryptic female choice.

These novel insights concerning post-copulatory sexual selection are the fruits of research conducted initially on insects. The discovery of sperm competition thus owes much to the yellow dung fly (*Scathophaga stercoraria*, Parker, 1970), whilst the concept of cryptic female choice derives from work on scorpion flies (*Harpobittacus nigriceps*, Thornhill, 1983). Indeed, since the 1980s, research on invertebrate taxa has continued to expand apace, whereas investigations of mammalian post-copulatory sexual selection have progressed much more slowly. This may be due, in part, to the practical difficulties inherent in conducting experiments on mammals. However, it is also the case that many mammalian reproductive physiologists were initially unaware of the invertebrate literature, or failed to appreciate its wider significance. That is no longer the case, and much has been accomplished to advance knowledge of post-copulatory sexual selection in mammals and in other vertebrate groups. Dobzhansky's dictum, that 'nothing in biology makes sense except in the light of evolution', most assuredly applies to mammalian reproductive physiology, just as it does to other branches of the biological sciences.

Thus, although reproductive physiologists have traditionally concentrated on tackling a host of complex proximate questions, such as the control of spermatogenesis, or the biochemistry of sperm and ova, in the nine chapters that follow my goal is to address the ultimate questions about the role played by copulatory behaviour, and by post-copulatory sexual selection, during mammalian evolution. Are the copulatory patterns displayed by male mammals subject to sexual selection, and how did they evolve in the various mammalian lineages? Phallic morphology exhibits considerable diversity, in some cases between closely related taxa. Why should this be the case? Why do mammals have such a complex and variable array of accessory reproductive glands, and what roles might their secretions play during post-copulatory sexual selection? What effects have sperm competition and cryptic female choice had upon the coevolution of the reproductive systems of both sexes, and how far might sexual conflict, as well as cooperation between the sexes, have influenced these matters? How did mating-induced and spontaneous patterns of ovulation come to exhibit their current phylogenetic distributions among the mammals?

With these questions in mind, Part II of this book focuses on the evolution of patterns of mammalian copulatory behaviour. Chapter 3 presents a phylogenetic analysis of mating behaviour, and examines the impact of modes of life and of natural selection upon copulatory traits in the Mammalia. Chapter 4 serves as an introduction to the concepts of copulatory courtship and post-copulatory sexual selection. This chapter also reviews current knowledge of the prevalence (or absence) of multiple-partner matings by mammals that have primarily polygynandrous, polygynous or monogamous mating systems. Part III comprises five chapters that explore connections between copulatory and post-copulatory sexual selection and the evolution of mammalian reproductive anatomy and physiology. Chapters 5–7 deal with the diversity of phallic structure and function, the testes and spermatozoa, and the accessory reproductive glands and ducts. Chapter 8 focuses on the anatomy and physiology of the female reproductive system in relation to mechanisms of cryptic choice and copulatory courtship. Chapter 9 considers the origins and evolution of mating-induced and spontaneous ovulation in female mammals. Part IV presents conclusions and suggestions for future research in this field, as well as a discussion of its relevance to understanding the evolution of human reproduction. I shall also say something about the decline of mammalian diversity, due to human overpopulation and the continued destruction of the planet's ecosystems.

Before embarking upon these tasks, however, it is essential to establish a firm basis for the comparative discussions of reproductive biology that follow. To this end, Chapter 2 reviews phylogenetic relationships between the various groups of extant mammals, and provides readers with an introduction to the enormous diversity displayed by the Class Mammalia.

2 Mammalian Classification and Evolution

Questions regarding character evolution among living mammals now have the decisive advantage of a relatively well-resolved tree.

Asher, Bennett and Lehmann (2009)

The last 25 years have seen significant developments in the fields of mammalian classification and evolutionary biology. Molecular genetic techniques have increasingly been applied to test traditional classifications that were based upon fossil evidence and comparative anatomical studies of extant taxa. As well as confirming many of the established tenets of mammalian classification, some fresh insights have emerged as a result of these endeavours. The following brief review of the phylogeny and basic biology of the 27 extant orders of mammals is designed to provide the reader with a sound basis for the discussions of copulatory behaviour, reproductive biology and evolution that unfold in the ensuing chapters.

How Many Species of Mammals Are There?

It might be imagined that all the various kinds of mammals were discovered long ago. In 1970, at the beginning of my research career, I thought that all the lemurs, monkeys and apes must be known to science. Surely, no new primates could remain concealed in the world's diminishing rainforests? Happily, I was wrong, and new species, not only of primates, but also of many other types of mammals, have steadily come to light during the last 50 years. In 1982 there were considered to be 4170 extant species of mammals, but this tally had risen to 5341 by the time that the third edition of *Mammal Species of the World* was published (Wilson and Reeder, 2005). A few years later, Schipper *et al.* (2008) included 5487 extant species in their analyses of mammalian diversity, and in 2018 Burgin *et al.* calculated that 6399 species of mammals currently exist (Table 2.1).

The number of species recognized by various authorities is affected by the penchant of taxonomists either to 'lump' taxa together or, more commonly, to 'split' existing taxa into separate species. Subspecies of certain well-known mammals are sometimes raised to specific rank, often on the basis of molecular genetic evidence. For example, the giraffe has long been been considered as a single species (*Giraffa camelopardalis*). However, a wide-ranging study of giraffe population genetics by Fennessy *et al.*

Table 2.1 Estimates of mammalian taxonomic diversity: 1982–2018 (based on Burgin *et al.*, 2018)

Taxa	1982	1993	2005	2017	2018
Orders	20	26	29	27	27
Families	135	132	153	159	167
Genera	1033	1135	1230	1267	1314
Species (extant)	4170	4631	5341	5475	6399

Data are from *Mammal Species of the World*, the IUCN Red List, and the Mammal Diversity Database (Burgin *et al.*, 2018).

(2016) led them to conclude that there are four species of giraffes. This has been disputed, however (Bercovitch *et al.*, 2017). Another example concerns an isolated population of orang-utans in a mountainous region in Sumatra that has been proposed to represent a new species (*Pongo tapanuliensis*: Nater *et al.*, 2017). Whether this truly is a new species or a subspecies of the Sumatran orang-utan (*P. abelii*) is debatable.

Yet, every so often, truly novel species of mammals come to light. Recent welcome surprises include a pygmy sloth (*Bradypus pygmaeus*) from Panamá (Anderson and Handley, 2001), new monkeys such as *Macaca munzala* from India (Sinha *et al.*, 2005) and the lesula (*Cercopithecus lomamiensis*) from the Democratic Republic of the Congo (Hart *et al.*, 2012), a previously unknown tapir (*Tapirus kabomani*) from the depths of the Amazon rainforest (Cuzzuol *et al.*, 2013) and a tree hyrax from western Nigeria (Bearder *et al.*, 2015). A new river dolphin has been discovered in Brazil (*Inia araguaiaensis*: Hrbek *et al.*, 2014) and there is even a new beaked-whale species, belonging to the Genus *Berardius* (Morin *et al.*, 2017). Such discoveries are not evenly distributed across the mammalian phylogeny. Thus, 323 of the 408 new mammals (i.e. 84 per cent of new species) described between 1993 and 2009 were bats, rodents, primates, or small insectivorous species belonging to the Order Eulipotyphla (Ceballos and Ehrlich, 2009). The bats and rodents combined comprise 65 per cent of all mammalian species. The great diversity represented by these two orders, and the fact that molecular studies are revealing that cryptic species are often concealed among morphologically similar taxa, makes it likely that many more new species of bats and rodents have yet to be described.

Subclasses of the Mammalia

There are three subclasses of living mammals: Monotremata, Marsupialia and Placentalia. The marsupials and placental mammals derive from common ancestors belonging to the Theria, a mammalian group that diverged from the egg-laying ancestors of monotremes (Prototheria) at some time between 161 and 217 million years ago (Mya). The Theria subsequently became separated (143–178 Mya) into two lineages: the Metatheria, which gave rise to the marsupials, and the Eutheria, which gave rise to the 'crown group' Placentalia (Figure 2.1). The latter comprises all extant eutherian mammals as well as their common ancestor and all extinct taxa that also share that common ancestor. All of today's eutherians thus belong to the Placentalia but, as we shall see, most of the fossil stem eutherians, which existed during the Cretaceous Period (145–66 Mya), are not considered to be members of the crown group Placentalia.

The Placentalia is the most diverse and successful of the three subclasses of living mammals in terms of its worldwide distribution, as well as its taxonomic and ecological diversity. Placental mammals currently comprise about 6000 living species belonging to 19 orders. They include diminutive representatives such as the mice, shrews and insectivorous bats, as well as megafauna such as elephants, whales, bears, sea lions, apes, buffalos and a host of others. Most agricultural livestock, such as pigs, cattle and sheep, as well as domestic pets, such as dogs, cats and hamsters, also belong to the Placentalia. By contrast, the Marsupialia or pouched mammals are represented currently by 350+ species; 3 orders of these are found in South America, and 4 orders occur in Australia, on New Guinea and some small neighbouring islands. The third and most ancient subclass is represented by the single order Monotremata, which comprises just five species of remarkable egg-laying mammals that are confined to Australia and New Guinea. The following sections describe the members of these three subclasses, focusing on their phylogenetic relationships, evolution and general biology.

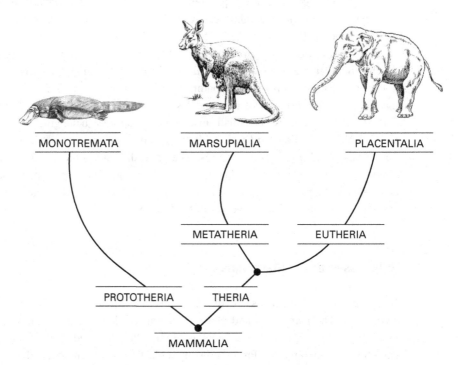

Figure 2.1 Phylogenetic relationships among the three subclasses of the Mammalia.

Subclass Monotremata

'Molecular clock' studies indicate that the earliest monotremes originated at some time between 161 and 217 Mya, during the Lower Jurassic (Phillips *et al.*, 2009). However, the earliest known fossil monotreme (*Teinolophus*) has been dated at 112–121 Mya, from the lower Cretaceous of Australia (Rich *et al.*, 2001). Both fossil and genetic evidence confirms that the monotremes were already established in Australia long before the arrival of marsupials there, at some time between 71 and 54.6 Mya (Beck, 2008; Godthelp *et al.*, 1992; Phillips *et al.*, 2009).

Only two types of echidna and a single species of the platypus have survived to the present day (Figure 2.2). The short-beaked echidna (*Tachyglossus aculeatus*) is very widely distributed throughout Australia. It is clothed in short hairs, interspersed with robust spines, and is equipped with long digging claws on its short, powerful limbs. The echidna is toothless, and it employs its long, sticky tongue to capture ants and other small invertebrates. Three species of a larger, long-beaked echidna, belonging to the Genus *Zaglossus*, occur on the Island of New Guinea. Long-beaked echidnas may weigh up to 15 kg, whereas adults of the short-beaked species vary from 2 to 7.5 kg in weight. Both types of echidna probably occurred in Australia until quite recently. This is known because a museum specimen of *Zaglossus bruijnii* originates from the Kimberley region of Western Australia; it was collected there in 1901 (Helgen *et al.*, 2012).

The extraordinary, amphibious, platypus (*Ornithorhynchus anatinus*) is the sole surviving representative of an ancient monotreme lineage. The limb bones and teeth of a platypus-like creature (*Monotrematum sudamericanum*), dated to approximately 61 Mya, have been discovered in Patagonia, and these fossils closely resemble those of a platypus (*Obdurodon*) which lived in Australia at around 25 Mya (Pascual *et al.*, 1992; Phillips *et al.*, 2009). Several species of *Obdurodon* have been described, and

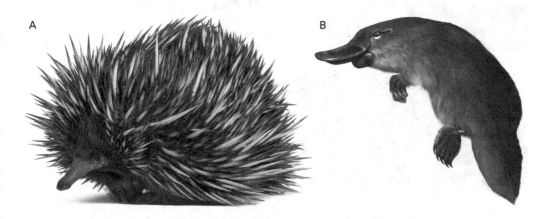

A   B

Figure 2.2 Australian monotremes. **A:** The short-beaked echidna (*Tachyglossus aculeatus*). **B:** The platypus (*Ornithorhynchus anatinus*). (Images: © Shutterstock.com.)

one of them was a giant of its kind, almost a metre in length and twice as large as today's platypus.

The distribution range of the platypus extends along the eastern seaboard of Australia, and includes the island of Tasmania in the south. It is found in rivers, lakes and streams, and is an adept swimmer, using its flattened, webbed forefeet for propulsion. The bill of the platypus is soft and leathery; it contains a battery of tactile and electro-receptors which assist the animal in locating the small aquatic invertebrates which form the bulk of its diet (Pettigrew, 1999). The adult is toothless, but a series of horny plates and ridges inside the bill allow it to grind up its food. The hind feet have claws and there is also a sharp hollow spur which, in adult males, receives the secretions of a venom gland situated in the thigh. The functions of these poison glands have been much debated. It is known that they enlarge during the breeding season, and they may play some role during inter-male competition, as males sometimes have puncture wounds in their tails at this time (Grant and Temple-Smith, 1998). Intra-sexual selection may also have influenced the evolution of body size in the platypus (adult males weigh 40 per cent more than females).

Like the echidna, the platypus is non-gregarious and each adult occupies its own burrow, close to the water's edge. During the breeding season the female platypus constructs a much longer burrow terminating in a nest chamber in which she deposits her eggs. Figure 2.3 shows the map of a platypus burrow made by Harry Burrell (1873–1945), a pioneering amateur naturalist and self-styled 'platypoditudinarian' who wrote an excellent book about his researches (Burrell, 1927). The female platypus usually lays two eggs in her nest chamber and incubates them for 1–2 weeks. Once they hatch, she feeds the young with milk from ducts that open directly onto the

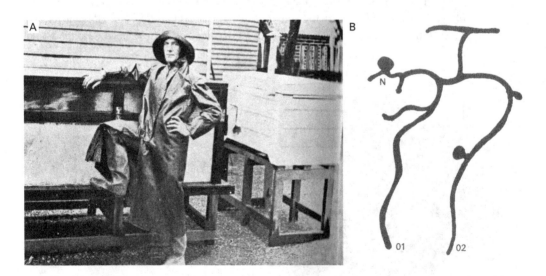

Figure 2.3 A: Harry Burrell (1873–1945), pictured beside his 'portable platypusary'. **B:** Map of a platypus breeding burrow, with two entrances (01 and 02). N = the female's nest chamber. (After Burrell, 1927.)

surface of her abdomen (female monotremes do not have nipples). Lactation lasts for 4–5 months, by which time the offspring are ready to leave the burrow.

The female echidna deposits her egg not in a nest chamber, but into a shallow, muscular pouch-like depression situated on her abdomen (Griffiths, 1998; Rismiller, 1999). Once hatched, the tiny offspring, which weighs barely one-third of a gram, remains in the pouch and begins to feed and to grow rapidly. Its body mass increases 100-fold during the first 14 days. The young echidna, which has been delightfully named the 'puggle' by field researchers (Rismiller, 1999) remains in the mother's pouch until it is between 50 and 60 days old. At this stage, the mother constructs a simple nursery burrow in which she leaves her offspring, but returns every 5 days in order to supply it with milk. The puggle feeds voraciously, increasing in body weight by up to 40 per cent during a single feed. By 3 months of age the infant is covered in soft hair, but short spines are also present. These emerge gradually and, by the time it is 7 months old, Rismiller records that the offspring has been weaned, and it weighs anywhere between 800 and 1300 g.

Despite obvious differences in their morphology and modes of life, the echidna and platypus share a great many anatomical traits, and they may be phylogenetically more closely related than was originally thought to be the case. The same kinds of specialized tactile and electro-receptors that have been identified in the bill of the platypus also occur, but at a lower density, in the beak of the echidna (Proske et al., 1998). There is a sharp spur on the back foot in both species, but it is atrophic in the echidna, and lacks the venom gland that is present in the male platypus. There are many skeletal similarities between these taxa and echidnas are also surprisingly good swimmers (Rismiller, 1999). Molecular genetic evidence now places the divergence between the echidna and platypus lineages at somewhere between 19 and 48 Mya (Phillips et al., 2009). These authors posit that echidnas 'had aquatically foraging ancestors that reinvaded terrestrial ecosystems'. These ancestors may have gained an ecological advantage when transitioning to terrestrial life by foraging on ants, because only one type of marsupial (the numbat) specializes in exploiting similar prey. The common ancestor of the platypus and echidna may also have prospered because it occupied a niche that was inaccessible to Australian marsupials, none of which is amphibious. Marsupial reproduction involves pouch infants remaining firmly attached to the mother's nipples for extended periods. These traits are not conducive to an aquatic life and, in fact, only one marsupial (the South American yapok) is known to forage in this way.

Some preliminary remarks are necessary regarding the reproductive organs of the monotremes. Given that all extant members of this infraorder reproduce by laying eggs, and that the platypus lineage is phylogenetically ancient, it seems likely that the Monotremata as a whole derives from oviparous ancestors (Temple-Smith and Grant, 2001). In the female echidna each ovary is enclosed within an infundibulum which leads to an oviduct, and uterus; both sides of the system open into a central urogenital sinus which connects, in turn, with the female's cloaca. However, in the platypus, only the left ovary is functional, as is also the case in most kinds of birds. In the male platypus and echidna, the testes are very large and are retained inside the abdomen (the testicond condition). In male monotremes the accessory reproductive glands consist of a single pair of bulbourethral (Cowper's) glands. Both the platypus and short-beaked echidna have large and morphologically complex penes. The significance of the unusual reproductive anatomy of monotremes, in relation to copulatory behaviour and post-copulatory sexual selection, is discussed in Chapters 3, 5, 6 and 8.

Subclass Marsupialia

The earliest known fossil metatherians are from the lower Cretaceous; *Sinodelphys szalayi*, from China, is the oldest example (dated at 125 Mya: Luo *et al.*, 2003, 2011). A diverse array of metatherian fossils has also been discovered in North America (Cifelli and Davis, 2003; Williamson *et al.*, 2014). However, no such early Cretaceous fossils have been found in either Australia or South America. A possible explanation for their absence is that North American mammals were unable to emigrate southwards before about 60–70 Mya, when the formation of an island chain, or perhaps a transitory land bridge, allowed them to enter South America (Muizon and Cifelli, 2001; Ortiz-Jaureguizar and Pascual, 2011). The earliest fully marsupial fossils known from South America are approximately 50 million years old (Woodburne *et al.*, 2014).

Ancestral marsupials reached Australia at some time between 71 and 54.6 Mya. This was possible because a huge southern super-continent (Gondwana), which included Australia, South America and Antarctica, existed at that time. The climate was also radically different then, and much milder; Antarctica was covered in forest. South American marsupials would thus have been able to disperse gradually across Gondwana to Australia, via Antarctica (Beck *et al.*, 2008; Simpson, 1980; Woodburne and Case, 1996; Woodburne and Zinsmeister, 1982).

South American Marsupials

Three orders of South American marsupials are currently recognized: Didelphimorphia, Paucituberculata and Microbiotheria. The Didelphimorphia includes the single Family Didelphidae, which contains 17 genera and approximately 87 species of opossums and mouse opossums. Most didelphids are arboreal omnivores with prehensile tails. Females of the larger species (>250 g in body weight) have a well-developed pouch (marsupium). However, in many didelphids a pouch is either lacking or is represented merely by skin folds that protect the female's nipples.

The only didelphid that occurs in North America is the Virginia opossum (*Didelphis virginiana*); it reached there via the isthmus of Panama. Formation of this isthmus during the late Pliocene, about 3 Mya, made it possible for mammals to cross in either direction between North and South America. Most of this 'Great American Interchange' involved a dramatic southerly migration of eutherian mammals. So ended the long period of splendid isolation that had characterized mammalian evolution in South America up to that point (Simpson, 1980). However, perhaps because of its omnivorous diet, largely terrestrial mode of life and extraordinary fecundity

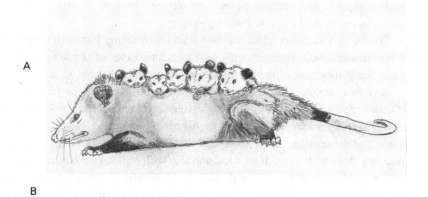

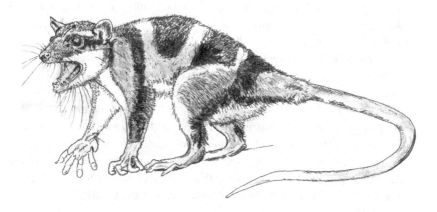

Figure 2.4 Examples of American opossums. **A:** The North American Virginia opossum (*Didelphis virginiana*). A female with her five offspring. **B:** The South American yapok (*Chironectes minimus*); the only amphibious marsupial. (Author's drawings, from photographs.)

(Figure 2.4A), *D. virginiana* was able to disperse northwards throughout much of southern and eastern USA. Indeed, its range is still expanding.

Mention should also be made here of an unusual didelphid, the yapok (*Chironectes minimus*), as it is the only amphibious marsupial. It uses its long tail and webbed hind feet for propulsion when swimming and its large mobile hands to catch small fishes and invertebrates such as crayfish (Figure 2.4B).

Few didelphids have been studied in the wild to determine their mating systems and patterns of sexual behaviour. However, it appears that adults of both sexes are usually non-gregarious, each individual having its own home range, and ranges overlap to varying degrees (e.g. in the Virginia opossum: Ryser, 1992). This is likely to represent the same type of dispersed social and sexual organization that occurs in many other non-gregarious, arboreal mammals, as for example in various nocturnal primates.

Scent-marking and vocalizations often play key roles in the social and sexual lives of such mammals, and multiple-partner matings, resulting in sperm competition, commonly occur in their dispersed mating systems.

The Order Paucituberculata contains a single surviving family of shrew opossums (the Caenolestidae). There are only seven extant species of shrew opossums, five of them being members of the Genus *Caenolestes*. One of these, *C. sangay*, was only discovered quite recently, in the high-altitude cloud forests of the Ecuadorean Andes (Ojala-Barbour *et al.*, 2013). Shrew opossums are small, cryptic, nocturnal creatures; almost nothing is known about their sexual behaviour or reproductive biology. We do know that the females lack a pouch and that the males have a bifid glans penis, traits that they share with many didelphids, and also with some of the Australian marsupials.

The third order of South American marsupials (Microbiotheria) is represented by a single living species, the mouse-sized marsupial known as *Dromiciops gliroides* or, to use its Spanish name, *monito del monte* ('little monkey of the mountains'). However, this group of marsupials was originally represented only by fossils of *Microbiotherium patagonium*, discovered in 1887 by Florentino Ameghino. *D. gliroides* was not described until 7 years later. The microbiotherians were long considered to be didelphids, but Szalay (1982) showed, on the basis of comparative studies of marsupial ankle bones, that *Dromiciops* is more closely related to Australian marsupials than it is to either the didelphids or the shrew opossums of South America. Despite some disputes concerning the phylogenetic position of *Dromiciops* (e.g. Hershkovitz, 1999), molecular genetic studies have confirmed the results of Szalay's insights. The Order Microbiotheria is now recognized as being an ancient lineage, dating back to the late Cretaceous, that is closely related to the earliest Australian marsupials (Mitchell *et al.*, 2014; Weisbecker and Beck, 2015).

Australasian Marsupials

For over 40 million years Australia has been physically isolated from the rest of the world's landmasses.This long period of isolation has given rise to a unique flora and fauna which is largely derived from a Gondwanan heritage. Only in Australia can one enjoy the sight of a waratah blooming amid rugged sandstone, or a kangaroo bounding away between stately eucalypts.

Tim Flannery (1994)

There are four orders of living Australasian marsupials: Notorictemorphia, Diprotodontia, Dasyuromorphia and Peramelemorphia (Figure 2.5). Much more is known about their behaviour and reproductive biology than is the case for the South American taxa considered thus far. However, the two species that constitute the Order Notorictemorphia provide an exception to this generalization. These are the marsupial moles (*Notorictes typhlops* and *N. caurinus*) that occur in the deserts of central and western Australia. They are blind and spend the greater part of their lives underground, burrowing through the sand and back-filling their tunnels as they do so (Benshemesh

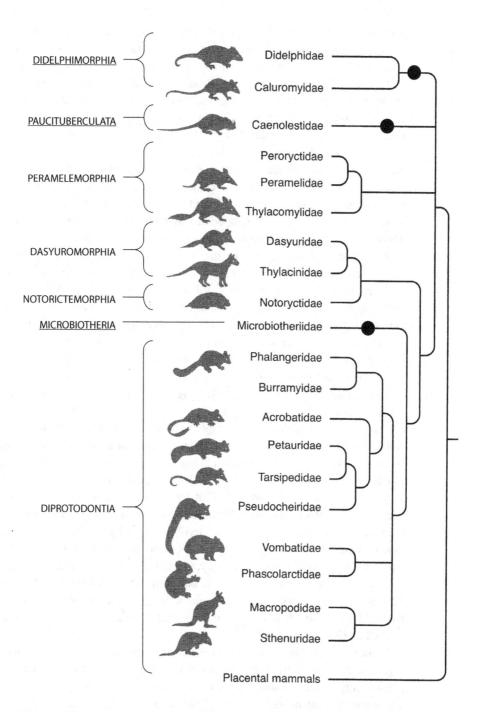

Figure 2.5 Phylogeny of the 7 orders and 20 recent families of marsupials. (Based upon Tyndale-Biscoe, 2005.) ● = the three South American lineages. Note that the South American order Microbiotheria is most closely related to the Diprotodontia, among the four orders of Australian marsupials. The Families Thylacinae (the marsupial wolf) and Sthenuridae (giant short-faced kangaroos) are extinct. The Family Caluromyidae is currently included in the Family Didelphidae, and the Peroryctidae in the Family Peramelidae by most taxonomists.

and Johnson, 2003). The opening of the female marsupial mole's pouch is situated at its posterior end, pointing backwards, as an adaptation to its fossorial way of life. Almost nothing is known concerning the reproductive biology of these enigmatic animals.

The Order Diprotodontia is by far the largest grouping; its 10 families include many of the best-known species, such as the koala, kangaroos, wallabies, wombats and possums. Diprotodonts all have a greatly enlarged pair of lower incisor teeth, whilst the upper jaw usually contains three pairs of smaller incisors. Canine teeth are lacking in these herbivorous marsupials. Their feet vary greatly in structure depending upon their modes of life, but they share one distinctive characteristic: the second and third toes are reduced in size and they are conjoined (i.e. syndactylous). Representatives of three diprotodont families that differ markedly in their ecology, anatomy and behaviour, the Phascolarctidae, Macropodidae and Phalangeridae, are discussed below. Then, brief descriptions of the remaining seven families are provided.

The koala (Figure 2.6A) is the sole living representative of the Family Phascolarctidae. Koalas are arboreal and folivorous; they subsist entirely on eucalypts. In the colder southern part of their distribution range (New South Wales), adult males weigh an average of 12 kg and females 8.5 kg, but both sexes are smaller in the northern (Queensland) populations. Although *Eucalyptus* leaves are readily available throughout the year, they are very low in nutritional value, and they contain toxic terpenes and phenols. However, koalas can consume amounts of eucalyptus oil that might prove fatal in humans.

The koala's diet is clearly a challenging one, and this has had numerous consequences as regards the evolution of its physiology and behaviour (Martin and Handasyde, 1999). Conserving energy is of paramount importance for this species. Koalas feed for only about 4 hours each night; the rest of the time they sleep. Their brains are also very small (in relation to body weight) when compared with the brains of other marsupials (Haight and Nelson, 1987). The digestive organs, by contrast, are very large indeed. Koalas are 'hind-gut fermenters' with a much-enlarged caecum, packed with symbiotic bacteria which break down plant cellulose. In this connection it is interesting to note the specialized behaviour shown by the female koala when it is time to wean her infant. She passes a pre-digested 'pap' consisting of caecal contents which the infant consumes. In this way, it acquires both nourishment and the symbiotic bacteria that it will need when it becomes fully independent (Minchin, 1937; Thompson, 1987). Koala infants continue to suckle for up to one year, remaining in the pouch for the first 6–8 months, and then gradually becoming independent and fully weaned at 12 months of age.

Koalas are non-gregarious and they have a dispersed type of social and mating organization. Each individual occupies its own home range, but their ranges overlap considerably and the animals communicate with one another by scent-marking and vocalizing. Dominant males have the largest home ranges and, during the mating season, they utter loud 'bellowing' calls, and mark trees with their urine and sternal glandular secretions. Inter-male competition is intense, but there is evidence that females sometimes engage in multiple-partner matings (Martin and Handasyde, 1999); post-copulatory sexual selection is thus likely to occur in this species.

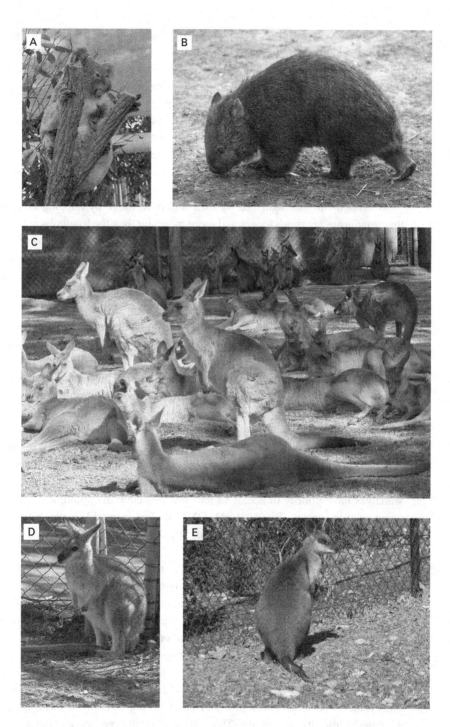

Figure 2.6 Some examples of diprotodonts. **A:** the koala (*Phascolarctos cinereus*). **B:** The common wombat (*Vombatus ursinus*). **C:** A group ('mob') of Eastern grey kangaroos (*Macropus giganteus*). **D:** Red-necked wallaby (*M. rufogriseus*). **E:** Swamp wallaby (*Wallabia bicolor*). (Photographs **A** and **C–E** byAmanda Dixson; **B:** © Shutterstock.com.)

The macropods (wallabies and kangaroos: Figures 2.6C–E), along with the much smaller rat-kangaroos, potoroos and bettongs, are members of the Superfamily Macropodoidea. There are approximately 73 species belonging to 16 genera in this superfamily. The tammar wallaby (*Macropus eugenii*) is one of the smaller species; adult males weigh 7.5 kg and females 5.5 kg on average. The adaptive radiation of kangaroos and wallabies in Australia has been compared to that of the ungulates in Africa (Lee and Cockburn, 1985). Thus, the macropods are also herbivores, grazing or browsing upon plants of various kinds, and they are foregut fermenters. Symbiotic bacteria that assist in digesting cellulose are contained in the elongated stomach (Dawson, 1995).

Macropods are distinguished by their ability to move by hopping bipedally, and their hindlimbs are much longer and more muscular than the forelimbs in the majority of species. Measurements of the activity of muscles and tendons controlling foot movements during saltatory (hopping) locomotion have shown that elastic energy recovery increases as the animal moves at greater speeds and is highly efficient (e.g. in the tammar wallaby: Biewener and Baudinette, 1995).

Most marsupials are either active at night, or at dawn and dusk (crepuscular). Tammar wallabies rest in scrubland during the day, but move into more open areas at night in order to graze and forage on a variety of plants (Tyndale-Biscoe, 2005). Again, like most marsupials, tammars do not form social groups; the only cohesive unit consists of a mother and her dependent offspring. However, the larger kangaroo species, such as *M. rufus* and *M. robustus*, do form unstable groups ('mobs') in which adult males compete for access to receptive females. Tammar wallabies occupy individual home ranges, which overlap extensively. This type of overlapping system is similar to that described above for the koala, and is sometimes referred to as 'overlap promiscuity'. However, the term 'dispersed mating system' is used in this book, for reasons that are discussed in Chapter 4. Although dominant male tammar wallabies have priority of access to females, it is clear that multiple-partner matings occur in this species (Rudd, 1994). DNA studies to establish paternity in captive groups have shown that dominant males sire approximately 50 per cent of offspring (Hynes *et al.*, 2005; Miller *et al.*, 2010a).

Tammar wallabies are unusual among the macropods in being seasonal breeders; most females give birth in January. Within hours of the tiny infant, or 'joey', making its ascent to her pouch, the female enters postpartum oestrus and is ready to mate with one or more partners. However, once she conceives, the zygote develops only as far as the early blastocyst stage. Then, its development is arrested and an extended period of embryonic diapause ensues. Embryonic diapause and ovarian quiescence are controlled by seasonal factors (long day length) in both the tammar and the red-necked wallabies (*M. rufogriseus*: Figure 2.6D). After the summer solstice (22 December), embryonic development resumes, and an offspring is born 40 days later, roughly 12 months after its conception. Thus, in tammar and red-necked wallabies, ovarian quiescence and embryonic diapause are governed by changes in photoperiod. In other macropods, however, the physiological mechanisms associated with lactation control these processes (Tyndale-Biscoe and Renfree, 1987).

The third example of variations of ecology and behaviour among the diprotodonts, the brushtail possum (*Trichosurus vulpecula*: Figure 2.7A), is one of the most widely distributed and adaptable marsupial species in Australia, often being found in urban environments. It is most abundant in forested areas, and its diet consists of leaves, flowers and fruits. Feeding occurs at night; each possum spends the daylight hours asleep in a den, such as a hollow log. Brushtail possums were brought to New Zealand in the middle of the nineteenth century, with the aim of farming them for the fur trade. However, escapees bred prolifically and (through no fault of its own) the species is now a major pest throughout the country.

Brushtail possums are non-gregarious; each animal occupies its own home range, and male ranges overlap extensively with those of females. DNA typing studies (Clinchy *et al.*, 2004; Taylor *et al.*, 2000) indicate that larger and older males tend to sire more offspring than others. However, these studies did not address the question of whether multiple-partner matings by females (and hence post-copulatory sexual selection) might occur in this species. Direct observations of mating behaviour

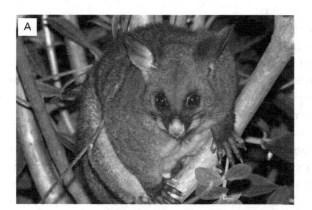
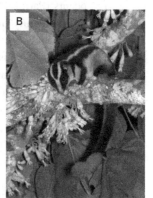
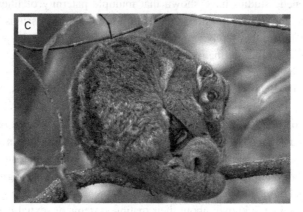

Figure 2.7 Some examples of possums discussed in the text. **A:** Brushtail possum (*Trichosurus vulpecula*). **B:** Striped possum (*Dactylopsila* sp.). **C:** Green ringtail possum (*Pseudocheirops archeri*). (Images: © Shutterstock.com.)

(Winter, 1976) have provided some useful answers. Winter observed that males sometimes spent 30–40 days forming a consortship with a female; under these circumstances aggression between the pair was reduced prior to copulation (females are the dominant sex). However, copulations also occurred in the absence of such consortships. In these cases a number of males gathered in proximity to a receptive female, and multiple-partner matings were observed. A close relative of the brushtail possum, the mountain possum or bobuck (*T. cunninghami*), forms pairs in the wild, and it has been presumed to have a monogamous mating system. However, extra-pair copulations must often occur, as genetic studies have shown that 35 per cent of offspring are sired by males other than a female's long-term partner (Handasyde *et al.*, 2007).

Turning now to brief descriptions of the remaining seven families of diprotodonts, the feathertail glider (*Acrobates pygmaeus*), which weighs just 10–14 g, is the world's smallest gliding mammal, and one of only two members of the Family Acrobatidae. It occurs in eastern Australia in tall mature forests and is nocturnal, feeding primarily on nectar, pollen and insects. Pygmy gliders build nests and sometimes sleep together in groups during the day. Females may have four young, and multiple paternity of litters occurs (Parrott *et al.*, 2005).

The Family Burramyidae contains five species of mouse-sized possums: the mountain pygmy possum (*Burramys parvus*) and four species of long-tailed pygmy possums (Genus *Cercartetus*). The mountain pygmy possum is unusual among marsupials because it hibernates during the winter (Broom and Geiser, 1995). Mountain pygmy possums are non-gregarious and occupy individual home ranges. Very little is known about their sexual behaviour. The sex ratio is heavily female-biased, however, and male mortality is high.

The honey possum (*Tarsipes rostratus*), the only member of the Family Tarsipedidae, is the sole survivor of an ancient lineage. Honey possums are tiny creatures, adult males weighing between 7 and 9 g and females 10–12 g. This crepuscular species occurs in South West Australia, and it is restricted to heathlands. Genetic studies have shown that multiple paternity of litters occurs in this species (Bryant, 2004; Wooller *et al.*, 2000). Male honey possums have very large testes in relation to their body weight (Rose *et al.*, 1997), and their spermatozoa are the longest recorded for any mammal (Cummins and Woodall, 1985). These traits are indicative of the occurrence of sperm competition in this species.

The Family Petauridae includes four striped possums, the rare and endangered Leadbeater's possum (*Gymnobelideus leadbeateri*) and seven glider species, all belonging to the Genus *Petaurus*. The striped possums (Genus *Dactylopsila*: Figure 2.7B) live in the rainforests of northern Queensland and lowland New Guinea. They are highly specialized feeders that use their strong incisor teeth to break open rotten logs, or to strip bark from trees, in search of grubs and insects (Lee and Cockburn, 1985). Striped possums are nocturnal and non-gregarious; unfortunately, very little is known about their mating systems or sexual behaviour.

Gliders resemble the group of rodents known as 'flying squirrels', as convergent evolution has resulted in both these groups developing similar volant specializations. Sugar gliders (*Petaurus breviceps*) glide by means of a cutaneous membrane (the patagium) that extends from wrist to ankle on each side of the body. They can travel 50 metres or more in this way, moving from tree to tree in search of nectar, pollen and tree saps or gums. Their distribution range includes northern and eastern Australia, as far southwards as Tasmania. Sugar gliders are nocturnal and more gregarious than most petaurids, so that up to seven adults and offspring spend each day huddled in a leafy nest. They mate during June/July; gestation lasts for 15–17 days and one or two infants are born. These develop rapidly, leaving the pouch at 70 days and becoming fully independent by 110–120 days of age. Some females may produce two litters in a season (Suckling, 1995; Tyndale-Biscoe and Renfree, 1987).

The Family Pseudocheiridae comprises six genera of ringtail possums as well as the greater glider (*Petauroides volans*). Ringtail possums are larger than the possums of the Genus *Petaurus* considered above; many of them weigh more than a kilogram. They have prehensile tails, and they are nocturnal and non-gregarious, browsing mainly on leaves. The caecum is enlarged and contains bacteria that break down the large amounts of plant cellulose consumed each night. With the exception of the common ringtail (*Pseudocheirus peregrinus*) most of these possums have very small distribution ranges and little is known about their reproductive biology. Examples include the green ringtail (*Pseudochirops archeri*: Figure 2.7C), the Daintree River ringtail (*P. cinereus*) and the Herbert River ringtail possum (*Pseudochirulus herbertensis*), all from the rainforests of north-eastern Queensland.

There are only three extant species in the Family Vombatidae: the common wombat (*Vombatus ursinus*, Figure 2.6B), the southern hairy-nosed wombat (*Lasiorhinus latifrons*) and the northern hairy-nosed wombat (*L. krefftii*), which is critically endangered. Wombats are semi-fossorial; they dig extensive burrows as refuges and nesting sites, but spend much of the time above ground in search of food. The pouch is protected during burrowing as its opening is situated at its posterior end, and points backwards. All three species are herbivorous and feed on grasses and roots. They are nocturnal, but they also graze during the day during colder periods of the year. Uniquely among marsupials, the wombats have teeth that grow continuously throughout life.

Common wombats occur in South East Australia, including the island of Tasmania. They are stocky, powerfully built creatures, weighing as much as 39 kg, although 26 kg is the average weight for adults of both sexes. They have sturdy limbs and strong claws. Home ranges vary in size from 5 to 23 hectares and each individual makes use of a number of burrows, scattered throughout its range. Wombats are non-gregarious creatures; they spend most of the time alone, except when mating occurs (McIlroy, 1976, 1995). Breeding may take place at any time of year, but tends to occur later in the more southerly, and colder, parts of the species range (Hogan *et al.*, 2013). Female wombats have two teats in the pouch, but only a single offspring is born. It remains in the pouch for 6 months and stays with its mother for a further 11 months before establishing its own home range.

The next order to be considered, the Dasyuromorphia, contains three Families: Dasyuridae, Myrmecobiidae and Thylacinidae. The last of these is extinct; the Tasmanian wolf (*Thylacinus cynocephalus*) was regarded as a danger to livestock, and it was ruthlessly exterminated during the early twentieth century. The Family

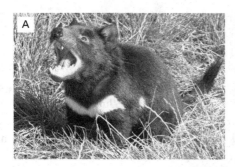
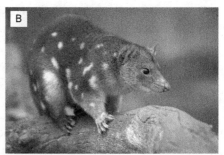
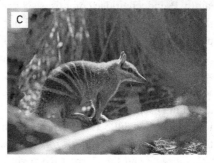

Figure 2.8 A: Tasmanian devil (*Sarcophilus harrisii*), largest of the surviving carnivorous marsupials. **B:** Tiger quoll (*Dasyurus maculatus*). **C:** Numbat (*Myrmecobius fasciatus*), the only marsupial which specializes in feeding on termites. (Images: © Shutterstock.com.)

Myrmecobiidae contains only a single species: the numbat (*Myrmecobius fasciatus*: Figure 2.8C), which is unusual in being diurnal, and unique among marsupials as it is the only species that specializes in feeding on termites. By far the largest family, the Dasyuridae, includes approximately 47 carnivorous and insectivorous species such as the Tasmanian devil and the native cats or quolls (Figure 2.8A,B) as well as a variety of much smaller-bodied taxa, including the dibblers, dunnarts and *Phascogale* and *Antechinus* species.

The Tasmanian devil (*Sarcophilus harrisii*) is the largest of the extant dasyurids; adult males weigh approximately 9 kg, and females 7 kg. It is a thick-set, broad-headed animal, covered in short black fur, but marked with a white blaze across the chest and the rump. The skull is robust, with strong jaws armed with large canine teeth and blade-like cutting molars and premolars. The Tasmanian devil is primarily nocturnal, and much of its diet consists of carrion. Although non-gregarious, individuals form part of a complex social network (Hamede *et al.*, 2009), and numbers of them will converge to compete for access to large carcasses. In recent years, the wild population has been decimated by an infectious facial cancer, which is transmitted when animals bite one another, as they often do when fighting over food or mating opportunities (Hawkins *et al.*, 2006; Wells *et al.*, 2017).

Tasmanian devils have a dispersed social organization and mating system; their home ranges overlap extensively, and vary in area between 2 and 20 km² (Jones,

1995). Multiple-partner matings occur, so that the mating system is polygynandrous. Copulations are prolonged (Eisenberg *et al.*, 1975), as is the case for many other dasyurids. Female dasyurids are polyovular, and Hughes (1982) reported that 11–56 ova and embryos were present in 6 female Tasmanian devils that he examined. There are only four nipples in the female's pouch in this species, however, and litter sizes are much smaller than the high ovulation rate might suggest (average litter size = 2.9: Tyndale-Biscoe and Renfree, 1987). Tasmanian devils are seasonal breeders; births occur in April, and offspring become independent by 40 weeks of age. Their average lifespan is about 6 years (Jones, 1995).

Most of the dasyurids except for the Tasmanian devil and the four quoll species are small animals; it has been estimated that 75 per cent of all species weigh less than 100 g. Superficially, they resemble rodents or shrews and they feed primarily on insects and other arthropods. Several of these taxa exhibit a remarkable type of mating system, known as semelparity, in which all the males in the population die at the close of the annual mating season. DNA typing studies have shown that multiple paternity within litters occurs in several species belonging to the Genus *Antechinus*. Males are highly aggressive and hyperactive throughout the mating season. Mortality is associated with stress-related suppression of the immune system, and associated debilitating effects (increased parasite loads, diseases and haemorrhagic ulceration of the gut: Bradley *et al.*, 1980). Semelparity in marsupials is discussed further in Chapter 4.

The Order Peramelemorphia contains at least 17 nocturnal and crepuscular species belonging to the Family Peramilidae, which comprises the Australian bandicoots and the greater bilby, as well as the spiny bandicoots of New Guinea and adjacent islands. These are medium-sized terrestrial insectivores and omnivores with body weights ranging from 0.5 to 2.5 kg. The spiny bandicoots occur in lowland rainforests, and new species are discovered from time to time (e.g. *Microperoryctes aplini*: Helgen and Flannery, 2004). One of the New Guinean species, the rufous spiny bandicoot (*Echimipera rufescens*), is also to be found in rainforests of the Cape York Peninsula in Australia. However, the majority of the Australian bandicoots and the greater bilby occur in much drier, open habitats. They have compact bodies and long, narrow heads. The hindlimbs are longer and more powerful than the forelimbs; this is especially the case in the greater bilby, which is also distinguished by having very long ears, and a long black and white tail. The feet of peramelids resemble those of macropods, and the second and third toes are syndactylous, as is the case for members of the Order Diprotodontia. However, the dentition of peramelids differs from that of diprotodonts and more closely resembles the dentition of dasyurids. Molecular studies of marsupial phylogeny also indicate that the Peramelemorphia and Dasyuromorphia may be phylogenetically more closely related to each other than they are to the Diprotodontia (Mitchell *et al.*, 2014).

Bandicoots are noted for their ability to reproduce rapidly. They nourish their developing young via a chorioallantoic placenta and their gestation periods are exceptionally short: just 12.5 days in the northern brown bandicoot (*Isoodon macrourus*) and long-nosed bandicoot (*Perameles nasuta*). This is the shortest gestation period recorded for any mammal (Tyndale-Biscoe and Renfree, 1987). The female's pouch contains eight teats, and litters usually contain up to four offspring. This makes it possible for females to raise two successive litters during a season; the second set of infants attaches to the four small teats that were not utilized by the previous litter.

Information concerning the social organization and mating systems of bandicoots is limited, especially as far as the New Guinea taxa are concerned. Australian species are typically non-gregarious, and individual home ranges overlap to form a dispersed type of social organization and mating system (e.g. in *P. nasuta*, *P. gunnii* and *Isoodon obesulus*: Lee and Cockburn, 1985; and in *P. bougainville*: Short *et al.*, 1998). Large relative testes sizes, indicative of sperm competition, occur in some species (Rose *et al.*, 1997; Short *et al.*, 1998).

In concluding this brief résumé of the extant marsupials, it should be noted that, with the exception of some macropods (e.g. the eastern grey kangaroo, Figure 2.6C), most of the extant taxa are small or medium-sized animals. Yet in the not so distant past, much larger marsupials existed in Australia, including the lion-sized predatory diprotodont (*Thylacoleo*), a 3-metre tall short-faced kangaroo (*Procoptodon goliah*) and a herbivore which was the size of a rhinoceros (*Diprotodon*: Figure 2.9). The first people to enter Australia, some 50,000 years ago, would have encountered a much more diverse marsupial fauna than exists today. The extinction of *Diprotodon*, and many other Australian marsupials, has been caused by *Homo sapiens* (Flannery, 1994). The South American marsupial fauna also contained some much larger representatives in

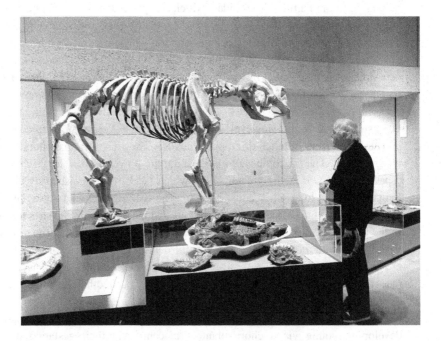

Figure 2.9 The skeleton of Diprotodon, largest of the marsupials, which became extinct after the first wave of humans reached Australia. (Photograph by Amanda Dixson.)

the past, belonging to the Families Borhyaenidae and Thylacosmilidae. *Thylacosmilus*, for example, was a formidable carnivore with greatly elongated upper canines, closely resembling the placental sabre-toothed cats. These large South American marsupials became extinct before human beings reached the Americas (Simpson, 1980).

Subclass Placentalia

Phylogeny of the Extant Placental Mammals

Most authorities currently recognize 19 orders of placental mammals, each of which can be assigned to one of four superordinal groupings or 'clades': Laurasiatheria, Euarchontoglires, Afrotheria and Xenarthra. On the basis of comparative molecular studies, the Laurasiatheria and Euarchontoglires derive from the same ancestral group of eutherians, the Boreoeutheria (meaning literally 'northern true beasts'). Phylogenetic relationships among the various superorders and orders of placental mammals are shown in diagrammatic form in Figure 2.10, and a brief overview of each of the four superorders is provided below.

The Superorder Laurasiatheria

The largest of the six orders that make up the Superorder Laurasiatheria, in terms of its overall size and diversity, is the Cetartiodactyla (Figure 2.11), which contains the artiodactyls, or even-toed, hoofed mammals (pigs and peccaries, ruminant ungulates, camelids and hippopotami), as well as the cetaceans (whales, dolphins and porpoises). Fossil evidence indicates that cetaceans arose from aquatic artiodactyl ancestors at some time during the Eocene (Thewissen *et al.*, 2007). However, the joining together of the extant Artiodactyla and Cetacea within a single order is primarily the result of molecular genetic studies indicating that the hippopotamus is more closely related to whales and dolphins than it is to other artiodactyls such as sheep or pigs (Nikaido *et al.*, 1999; Ursing and Arnason, 1998). Hippos are amphibious, as were the earliest quadrupedal precursors of cetaceans. Behavioural research has revealed that the larger of the two hippo species (*Hippopotamus amphibius*) vocalizes while it is under the water. For example, hippos produce trains of clicking sounds, very similar to those used by whales and dolphins for echolocation and social communication (Barklow, 2004; Maust-Mohl *et al.*, 2018). Hippos also exhibit morphological specializations of their genitalia that resemble those that occur in the Cetacea, as will be discussed in Part III of this book.

The odd-toed ungulates (Order Perissodactyla) comprise 17 species belonging to 3 families (the rhinoceroses, tapirs and equids: Figure 2.12), as compared with the more than 220 species and nine families of artiodactyls that are alive today. Historically, the perissodactyls were much more diverse than is currently the case. Fossil evidence shows that they were the dominant ungulates in America and Eurasia between 55 and 25 Mya, but their numbers have declined since the late Oligocene and

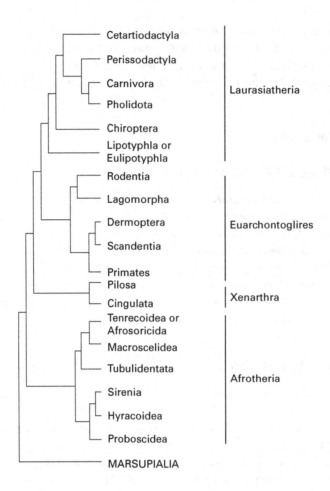

Figure 2.10 Phylogenetic relationships among the 4 superorders and 19 orders of the placental mammals. Redrawn and modified from Archibald (2011).

the Miocene. Currently, there are only five species of tapirs: four in South America and one in Malaysia, and five species of rhinoceros, in Africa, Asia and South-East Asia. Most of these animals are highly endangered; the black rhinoceros (*Diceros bicornis*), for example, has been reduced to a few thousand survivors in Africa, whilst the Javan rhino (*Rhinoceros sondaicus*) is the world's most endangered large mammal. Fewer than 80 of them remain in the Ujung-Kulon National Park in Western Java.

The earliest equids occurred in the Eocene, and they were small, browsing species that weighed less than 50 kg. Fossils of much larger taxa are known from the Miocene, and they flourished in North America as grazers in more open grassland habitats. The Genus *Equus*, to which all the extant species belong, first appeared in North America about 4 Mya, and by the close of the Pliocene and early Pleistocene its members had spread to the Old World. Their descendants include today's zebras, wild asses and

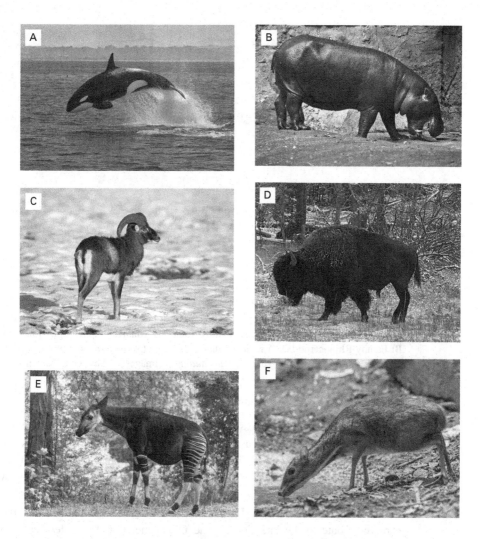

Figure 2.11 Examples of species that belong to the Order Cetartiodactyla. Family Delphinidae: **A:** orca (*Orcinus orca*). **B:** Family Hippopotamidae: pygmy hippo (*Choeropsis liberiensis*). **C:** Family Bovidae: mouflon (*Ovis orientalis*); **D:** American bison (*Bison bison*). **E:** Family Giraffidae: okapi (*Okapia johnstoni*). **F:** Family Tragulidae: lesser mouse-deer (*Tragulus kanchil*). (Photograph of the American bison is by courtesy of Professor Charles Daugherty; other images: © Shutterstock.com.)

wild horses of Africa and Asia (MacFadden, 2005; Vaughan *et al.*, 2015). The African wild ass (*Equus asinus*) is considered to be the ancestor of the domestic donkey, whilst Przewalski's horse is a member of the same species as the domestic horse (*E. caballus*).

The Order Carnivora contains more than 280 species, and its representatives are found throughout most of the world. They vary in size from tiny mustelids (such as the

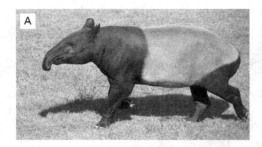
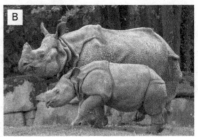
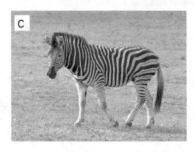

Figure 2.12 Order Perissodactyla. **A:** Family Tapiridae. Malayan tapir (*Tapirus indicus*).
B: Family Rhinocerotidae. An adult Indian rhinoceros (*Rhinoceros unicornis*) with its calf.
C: Family Equidae. Plain's zebra (*Equus quagga*). (Images: © Shutterstock.com.)

least weasel, which weighs less than 250 g) to bull elephant seals weighing in excess
of 2500 kg. Not all of the carnivores are exclusively predatory animals. Bears and
raccoons, for example, are omnivorous, and the giant panda subsists exclusively on a
diet of bamboo. The aardwolf (*Proteles cristatus*) feeds mostly on termites, while the
walrus scours the sea floor for molluscs which it opens by using its muscular lips and
tongue, rather than its teeth. The earliest fossil representatives of living families of
carnivores date to the late Eocene and Oligocene. Fossils of stem carnivores (the
Miacoidea and Viverravidae) are known from earlier Paleocene and Eocene deposits.
Fossil evidence indicates that it was the Miacoidea that gave rise to the various
families of the Carnivora that exist today (Goswami and Friscia, 2010).

The extant carnivores are usually divided into two suborders: Caniformia and
Feliformia (Figures 2.13 and 2.14). The Caniformia includes the wolves, dogs, jackals
and foxes (Canidae), the bears (Ursidae) and giant panda (Ailuridae), skunks
(Mephitidae), raccoons (Procyonidae) and the weasels, otters and their allies
(Mustelidae). In addition, three families of aquatic pinnipeds, the earless seals
(Phocidae), eared seals and sea lions (Otariidae) and the walrus (Odobenidae), are
included in the Caniformia (Koretsky *et al.*, 2016). The Feliformia is composed of six
families. The most basal of these (Nandiniidae) contains a single species, the African
palm civet (*Nandinia binotata*). This small, arboreal and largely frugivorous civet is
genetically distinct from other feliforms and certain features of its auditory anatomy
are more primitive (Flynn and Nedbal, 1998). The Family Felidae contains 40 species

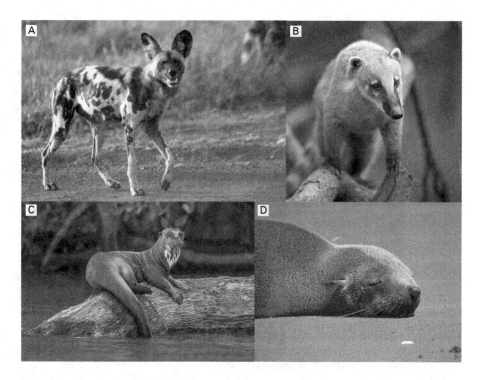

Figure 2.13 Carnivores of the Suborder Caniformia. **A:** African wild dog (*Lycaon pictus*). **B:** Coatimundi (*Nasua narica*). **C:** Giant otter (*Pteronura brasiliensis*). **D:** New Zealand fur seal (*Arctocephalus forsteri*). (Images **A–C**: © Shutterstock.com; **D**: photograph by Amanda Dixson.)

of cats, ranging in size from small taxa, such as the domestic cat, margay, jaguarundi and serval, up to very large and formidable predators, including the lion and leopard of Africa and Asia, and the jaguar of South America. The Old World civets and genets of the Family Viverridae are mostly small or medium-sized mammals that prey upon small vertebrates and insects. They are nocturnal ambush hunters, and most are forest-dwelling and arboreal. Exceptions include the semi-aquatic otter civet (*Cynogale bennettii*) and the largest member of this family, the African civet (*Civettictis civetta*), which weighs 20 kg and is predominantly terrestrial. Four species of hyenas constitute the Family Hyaenidae: the spotted hyena, brown hyena, striped hyena and the aardwolf. The spotted hyena of Africa is an active predator as well as a scavenger of lion kills and a carrion eater. It lives in large social groups ('clans') in which adult females occupy the top-ranking positions (Kruuk, 1972). Female spotted hyenas have a greatly enlarged clitoris and, uniquely among mammals, they copulate and give birth via the clitoral canal.

The two remaining families of the Feliformia are the Herpestidae and Eupleridae. The herpestids are better known as the mongooses. These are lithe creatures with long bodies and tails (the largest weighs about 5 kg), 33 species of which occur mainly in Africa, the Middle East and parts of Asia and South-East Asia. Some mongooses live

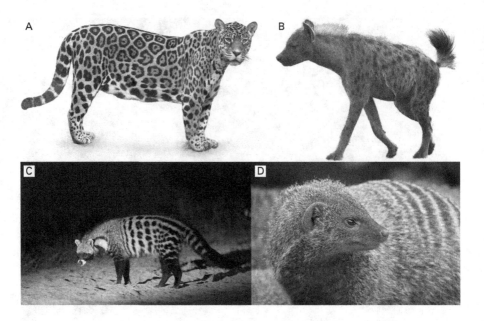

Figure 2.14 Carnivores of the Suborder Feliformia. **A:** Jaguar (*Panthera onca*). **B:** Spotted hyena (*Crocuta crocuta*). **C:** African civet (*Civettictis civetta*). **D:** Banded mongoose (*Mungos mungo*). (Images: © Shutterstock.com.)

in complex social groups, as for example the meerkat (*Suricata suricatta*), which has been the subject of a long-term programme of field research conducted in the Kalahari Desert (Clutton Brock, 2016). The euplerids are considered to be descendants of an African herpestid ancestor that reached Madagascar at some point around 23 Mya. There are seven extant species in the Family Eupleridae, the largest of which is the fossa (*Cryptoprocta ferox*). The fossa is arboreal and nocturnal; it is a major predator of lemurs. Fossas display some unusual features of their genital anatomy and copulatory behaviour that are discussed later in this book, in relation to possible effects of post-copulatory sexual selection.

The Order Pholidota contains seven species of pangolins, or scaly anteaters, all of which belong to the Family Manidae (Figure 2.15). Surprisingly, molecular research indicates that the pangolins may be phylogenetically most closely related to carnivores (e.g. Murphy *et al.*, 2001a). Yet, they are markedly different morphologically, as they lack teeth, and use their greatly elongated tongues to capture ants and termites. Their bodies and long tails are covered in hard, overlapping scales. Convergent evolution has resulted in pangolins exhibiting specializations that are more typical of some xenarthrans, such as the South American anteaters and armadillos, but they are no longer considered to be closely related to them.

Pangolins occur in Africa and Asia (Figure 2.15), although one extinct genus (*Patriomanis*) is known from the Eocene of North America. The largest extant species, the giant pangolin (*Smutsia gigantea*), occurs in Africa. It weighs over 30 kg, and it

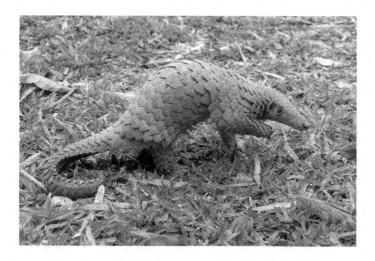

Figure 2.15 Order Pholidota: Sunda pangolin (*Manis javanica*). (© Shutterstock.com.)

uses its powerful limbs and claws to dig extensive burrows. Other more gracile species, such as the long-tailed pangolin (*Phataginus tetradactyla*), are arboreal and have prehensile tails. Pangolins are relatively solitary creatures that occupy individual ranges and communicate primarily by means of olfactory cues. Relatively little is known about their sexual behaviour, and several species are becoming increasing rare, due largely to their use in traditional medicine in China and elsewhere.

One in every 5 mammalian species is a bat; the Order Chiroptera contains 202 genera and more than 1120 species. New bats are still being discovered, due in large measure to the occurrence of cryptic species that are morphologically almost indistinguishable but differ significantly in their behaviour and genetic constitution. A celebrated example concerns *Pipistrellus pipistrellus*, the commonest and most widely distributed of the European bats. Studies of its vocalizations and cytochrome-b sequences have revealed that the common pipistrelle actually consists of two distinct species, *P. pipistrellus* and *P. pygmaeus* (Barratt *et al.*, 1997; Jones and Barratt, 1999). Although closely related species of bats are often very difficult to distinguish morphologically, one trait that is useful concerns their penile morphology (for example, in identifying cryptic species of vespertilionids: Fasel *et al.*, 2020). Diversification of penile morphology due to post-copulatory sexual selection will be discussed in Chapter 5.

The fossil record of bat evolution extends back to the early Eocene, approximately 55 Mya, although molecular studies indicate that the Chiroptera might have originated somewhat earlier than this (Teeling *et al.*, 2005). Fossil bats have been discovered in Europe, India, Australia and the Americas. For example, Simmons *et al.* (2008) have described a primitive bat from the early Eocene of Wyoming (*Onychonycteris finneyi*) which was probably capable of quadrupedal locomotion as well as fluttering flight. Simmons *et al.* did not consider that this species was able to echolocate. However, studies of the anatomy of the inner ear (cochlea) of some other Eocene bats indicate that they were echolocators (Fenton and Simmons, 2014).

Traditionally, the Order Chiroptera has been divided into two suborders: the Megachiroptera and the Microchiroptera (e.g. Altringham, 1996; Nowak, 1999). The Megachiroptera is represented by the single Family Pteropodidae: the Old World fruit bats or flying foxes. The largest bats belong to this family; some have wingspans of up to 1.7 metres (e.g. in the Genus *Pteropus*). The Suborder Microchiroptera contains all the echolating bats, of which there are 17 families; they occur throughout the world and are found on every continent except Antarctica. An example of each suborder is shown in Figure 2.16.

Molecular studies have impacted chiropteran phylogeny as is the case for many other groups of placental mammals. Thus, phylogenomic analyses place the fruit bats (Pteropodidae) along with five families of echolocating species in the same suborder, separate from the other families of echolocating bats (Teeling *et al.*, 2005; Tsagkogeorga *et al.*, 2013). This newer phylogenomic arrangement indicates that echolocation either evolved separately in the two suborders, or that it evolved once but was secondarily lost in the Pteropodidae.

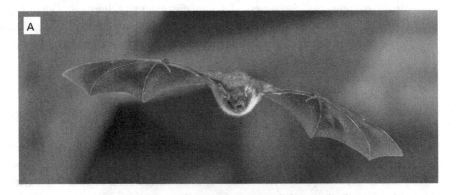

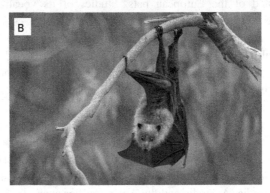

Figure 2.16 Order Chiroptera. **A:** Suborder Microchiroptera, Family Vespertilionidae: natterer's bat (*Myotis nattereri*). **B:** Suborder Megachiroptera, Family Pteropodidae: grey-headed flying fox (*Pteropus poliocephalus*). (Images: © Shutterstock.com.)

The mating systems and reproductive specializations of bats will be discussed later, in Part III of this book. It is sufficient at this point to note that multiple-partner matings by females are known to occur in some taxa, and that large relative testes sizes (indicative of sperm competition) characterize certain families of bats (e.g. the Pteropodidae, Rhinopomatidae and Vespertilionidae: Wilkinson and McCracken, 2003). Also, females of a number of bat species possess a remarkable ability to store viable sperm within their reproductive tracts for months prior to the occurrence of fertilization (Racey, 1979). These specializations may be associated with occurrences of post-copulatory sexual selection via cryptic female choice and/or sperm competition.

The Order Eulipotyphla currently contains four families: the hedgehogs, shrews, moles and solenodons (i.e. the Erinaceidae, Soricidae, Talpidae and Solenodontidae: Douady *et al.*, 2002a). There are 54 genera and 441 species in the Eulipotyphla and, of these, the Soricidae is by far the largest family: 85 per cent of all species of the Eulipotyphla are shrews (Vaughan *et al.*, 2015). The selenodons, by contrast, are represented by two primitive relict species that survive only on the islands of Haiti (*Solenodon paradoxus*) and Cuba (*S. cubanus*).

The available fossil evidence indicates that, like other Laurasiatherians, the Eulipotyphla originated in the northern hemisphere. Thus, the earliest fossils of hedgehogs, such as *Litolestes* and *Oncocherus*, date from the Paleocene of North America (Novacek *et al.*, 1985; Scott, 2006), whilst ancestral shrews occurred in Eurasia, Africa and North America during the Eocene (Vaughan *et al.*, 2015). The solenodons are thought to be related to extinct North American insectivores, of the Family Apternodontidae, that were widely distributed in North America from the late Paleocene until the early Oligocene (Asher *et al.*, 2002).

Eulipotyphlans are typically nocturnal, insectivorous or omnivorous animals. However, many shrews are active by both day and night. Among the Talpidae, the moles are highly specialized for a fossorial existence, and feed upon a variety of invertebrates, including earthworms, while the desmans are amphibious hunters that include fish and frogs in their diet. Although members of all four families of the Eulipotyphla are usually considered to be 'solitary' (i.e. non-gregarious in their habits), the social and sexual lives of very few species have been studied in detail. Some evidence of pairing, or of larger social groupings, exists for a small number of moles and shrews (Valomy *et al.*, 2015).

Originally, the taxa discussed here, and currently assigned to the Eulipotyphla, formed part of a much larger assemblage which constituted the Order Insectivora. Over the course of time, however, the Insectivora gradually became 'a catch-all repository for taxa of doubtful affinities' (Vaughan *et al.*, 2015). This situation caused significant problems for mammalogists and evolutionary biologists (e.g. Nowak, 1999). Fortunately, the advent of phylogenomic techniques has resolved the confusion surrounding the phylogeny of the Insectivora. Various groups that were previously placed in the Insectivora are now accorded ordinal status, and have been removed from the Superorder Laurasiatheria. Thus, the elephant shrews (Macroscelidea), golden moles (Chrysochloridae) and tenrecs (Afrosoricida) are now included in the

Afrotheria. The treeshrews (Scandentia) and 'flying lemurs' or colugos (Dermoptera) are placed in the Superorder Euarchontoglires.

The Superorder Euarchontoglires

This superorder contains five orders: the Rodentia, Lagomorpha (rabbits and pikas), Primates (lemurs, monkeys, apes and humans), Dermoptera (colugos) and Scandentia (treeshrews).

The Rodentia is by far the largest mammalian order. Wilson and Reeder reported in 2005 that there are 2277 species of rodents (equivalent to 42 per cent of all the mammals). Rodents share a suite of dental specializations, including a pair of chisel-like incisor teeth in each jaw which grow continuously throughout life. These enable species such as squirrels to gnaw nuts and seeds, beavers to cut through timber and build their lodges, and naked mole-rats to tunnel in search of the tubers that sustain their large colonies (Figure 2.17).

Rodents have a worldwide distribution and their earliest fossils date back to the Paleocene and the dawn of the Eocene approximately 60–56 Mya. By the early Oligocene most of the modern families of rodents were already established. Although extensive pruning of the phylogenetic tree, due to extinctions, has reduced the diversity of some orders of mammals (e.g. the Perissodactyla), this has not been the case where the rodents are concerned.

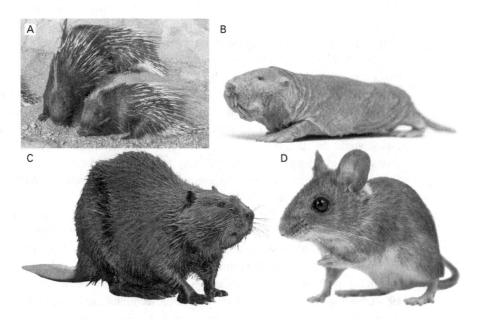

Figure 2.17 Rodents. **A:** Malayan porcupine (*Hystrix brachyura*). **B:** Naked mole-rat (*Heterocephalus glaber*). **C:** North American beaver (*Castor canadensis*). **D:** Woodmouse (*Apodemus sylvaticus*). (Images: © Shutterstock.com.)

The extant rodents are divisible into the following five suborders (Vaughan *et al.*, 2015):

Histricomorpha Histricomorphs occur in Africa and South America; the South American taxa are the descendants of African precursors. This suborder includes the Old World porcupines and African mole-rats, the South American porcupines, guinea pigs and capybara (which is the largest rodent of all, weighing 50 kg), as well as the tuco tucos and degus.

Castorimorpha This suborder includes the beavers (two species of the Genus *Castor*), as well as the pocket gophers (Geomyidae) and kangaroo rats (Heteromyidae).

Anomaluromorpha The anomalures, or scaly-tailed squirrels, occur in the forests of Western and Central Africa. They are nocturnal arboreal gliders that roost in small groups in tree hollows during the day. This suborder also includes two species of African springhares (Genus *Pedetes*).

Myomorpha The two largest families of the Mammalia (the Muridae and Cricetidae) belong to this suborder. The Muridae includes the Old World rats, mice and gerbils. The Cricetidae comprises many New World species of rats and mice, as well as voles, lemmings and hamsters that are found throughout Europe and Asia.

Sciuromorpha includes 278 species of diurnal squirrels, chipmunks, marmots and prairie dogs (Family Sciuridae) which originated in North America during the late Eocene, and 28 species of dormice (Family Gliridae) which are found only in the Old World. The Sciuromorpha also includes an unusual relict species: the mountain 'beaver' (*Aplodontia rufa*). *A. rufa* is the only surviving member of the Family Aplodontiidae. It is a compact, short-limbed fossorial animal, weighing 600–700 g, that lives only in the mountain forests of the Pacific Northwest of America (Carraway and Verts, 1993). It has a remarkably large penile bone (baculum), as is discussed in Chapter 5, which deals with effects of sexual selection on the evolution of phallic morphology.

Diverse mating systems are represented among the various suborders of rodents (Waterman, 2007). For example, monogamy occurs in a number of taxa, as in both species of the beaver. Naked mole-rats (*Heterocephalus glaber*) have a remarkable eusocial system in which groups of 70–80 members include only one reproductive female (Jarvis, 1991). In many taxa, females commonly engage in multiple-partner matings; as, for example, among the squirrels, chipmunks and prairie dogs (Family Sciuridae) and the rats and mice of the Suborder Myomorpha. The potential for sperm competition and cryptic female choice to occur is thus widespread in the Rodentia (Solomon and Keane, 2007; Waterman, 2007), as is discussed in Chapter 4 and in Part III of this book.

Closely related to the rodents are the rabbits and hares (Family Leporidae) and the smaller pikas (Family Ochotonidae) of the Order Lagomorpha (Figure 2.18). They are widely distributed throughout the Old World, and also occur in North America. The European rabbit (*Oryctolagus cuniculus*) has been translocated to Australia and New Zealand, with disastrous ecological consequences. Approximately 91 recent species of lagomorphs are currently known, of which the rabbits and hares account for 12 genera

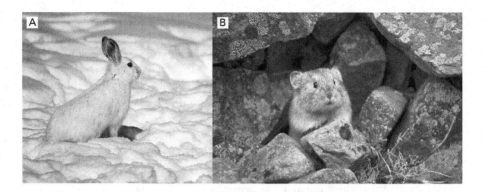

Figure 2.18 Lagomorphs. **A:** Family Leporidae: snow-shoe hare (*Lepus americanus*). This species grows a white coat of hair during the winter months. **B:** Family Ochotonidae: the northern pika (*Ochotona hyperborea*), which occurs in mountainous areas of Northern Asia. (Images: © Shutterstock.com.)

and 61 species, as compared to one genus and 30 species of pikas (Vaughan *et al.*, 2015). Fossils of forms belonging to both the extant families date from the Eocene.

Lagomorphs feed primarily on grasses and herbaceous plants. As an adaptation to extract the maximum nutritional value from their vegetarian diet, they exhibit coprophagy. Soft faecal pellets are produced and these are consumed for a second passage through the digestive tract. This order is also distinguished by the high rates of reproduction exhibited by many taxa. As an example, in the domestic rabbit, females (does) may become pregnant at 3 months of age and they produce a litter of 5–6 offspring after a gestation period of between 28 and 33 days. Does become sexually receptive shortly after giving birth, so that multiple litters are possible during each year, especially in captive animals (Nowak, 1999). Experimental research using domestic rabbits has shown that induced ovulation occurs in this species, in response to a variety of stimuli provided by the male (Brooks, 1937). It is likely that most other lagomorphs are also induced ovulators. The phylogenetic distribution and evolution of induced ovulation in mammals are examined in Chapter 9.

The Order Dermoptera contains two genera, and at least two species of the colugos or 'flying lemurs' (*Galeopterus variegatus* and *Cynocephalus volans*, Figure 2.19A). Colugos do not fly; they glide by means of the patagial membranes that extend between the limbs on each side of the body and attach to the tip of the tail. Nor are colugos lemurs, although the Dermoptera and the Primates are currently considered to be sister taxa (Figure 2.10). Molecular and morphological studies also indicate that *G. variegatus* populations of the Malaysian peninsula, Borneo and Java may represent three separate species (Janeca *et al.*, 2008). The earliest ancestor of the colugos (Genus *Dermotherium*) was initially described on the basis of a late Eocene jaw fragment, discovered in Thailand (Ducrocq *et al.*, 1992).

Adult colugos weighing between 1.0 and 1.75 kg are able to glide for over 100 metres between trees, in order to feed on leaves, flowers, fruits and sap. In association with their vegetarian diet, the stomach, intestine and caecum are very

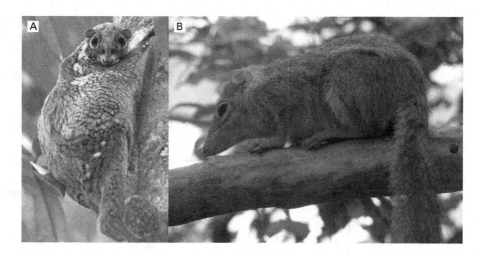

Figure 2.19 A: Order Dermoptera: a colugo or 'flying lemur' (*Galeopterus variegatus*). **B:** Order Scandentia: common treeshrew (*Tupaia glis*). (Images: © Shutterstock.com.)

large in these animals. Wharton (1950), for instance, recorded that a colugo 'which has a head and body length of about 16 inches, has an intestinal tract 11 feet long'. Colugos are nocturnal and non-gregarious. Males perform more glides and travel longer distances than females each night. Byrnes *et al.* (2011) reported that this was not due to a sex difference in feeding behaviour, but might possibly be due to males patrolling their territories or searching for mates.

The Order Scandentia contains 5 genera and 20 species of treeshrews. These small and superficially squirrel-like mammals occur in India, Burma and throughout much of South-East Asia. Nineteen species belong to the Family Tupaiidae (Figure 2.19B). These are highly active diurnal or crepuscular animals; they are omnivorous and include small vertebrates and insects as well as fruits in their diet. A single species belonging to the Family Ptilocercidae, the pen-tailed treeshrew (*Ptilocercus lowii*), is arboreal and nocturnal.

For many years the treeshrews were considered to be members of the Order Primates (e.g. Clark, 1962; Napier and Napier, 1967; Simpson, 1945). There was gradual acceptance, however, that 'most of the similarities shared by the tree-shrews and primates are attributable to retentions from the ancestral placental stock' (Martin, 1990). Thus the treeshrews were removed from the Primates and placed in the Order Scandentia. Modern phylogenomic studies confirm that the treeshrews should be accorded ordinal status. Some authorities consider that the Scandentia, Dermoptera and Primates represent a monophyletic 'clade' (the Euarchonta). This is not universally accepted, however. Fossil evidence of treeshrew evolution is of limited value in resolving this question, as the only known Eocene fossils closely resemble extant members of the Scandentia.

The Order Primates is represented by approximately 400 extant species, which are assigned to 6 superfamilies: the lemurs of Madagascar, the galagos and lorises of

Africa and Asia, the South-East Asian tarsiers, New World monkeys, Old World monkeys, and the apes and humans (Figure 2.20). Some representatives of these superfamilies are shown in Figure 2.21. Two classification schemes for the Order Primates are used in various texts. First, the Superorders Lemuroidea, Lorisoidea and

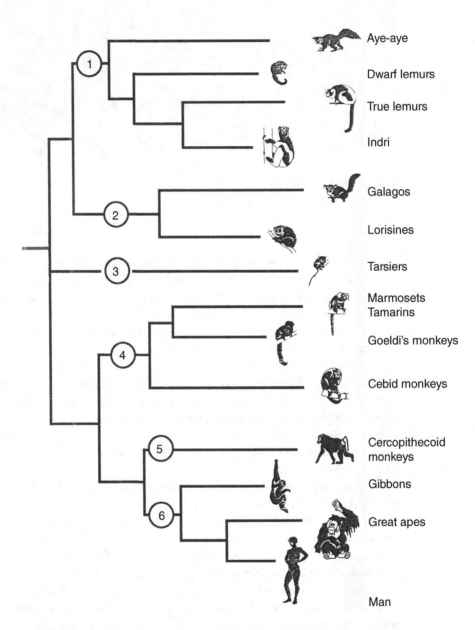

Figure 2.20 Phylogenetic relationships among the six superfamilies of extant primates: (**1**) Lemuroidea; (**2**) Lorisoidea; (**3**) Tarsioidea; (**4**) Ceboidea; (**5**) Cercopithecoidea; (**6**) Hominoidea. (From Dixson, 2012, after Martin, 1995.)

Prosimians   Anthropoids

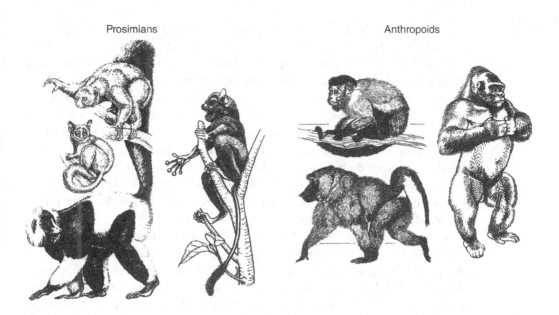

Figure 2.21 Examples of prosimians and anthropoids belonging to the six superfamilies of extant primates. Suborder Prosimii – lower left: ruffed lemur (*Varecia variegata*); upper left: potto (*Perodicticus potto*) and immediately below it, a lesser galago (*Galago senegalensis*); right: tarsier (*Tarsius spectrum*). Suborder Anthropoidea – lower left: an Old World monkey, the baboon (*Papio* sp.); upper left: a South American capuchin (*Cebus* sp.); right: a silverback male gorilla (*Gorilla gorilla*) beating its chest. (From Dixson, 2015a, after Clark, 1962, and Schwartz, 1987.)

Tarsioidea have traditionally been included within a single suborder, the Prosimii, whilst the remaining three superorders are grouped together as the simians or anthropoids (monkeys, apes and humans: Suborder Anthropoidea; Simpson, 1945). Prosimians, such as the lemurs, lorises and galagos, are anatomically more similar to stem forms which gave rise to the modern primates and for this reason they are sometimes (misleadingly) referred to as 'lower primates'. A second valid arrangement divides the primates into the Suborders Haplorhini and Strepsirhini. This takes account of the peculiar mixture of anatomical traits displayed by the tarsiers, some of which they share with the extant prosimians and others with the anthropoids. The tarsiers are accordingly often included with the anthropoids as members of the Suborder Haplorhini, whilst the lemurs and the lorisoids are placed in the Suborder Strepsirhini.

Unlike most orders of mammals discussed so far, the primates are defined by their possession of a suite of generalized traits, rather than by any single adaptation. Thus, they have forward-pointing eyes and excellent stereoscopic vision, as well as grasping hands and feet with flattened nails (rather than claws) on at least some digits. These traits probably derive from arboreal ancestors that hunted actively for insects and other small animals. Fossils of such possible ancestors, belonging to the Adapidae and Omomyidae, date from the Eocene 56–34 Mya. Primates are also large-brained animals, which reproduce relatively slowly, and extended periods of infant and juvenile life are typical, especially so among the apes and in *Homo sapiens*.

Most prosimians are nocturnal, relatively small-bodied animals (e.g. the potto, and Senegal galago in Figure 2.21). Some of the larger lemurs are diurnal and live in social groups (e.g. the ruffed lemur in Figure 2.21). All the extant lemurs share a nocturnal ancestry, however, so that even the diurnal forms retain traits (such as a reflecting layer or *tapetum lucidum* behind the retina of the eye) that arose in nocturnal environments. Many of the nocturnal prosimians are non-gregarious, and adults occupy individual, overlapping home ranges. They make extensive use of olfactory communication in sexual and social contexts, and fieldwork on a number of species (e.g. lesser galagos, mouse lemurs and the aye-aye) has confirmed that females mate with a number of males during restricted periods of sexual receptivity.

Among the anthropoids, the New World and Old World monkeys show many similarities of morphology and behaviour, owing to their similar modes of life and the effects of convergent evolution. Thus, they all live in groups, with complex social organizations and diverse mating systems. With the exception of the owl monkeys (Genus *Aotus*) they are diurnal and possess excellent colour vision. All the New World monkeys are arboreal, and they make use of urine and cutaneous secretions for communication in social and sexual contexts. The Old World monkeys of Africa and Asia constitute a more diverse array of terrestrial species (e.g. geladas, macaques and baboons) as well as arboreal forms, such as the colobus monkeys and guenons. Scent-marking behaviour is very rare among the Old World anthropoids, visual cues being more important, so that adult females of some species develop large pink or reddish sexual skin swellings during the follicular phase of the menstrual cycle. This is the case, for example, in some macaques, baboons and mangabeys, while, among the apes, female chimpanzees and bonobos also develop sexual skin swellings.

Turning to the Hominoidea, it has long been recognized that the apes, and especially the chimpanzee and gorilla, might be most closely related to *Homo sapiens*. Modern research has confirmed the insights of Darwin and Huxley concerning these matters; indeed, molecular studies indicate that humans and chimpanzees share a common ancestor, and an African origin, at approximately 7–8 Mya. The social and sexual lives of apes are diverse, so that the chimpanzee and its close relative the bonobo live in flexible fusion–fission communities with a multimale–multifemale mating system. Female chimpanzees mate with many partners during the fertile period, and likewise males will mate with a number of females. Sexual relationships are highly labile and short-term in nature, which is very different from those of most human beings. Gorillas, by contrast, are polygynous, so that adult ('silverback') males compete to lead small groups ('harems') of females. Successful males have considerable mating and reproductive success; DNA typing studies of mountain gorillas show that dominant males sire 85 per cent of the offspring born into their groups (Bradley *et al.*, 2005). In South-East Asia, the orang-utan is most unusual among the anthropoids in being non-gregarious; adults of both sexes occupy large individual home ranges in the rainforests of Borneo and Sumatra. Male orang-utans are massive creatures and, at 100 kg in weight, they are among the world's largest arboreal mammals. By contrast, the Asiatic gibbons, which are much smaller and are sometimes referred to as the 'lesser apes', live in small, highly cohesive family groups. They are monogamous and while occasional extra-pair copulations occur, the available evidence indicates that most offspring are sired by resident males in these family units.

The Superorder Afrotheria

The Afrotheria comprises a morphologically diverse assemblage of six orders of mammals which, at first sight, would seem unlikely to be closely related (Figure 2.22). Yet the validity of the Afrotheria as a taxonomic group is strongly

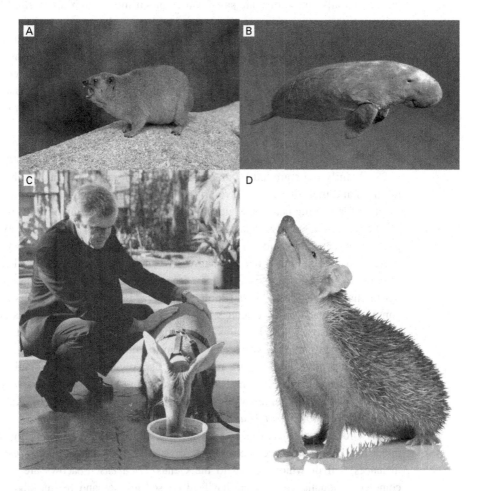

Figure 2.22 Examples of Afrotherians. **A:** Rock hyrax (*Procavia capensis*). **B:** Dugong (*Dugong dugon*). **C:** Aardvark (*Orycteropus afer*). **D:** Lesser hedgehog tenrec (*Echinops telfairi*). (Images **A**, **B** and **D**: © Shutterstock.com; C: photograph by Amanda Dixson.)

supported by the results of phylogenomic research, as well as by anatomical evidence (Asher *et al.*, 2009; Seifert, 2007; Tabuce *et al.*, 2008). One of its two major divisions, containing the Proboscidea (elephants), Sirenia (manatees and dugongs) and Hyracoidea (hyraxes), has historically been recognized under another name: the Paenungulata. The other major division of the Afrotheria consists of three orders: Tubulidentata (the aardvark), Afrosoricida (tenrecs, otter shrews and golden moles) and Macroscelidea (elephant shrews).

The Order Proboscidea contains three extant species of the Family Elephantidae: the African savannah elephant (*Loxodonta africana*), the smaller forest elephant (*L. cyclotis*) and the Asian elephant (*Elephas maximus*). These are the last survivors of a geographically widespread group which had its origins during the early Eocene (Shoshani and Tassy, 1996). Elephants are the largest land mammals; an adult male savannah elephant may weigh up to 7500 kg. One pair of the upper incisor teeth is greatly elongated to form tusks, whilst the premolar and molar teeth are adapted to grind up tough vegetation. Adult elephants consume approximately 200 kg of forage each day. Their massive grinding teeth erupt slowly in sequence so that, when one tooth is worn down, it is replaced by the next. Once the final (sixth) set of teeth emerges these must last for the remainder of an elephant's lifespan; some exceptional individuals may reach 70–75 years of age (Stansfield, 2015).

Long-term fieldwork on African elephants has shown that they have a matriarchal, fusion–fission type of social organization (Archie *et al.*, 2006; Moss, 1988). Family units are led by an older dominant female, and include her female relatives and their offspring. Several family groups may sometimes unite and stay together for varying periods. Males, by contrast, leave their natal groups when they are between 10 and 18 years old and become solitary foragers. They lead a peripatetic existence and, as adult 'tuskers', they periodically enter a state of musth, during which they become aggressive and unpredictable in their behaviour. During musth, testosterone levels increase and an odiferous secretion is produced by the male's temporal glands (Poole and Moss, 1981). Tuskers in this condition compete with each other to mate with females during their brief periods of sexual receptivity (Moss, 1983). It is now known that elephants are able to emit very-low-frequency vocalizations, which enable them to communicate over long distances. Sexually receptive females are thought to use such infrasonic vocalizations to communicate with breeding males. The fascinating story of the discovery of this unusual form of communication among elephants is described by Katy Payne (1998) in her book *Silent Thunder*.

The Order Sirenia contains four extant species of seacows: the dugong (*Dugong dugon*) and three manatee species (the Amazonian, West Indian and West African manatees), all of which belong to the Genus *Trichecus*. Seacows are very large, completely aquatic vegetarians that feed on sea grasses and marine algae that are low in nutritional value. Their forelimbs are shaped like paddles, they lack hindlimbs and their tails are flattened horizontally, like those of whales and dolphins. As an example, Figure 2.22B shows the dugong; this species has been recorded as reaching a maximum weight of 908 kg. Dugongs and other sirenians have low metabolic rates and, despite their large size and possession of a layer of blubber, they do not retain heat effectively under colder conditions. Hence the seacows are mainly to be found in tropical waters.

Fossil Sirenians are known from Eocene deposits in Africa, Europe and Jamaica. Figure 2.23 shows a reconstruction of the skeleton of one of the Jamaican fossils, *Pezosiren portelli*. This is the oldest known ancestral sirenian which was fully quadrupedal. *Pezosiren* was thus probably still capable of an amphibious existence rather than being exclusively aquatic (Domning, 2001).

Sirenians have long lifespans, and they reproduce slowly; dugongs, for example, may live for 70 years and females give birth to a single offspring every 3–7 years (Marsh, 1980; Marsh *et al.*, 1984). Dugong mating systems are not well understood, and they may vary geographically. Anderson (1997) described a possible type of lek mating system for the dugong population of Shark Bay in Western Australia, where individual males patrolled 'small exclusive zones of activity' and courted passing females. By contrast, Hartman (1979) reported that groups of male manatees (*T. manatus*) in Florida may follow a receptive female for extended periods and that multiple-partner matings occur in these aggregations. Post-copulatory sexual selection would be expected to occur in these circumstances.

Seacow populations are under threat due to hunting, habitat destruction, marine pollution and other human activities that put the animals at risk, such as collisions with speed boats. It is worth noting here that the largest of all the seacows (*Hydrodamalis gigas*) is already extinct; it was exterminated during the eighteenth century. Estimated to have reached 8 metres in length and to have weighed 10 metric tons, these innocuous giants once grazed in shallow waters around the North Pacific rim. The last recorded population to escape the hunters' notice was discovered in the Bering Sea by a Russian expedition in 1741. The appalling fate of this remnant population was recorded at the time by the German naturalist after whom the species gets its name: Steller's seacow.

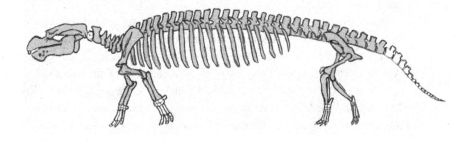

Figure 2.23 Reconstruction of the skeleton of the fossil sirenian *Pezosiren portelli*, a quadrupedal ancestor of the extant seacows. (From Domning, 2001.)

Their capture was effected by a large iron hook, . . . the other end being fastened by means of an iron ring to a very long, stout rope, held by thirty men on shore. The harpooner stood in the bow of the boat with the hook in his hand and struck as soon as he was near enough to do so, whereupon the men on shore grasping the other end of the rope pulled the desperately resisting animal laboriously towards them . . . it was attacked with bayonets, knives and other weapons and pulled up on land. Immense slices were cut from the still living animal, but all it did was shake its tail furiously.

The Order Hyracoidea consists of the single Family Procaviidae, which contains three genera and four species of the hyraxes (*Procavia capensis*, *Heterohyrax brucei*, *Dendrohyrax dorsalis* and *D. arboreus*). The earliest representatives of the hyraxes lived in Africa during the Eocene, and the Order Hyracoidea was once much larger than is now the case.

Hyraxes are agile, rodent-like herbivores that weigh about 4 kg (Figure 2.22A). All four species have African distributions, but *P. capensis* also occurs in parts of the Middle East and the Arabian Peninsula. Ecologically they are broadly divisible into two types: the tree hyraxes (*Dendrohyrax* spp.) and rock hyraxes (*Procavia* and *Heterohyrax*). Tree hyraxes are nocturnal, highly arboreal and non-gregarious. Adults occupy individual home ranges and the larger male ranges overlap with those of a number of females. During the night, adults of both sexes emit loud, prolonged vocalizations that gradually increase in amplitude and end in a marked crescendo (Shultz and Roberts, 2013). Rock hyraxes are mainly diurnal and inhabit rocky outcrops, cliffs and similar habitats where they can obtain shelter as well as food. They live in mixed sexed groups and have a multimale–multifemale (polygynandrous) mating system (Bar Ziv *et al.*, 2016).

The Order Tubilidentata contains a single extant representative, the aardvark (*Orycteropus afer*). This species is widely distributed in Africa, south of the Sahara desert. The name 'aardvark' derives from the Afrikaans word for 'earth pig', and it is a most unusual-looking animal (Figure 2.22C). Adults weigh between 50 and 70 kg and with their compact bodies, powerful limbs and strong flattened claws they are able to burrow rapidly and to break into termite mounds and ant nests in pursuit of their prey. The aardvark has large ears and a tubular snout; the entrance to its nostrils is guarded by thick hairs, and its long, sticky tongue can be protruded to capture ants and termites.

Although convergent evolution has resulted in superficial resemblances between the aardvark and some other mammals that specialize in eating ants or termites, it is not closely related to either the pangolins of Africa and Asia or the anteaters of South America. The position of the aardvark as a member of the Afrotheria is now well established (Tabuce *et al.*, 2008). Fossil relatives of the aardvark are known from the Miocene and the Miocene–Pliocene boundary of Eurasia and Africa (e.g. *Orycteropus abundulafus* from the Mio-Pliocene of Chad in Northern Africa: Lehmann *et al.*, 2005).

The aardvark is non-gregarious and is mainly active at night; it spends the daylight hours concealed in a burrow. Aardvarks are noted for their ability to dig very rapidly and they construct a number of temporary burrows throughout their home ranges.

Field studies of aardvarks fitted with radio transmitters (Taylor and Skinner, 2003) showed that their home ranges are very large and overlap one another, so that eight individuals may occupy a total area of about 10 km². This indicates that the aardvark might have a dispersed type of mating system, similar to that of some other nocturnal, non-gregarious mammals; but, in truth, nothing is known about the sexual behaviour of the aardvark.

The Order Afrosoricida is divided into two suborders: the Chrysochloridea (golden moles) and the Tenrecomorpha (tenrecs and otter shrews). Golden moles are found only in Africa; 9 genera and 21 species are currently recognized (Bronner, 2013). They are highly adapted for a fossorial existence and, although completely blind, they are acutely sensitive to vibrations and able to 'swim' through the sand in search of insect prey. Unfortunately, very little is known about their reproductive biology, including their sexual behaviour.

There are 34 species of the Tenrecomorpha, 31 of which occur in Madagascar (the tenrecs) and 3 species (the otter shrews) are African in their distribution. Few fossils of tenrecs have been discovered. However, molecular phylogenetic studies by Douady *et al.* (2002b) suggest that the ancestors of tenrecs and the African otter shrews split at around 53 Mya, and that tenrecs had colonized Madagascar at some time before 37 Mya. A wide adaptive radiation of the Madagascan forms has resulted in convergent evolution, so that some tenrecs closely resemble moles (*Oryzorictes* spp.: rice tenrecs), shrews (*Microgale* spp.) and hedgehogs (e.g *Setifer setosus* and *Echinops telfairi*, the lesser hedgehog tenrec, Figure 2.22D).

Much more is known about the behaviour and reproductive biology of tenrecs than is the case for the golden moles. In the streaked tenrec (*Hemicentetes semispinosus*), a remarkable 'stridulating organ' consisting of a small group of quills is situated in the centre of the back. These spines are under muscular control, and when rubbed together they produce sounds that are thought to maintain contact between group members (Gould and Eisenberg, 1966). The communicatory biology and sexual behaviour of captive tenrecs has been studied in some detail, and prolonged patterns of copulation occur in a number of species (Eisenberg, 1975; Eisenberg and Gould, 1970). The evolution of copulatory durations is covered in Part II of this book, and also in Chapter 9 which deals with the origins of induced and spontaneous ovulation in the Mammalia.

The final order of Afrotherians to be considered is the Macroscelidea, commonly referred to as the elephant shrews or sengis. There are 15 species of sengis belonging to 4 genera, and all of them occur in Africa. Fossil evidence of this order is also confined to Africa and dates back to the Eocene (Holroyd and Mussell, 2005).

The name 'elephant shrew' refers to the long and highly mobile snout which is used to locate and capture insects. They are small, long-limbed animals; even the largest 'giant' sengis (Genus *Rhynchocyon*) weigh only about 500 g. The sengis are diurnal or crepuscular in their activity patterns and they have a remarkable ability to run extremely fast when avoiding predators. For example, the rufus elephant shrew

(*Elephantulus rufescens*) maintains a complex network of trails throughout the under-brush that constitutes its territory; it constantly patrols and clears away any potential obstacles (Rathbun, 1979). An intimate knowledge of these trails makes it possible for these mammals to flee at high speed when threatened.

Sengis are often considered to be monogamous; a male and female jointly defend a territory as, for example, in the golden-rumped sengi (*Rhynchocyon chrysopygus*: FitzGibbon, 1997), the round-eared sengi (*Macroscelides proboscideus*: Schubert *et al.*, 2009) and the eastern rock sengi (*Elephantulus myurus*: Ribble and Perrin, 2005). However, these studies, and others, indicate that, in practice, male sengis find it difficult to mate guard and defend the territory of more than one female (Rathbun and Rathbun, 2006). Indeed, it is not yet known whether the social system, and pairing between the sexes, equates to the genetic mating system in these interesting mammals.

Despite the fact that female sengis usually give birth to just one or two offspring, at least five species are known to exhibit polyovulation, whereby very large numbers of ova are released during each ovarian cycle (Birney and Baird, 1985; Van Der Horst and Gillman, 1940). In the eastern rock sengi, for example, females may ovulate anywhere between 25 and 85 ova. Polyovulation is uncommon among mammals, but cases have also been identified among a few species belonging to the Afrosoricida, Chiroptera, Rodentia, Artiodactyla and Dasyuromorphia.

The Superorder Xenarthra

Armadillos, anteaters and sloths look so unlike and act and live so differently that it might hardly occur to anyone to classify them together without more anatomical study. Such study reveals that they do share peculiarities that undoubtedly indicate a common origin, although one in the remote past.

George Gaylord Simpson (1980)

Skeletal peculiarities shared by the armadillos (Order Cingulata) and the anteaters and sloths (Order Pilosa) include the presence of additional vertebral projections which strengthen the lumbar region of the spinal column. There is also an important difference in the way that the pelvic girdle is joined to the sacrum of the backbone. In xenarthans, the ilia and ischia of the pelvic girdle articulate with the sacrum, whereas in other placental mammals only the ilia are joined to the sacrum.

Some examples of the various types of xenarthrans that are alive today are shown in Figure 2.24. There are 20 species of armadillos, 4 species of anteaters and 6 species of sloths, all of which are native to South and Central America. However, one species, the nine-banded armadillo (*Dasypus novemcinctus*: Figure 2.24A), has extended its range beyond Central America to include Texas and other southern states of the USA. This northward extension of the nine-banded armadillo's range from Mexico into the USA may have occurred relatively recently (Loughry and McDonough, 2013).

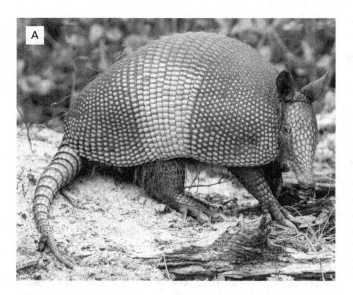

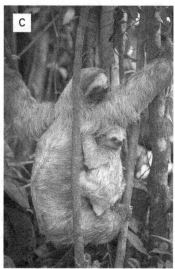

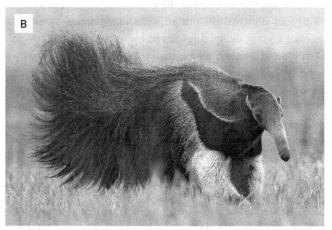

Figure 2.24 Superorder Xenarthra. **A:** Nine-banded armadillo (*Dasypus novemcinctus*). **B:** Giant anteater (*Myrmecophaga tridactyla*). **C:** A female Hoffmann's two-toed sloth (*Choloepus hoffmanni*) with her infant. (Images © Shuttlestock.com.)

The armadillos (Dasypodidae) are notable for their covering of boney armour, which is jointed in the mid-section of the body, allowing some flexibility of movement and the ability, in some species, to curl up into a ball as a defensive measure. Armadillos vary greatly in size, the largest being the giant armadillo (*Priodontes maximus*), well-fed captive specimens of which can reach 60 kg in weight. However, in the wild, weights of between 18.7 and 32.3 kg are the norm (Redford and Eisenberg, 1992). At the opposite end of the scale, the pink fairy armadillo (*Chlamyphorus truncatus*) may weigh as little as 85 g (Nowak, 1999). It is one of the fossorial armadillo species, but all armadillos are equipped with strong limbs and stout claws for digging. They feed mainly on insects including ants and termites, as well as other invertebrates, but sometimes include small vertebrates and carrion in their diet.

Armadillos, like other xenarthrans, are non-gregarious (Desbiez *et al.*, 2018; Loughry and McDonough, 2013). The social organization of the nine-banded armadillo has been studied in Texas by McDonough (1997, 2000). Both sexes occupy individual home ranges, and the larger ranges of breeding males overlap extensively with those of multiple females. During the annual mating season, which peaks between June and August, the largest and oldest males associate for varying periods with a series of females. These serial 'pairings' appear to be a form of mate-guarding by males, and the mating system has been described as polygynous. In the six-banded armadillo (*Euphractus sexcinctus*), Tomas *et al.* (2013) have described a different system that involves mating chases by groups of males and single females. Whether females mate with multiple partners is not known.

One of the reproductive peculiarities of the nine-banded armadillo, which it shares with other members of the Genus *Dasypus*, concerns the occurrence of polyembryony, so that females give birth to four identical offspring. In the nine-banded armadillo, implantation of the single blastocyst is delayed for several months after conception. Once implantation has taken place, however, the blastocyst divides, and gives rise to four genetically identical embryos (Enders 2002; Loughry *et al.*, 1998). Galbreath (1985) proposed that the morphology of the simplex uterus of armadillos may have influenced the evolution of polyembryony. He noted that only a very small area of the uterine wall is available for implantation to occur, and that most armadillos generally produce single offspring. In members of the Genus *Dasypus*, such as the nine-banded armadillo, the evolution of polyembryony has made it possible for four offspring to develop at a single implantation site (however, see Enders, 2002, for a critique of Galbreath's hypothesis).

The fact that a female nine-banded armadillo's quadruplet offspring are genetically identical raises the possibility that kin selection might favour their cooperative or altruistic behaviour and increase their chances of survival. There can be no doubt that the nine-banded armadillo is a very successful species, with an enormous distribution range. For whatever reason, its ability to produce multiple offspring via polyembryony has clearly proven advantageous.

Turning now to the Order Pilosa, this includes two families of anteaters and two families of sloths. Anteaters, with the exception of the largest species (*Mymecophaga tridactyla*: Figure 2.24B) are partly or entirely arboreal. The giant anteater is terrestrial in its habits and occurs in savanna and grassland habitats in Central and South America. Adults weigh 18–39 kg and they are covered in long coarse hair, with a large plumed tail that can be folded across the animal when it is at rest. Giant anteaters have powerful claws on their forelimbs that are used to break open termite and ant mounds. The tongue is highly mobile, and can be protruded for up to 60 cm when capturing its prey. The giant anteater, along with two much smaller *Tamandua* species (*T. mexicana* and *T. tridactyla*), is placed in the Family Myrmecophagidae. The fourth anteater species, the silky anteater (*Cyclopes didactylus*), has been assigned to a separate Family, the Cyclopedidae, on the basis that its ancestors diverged from the myrmecophagids roughly 54 Mya during the early Eocene (Delsuc *et al.*, 2001). It is a small nocturnal anteater, weighing less than 400 g, which uses its prehensile tail when climbing and hunting for insects in the rainforest canopy.

The two sloth families are the Bradipodidae (Genus *Bradypus*: four species of three-toed sloths) and the Megalonychidae (Genus *Choloepus*: two species of two-toed sloths). Sloths use the long curved claws on their fore- and hindlimbs to suspend themselves below branches whilst on the move (Figure 2.24C). They are highly arboreal and folivorous, the large stomach acting as a fermentation chamber for the digestion of leaves. The slow-moving way of life of sloths is partly a reflection of their low metabolic rates and very limited ability to control their body temperature, as well as the need to conserve energy given the poor nutritional quality of their diet. Sloths find it very difficult to move about at ground level, but once every week or so they descend briefly from the trees in order to defecate.

It is likely that the unusual physiological adaptations and slow mode of life displayed by sloths must affect their social and sexual interactions. Sloths are relatively solitary (i.e. non-gregarious) animals, as are other members of the Xenarthra. It is known that each individual occupies a home range, and that the larger home ranges of adult males overlap those of a number of females. Adult males are sometimes antagonistic to each other, but it is probably only the 'core' of each male's range that is defended. Fieldwork involving DNA typing to determine parentage of offspring has been conducted on *Bradypus variegatus* and *Choloepus hoffmanni* (Garcés-Restrepo *et al.*, 2017; Pauli and Peery 2012; Peery and Pauli 2012). Female sloths give birth to single offspring and these may be sired by different males during successive years (e.g. in *C. hoffmanni*: Garcés-Restrepo *et al.*, 2017). There is no evidence that sloths are monogamous, but neither is there firm evidence that females mate with multiple partners during a single mating season. Some males sire more offspring than others, so that a polygynous mating system is a possibility (in *B. variegatus*: Pauli and Peery, 2012), although a lack of fine-grained data on sexual interactions limits interpretation of the paternity data.

The small number of extant xenarthran species described here represents only a fraction of the taxa that have existed in the past. The earliest known xenarthran fossils are fragments of the boney armour plates of armadillos dating from the early Eocene or the Paleocene of South America (Simpson, 1980; Vaughan *et al.*, 2015). However, prior to the formation of a land bridge with North America during the Pliocene, a vast adaptive radiation of xenarthrans had occurred in South America. Some of these, including tank-like glyptodonts and huge ground sloths (Figure 2.25) survived well into the Pleistocene epoch and their fossils have also been discovered in parts of North America.

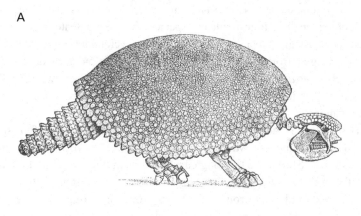

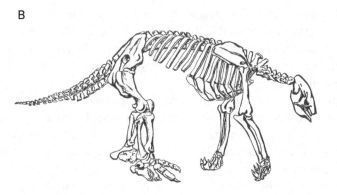

Figure 2.25 Examples of fossil xenarthrans. **A:** *Glyptodon*, from the Pleistocene of South America. This massive relative of the extant armadillos was about 9.5 feet long. **B:** Skeleton of an extinct ground sloth (*Nototherium*) which, in life, was about 7.5 feet long. (From Romer, 1962.)

Dating the Origins of Placental Mammals

Few other episodes in the history of life have rivaled the dramatic extinction of the non-avian dinosaurs and the rapid radiation of mammals. Unquestionably, without the former's extinction, the latter's diversification into clades as different as bats and whales would never have occurred.

David Archibald (2011)

When did the earliest members of the 19 orders of the Placentalia described in the foregoing sections make their appearance? Despite the fact that fossils of mammals are known from the Cretaceous period (145–66 Mya), none of them can be assigned with certainty to the Subclass Placentalia. Most of these fossils are fragmentary in nature,

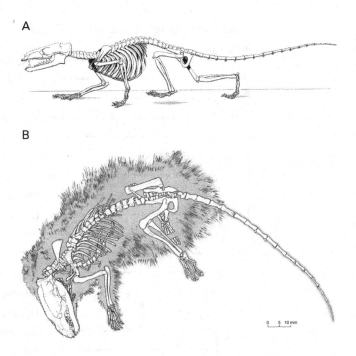

Figure 2.26 The skeleton of the small 125 million-year-old Cretaceous mammal *Eomaia scansoria*. **A:** Reconstructed in its entirety. **B:** As originally discovered, to show the 'halo' effect of the fur surrounding the fossilized bones. The scale is in 5-mm divisions. (From Ji *et al.*, 2002.)

consisting only of the jaws and teeth of animals that were probably no larger than shrews or rats (Archibald, 2011; Kemp, 2005; Rose and Archibald, 2005; Wible *et al.*, 2007). A rare example of a complete fossil skeleton is provided by *Eomaia scansoria*, from Liaoning Province in China (Ji *et al.*, 2002). This 125 million-year-old specimen even retains traces of its fur, in the form of a 'halo' that surrounds the skeleton (Figure 2.26). However, fossils of crown group placentals do not appear until the Paleocene and Eocene epochs (66–34 Mya), during which time representatives of all but 1 of the 19 extant placental orders make their first appearance in the fossil record (Figure 2.27). The Tubilidentata is the sole exception, as the earliest fossils of aardvarks date to 24 Mya, at the end of the Oligocene.

The fossil record thus indicates that the diversification of placental mammals took place after the mass extinction event which occurred at the close of the Cretaceous some 66 Mya. A huge meteor collided with the Earth at this time, causing major environmental changes at what is usually referred to by geologists as the K/T or K/Pg boundary. Some other geological events also occurred during this period. There were widespread marine regressions (falling sea levels) and prolonged massive volcanic eruptions in the Deccan Traps of Western Central India. These events may have contributed to climatic and ecological changes that accelerated the extinction of the

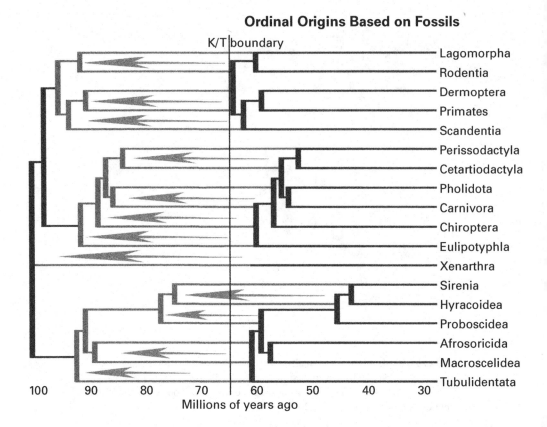

Figure 2.27 Origins and diversification of the various orders of placental mammals, contrasting datings based upon the fossil record (post K/T boundary: 66 Mya) with the much earlier datings derived from molecular data, as indicated by the arrows. (From Archibald, 2011.)

non-avian dinosaurs. The disappearance of so many dinosaur taxa would have opened up a wide variety of ecological niches for exploitation by mammals (Archibald, 2011).

A number of molecular studies have produced substantially earlier estimates for the origin and inter-ordinal diversification of placental mammals than those based upon the fossil record (Figure 2.27). They push these events back into the Cretaceous, well prior to the K/T boundary (e.g. Bininda-Emonds *et al.*, 2007). Possible reasons for discrepancies between the molecular and fossil estimates are discussed by David Archibald in his book *Extinction and Radiation: How the Fall of the Dinosaurs Led to the Rise of Mammals*. He suggests that difficulties in calibrating molecular clocks accurately, with respect to the fossil record, and assumptions about consistent rates of molecular evolution may have led to inaccurate estimates. For example, it is possible that rates of molecular evolution may have accelerated among the placental mammals after the K/T extinction event as they diversified rapidly in the absence of competition from the non-avian dinosaurs. The early fossil record of some of the orders of placental mammals is far from complete (e.g. for the Afrosoricida and Tubilidentata). Yet, thus far, discoveries of the earliest fossils of the various orders of placental mammals have all been made at post K/T boundary sites.

Part II

The Act of Mating

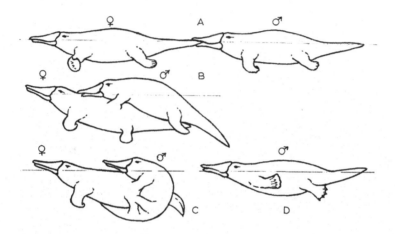

Aquatic courtship in the platypus
Strahan and Thomas, 1975

3 Copulatory Patterns: Phylogeny and Modes of Life

Nature rarely deals with discrete categories. Only the human mind invents categories and tries to force facts into separated pigeon-holes.

Kinsey, Pomeroy and Martin (1948)

So great is mammalian ecological and anatomical diversity that mating can take place under widely differing conditions depending upon which species is considered (e.g. in the water, on land, in the rainforest canopy, in burrows and on ice floes). This chapter focuses on the phylogenetic distribution of copulatory and associated behavioural traits throughout the Mammalia. The goal of this exercise is to determine, as far as possible, the degree of homology or convergent evolution that might exist between the various taxa, regarding their patterns of copulatory behaviour. As part of this exercise, it is important to consider the extent to which copulatory traits might have been moulded by ecological factors and by natural selection. This will pave the way for the discussions of the role played by sexual selection, in the next chapter.

Defining and Classifying Copulatory Patterns

Donald Dewsbury (1972) devised a system for classifying mammalian copulatory patterns depending upon the presence, or absence, of four components:

1. A 'lock' or 'tie' between the male and female genitalia.
2. Pelvic thrusting movements by the male partner.
3. Multiple intromissions prior to ejaculation.
4. A capacity to exhibit multiple ejaculations.

This system which, it should be noted, deals with copulatory behaviour exclusively from the male partner's perspective, results in 16 possible masculine copulatory patterns, as is shown in Figure 3.1A. Dewsbury did not regard this as a 'finished system'. He noted that 'as work proceeds, some attributes may prove to be unimportant or unworkable, while additional attributes may prove to be of value'.

One problem that has emerged when using this scheme, for example in studies of primate sexual behaviour (Dixson, 2009, 2012), concerns the lack of any measure of the duration of copulation. Intromission times vary tremendously in mammals, from less than one second in laboratory rats (*Rattus norvegicus*; Beyer *et al.*, 1982) to 5–12

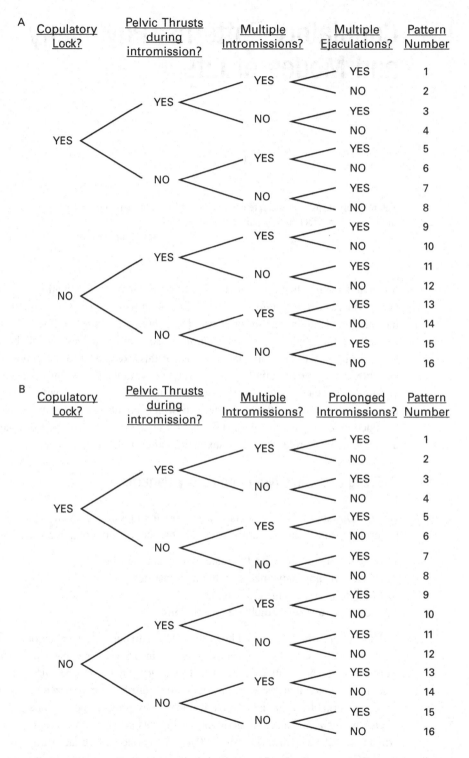

Figure 3.1 A: Dewsbury's schema for classifying masculine patterns of copulatory behaviour in mammals. (Redrawn from Dewsbury, 1972.) **B:** The modified version of Dewsbury's schema used in the current study. (From Dixson, 2012.)

hours in some dasyurid marsupials (e.g. *Antechinus* spp.; Shimmin *et al.*, 2002; Woolley, 1966). Indeed, prolonged copulations are not unusual among mammals; interested readers will find a list of average intromission durations for 170 genera of mammals in Appendix 2 of this book. At the species level, examples (in minutes) include the echidna: 30–180; eastern quoll: 300; black rhinoceros: 32, grey wolf: 120; black-footed ferret: 118, and alpaca: 6–46.

Intromission duration is likely to represent an important evolutionary trait among mammals. For example, it has been suggested that prolonged copulations might represent the ancestral condition for the Mammalia as a whole (Eisenberg, 1981; Ewer, 1968). For this reason, as in earlier studies (Dixson, 2009, 2012), I have added the presence, or absence, of prolonged intromissions to Dewsbury's original classification system. His fourth measure (multiple ejaculations) has been removed, however. This measurement, which records whether males are capable of mating and ejaculating twice within 60 minutes, has proven to be widespread, perhaps because of the arbitrary nature of the time criterion used. The modified version of Dewsbury's scheme adopted here thus replaces 'multiple ejaculations' with the new category 'prolonged intromissions', to produce the 16 possible copulatory patterns shown in Figure 3.1B. This should not be interpreted as discounting the importance of knowing whether males exhibit multiple ejaculations during copulatory bouts. Both sperm competition and cryptic female choice are influenced by such behaviour, as is discussed in Chapters 4, 8 and 9.

Dewsbury's (1972) report in the *Quarterly Review of Biology* included 118 species, of which the copulatory patterns of just 40 species could be classified in full. Thus, as well as modifying his classification scheme, I have attempted to assemble a larger data set, because this is essential if progress is to be made in examining the comparative biology and evolution of mammalian copulatory behaviour. I hope that readers will bear with me, if I describe briefly the methods used to collect additional data, and some of the problems that arose during that process.

There is an enormous literature dealing with mammalian reproduction and with various aspects of reproductive behaviour. Nowadays the availability of search engines and online access to scientific journals makes it much simpler to track down information than was the case in Dewsbury's time. However, when conducting searches, I soon discovered that even reports with promising titles frequently contained no useful information whatsoever about copulatory traits. It was a relief to read contributions by biologists who had taken the trouble to record mating patterns in detail; some of them (a minority) had even adopted Donald Dewsbury's classification scheme.

There still remain many groups of mammals for which very little has been published concerning their mating habits. The bats (Chiroptera) provide a good example. I have read field studies of bats where the authors say that they saw the animals mating, and then dash my hopes by providing no further information. Such tantalizing omissions are also commonplace in published accounts of other mammals. I very much hope that mammalogists, and behavioural ecologists in particular, will seek to rectify this situation in the future. Those who work in zoological gardens also have unique opportunities to observe mating in exotic species. Some reports certainly do originate from zoo research; examples include valuable contributions by Eisenberg, Wemmer, Kleiman and their colleagues at the National Zoo in Washington, DC. I am also especially grateful to Dr Gabriela Flack for sharing with me her observations of the mating behaviour of the pygmy hippopotamus (*Choeropsis liberiensis*). However, the most frustrating account I have read involved another unusual African mammal, the aardvark (*Orycteropus afer*, sole member of the Order Tubilidentata). The authors stated that they 'often saw the aardvarks copulating'. Alas, they included no description of mating behaviour in their report. As a result, the Tubilidentata remains one of very few orders of mammals for which I have been unable to locate any information about mating behaviour.

One further useful source of data which was not available to Donald Dewsbury concerns online postings of videos by members of the general public, who have observed exotic species mating while visiting zoos or National Parks in various parts of the world. Their recordings have made it possible for me to observe and classify copulatory patterns for a number of unstudied species at first hand, or to confirm information derived from the published literature. Perhaps my most pleasant surprise was to find a video showing colugos (*Cynocephalus variegatus*) mating in a rainforest in Borneo! This provided the only information I have been able to locate concerning the mating behaviour of the peculiar 'flying lemurs' of the Order Dermoptera.

Trials and tribulations set aside, it proved possible to classify copulatory patterns for 306 species of mammals and to obtain incomplete profiles for a further 126 species (for full details, see Appendix 1). Although this greatly expands upon Dewsbury's original listings, it still constitutes but a small fraction of current mammalian diversity. Thus, information on the marsupials is quite limited; only species belonging to the Diprotodontia and Dasyuromorphia are represented in meaningful numbers. Among the placental mammals, some information is now available for 18 of the 19 orders, but numerous gaps occur, as for example for many members of the Superorders Xenarthra and Afrotheria.

Finally, it is important to emphasize that the modified version of Dewsbury's scheme deals with patterns of copulatory behaviour solely from the male partner's perspective. In reality females can, and often do, exert important effects on the progress and coordination of copulation. Some examples of such female influences will be included here, as a prelude to the more detailed discussions of cryptic female choice in Chapter 4, and also in Part III of this book (in Chapters 8 and 9). With these caveats in mind, phylogenetic variations in patterns of copulatory behaviour are described in the sections that follow.

The Phylogenetic Distribution of Copulatory Patterns

The Five Major Patterns

Of the 16 possible copulatory patterns that might, in theory, occur in male mammals (Figure 3.1B), just five patterns (nos. 3, 10, 11, 12 and 16) account for 92 per cent of all species for which I have been able to obtain information. Only one of these patterns (no. 3) involves a 'lock' or 'tie' between the genitalia of both sexes and it is the least frequently represented of the five major patterns.

Pattern No. 3

This copulatory pattern involves a single prolonged intromission, with pelvic thrusting and a pronounced anatomical tie, or lock, between the genitalia of the participants. Most of the species that mate in this way are carnivores, and especially members of the Family Canidae; 10 species of foxes, dogs, wolves and dholes are known to exhibit this pattern. The lock between the genitalia is, in some cases, so strong that the partners remain tied together after the male dismounts, and turns to face in the opposite direction (Figure 3.2). This pattern has been studied in detail in the domestic dog (Hart, 1967; Hart and Kitchell, 1966). Intromission is followed by an 'intense ejaculatory reaction' lasting for 15–30 seconds, during which stepping movements of the hindlimbs and very rapid pelvic oscillations occur. A copulatory lock then ensues, and is maintained for 10–30 minutes due to engorgement of the *bulbus glandis* at the base of the glans penis. Seminal transfer continues during the lock. Hart and Kitchell's experiments also showed that these processes are largely under the control of complex spinal reflexes. It is important to note that spinal reflexes also occur in female dogs, including an oestrogen-sensitive reflex which results in lateral curvature of the hindquarters and vertical orientation of the vulva in response to the male's (pre-intromission) pelvic thrusts. These responses augment the female's receptive posture and increase the likelihood that a complete intromission will occur (Hart, 1970, 1978).

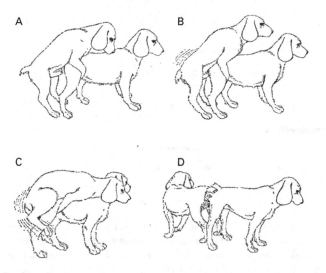

Figure 3.2 Stages during copulatory behaviour of the domestic dog. **A:** Mounting and clasping. **B:** Pelvic thrusting. **C:** Intense ejaculatory reaction. **D:** Copulatory lock. (From Hart, 1967.)

In the second major lineage of the Carnivora, the Feliformia, the spotted hyena (*Crocuta crocuta*) exhibits pattern no. 3, but in this case the male achieves intromission via the clitoral canal of the female, and the resulting tie between the genitalia is not as pronounced as in the canids. Spotted hyenas often maintain intromission for some minutes after ejaculation has occurred (Szykman *et al.*, 2007). Thus, even within the same order of mammals copulatory locks can involve genital specializations that have developed independently, and that are clearly not homologous. This also applies to many other cases of locking mechanisms, as is discussed in Chapter 5, where the evolution of phallic morphology is examined in detail.

Pattern No. 16

Pattern number 16 involves the male making a single rapid 'copulatory thrust' during an intromission which lasts for a few seconds at most (Figure 3.3). There are currently 91 species of placental mammals that are known to exhibit this rapid mating pattern, and most of them (*n* = 69) belong to the Cetartiodactyla. Among the terrestrial

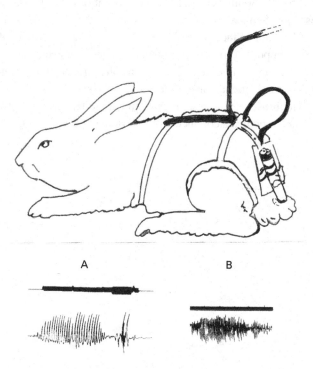

A   B

Figure 3.3 A male New Zealand white rabbit fitted with a harness and accelerometer to measure the extremely rapid pelvic movements that occur during mounting. **A:** Once mounting begins the male makes a rapid series of pelvic thrusts prior to intromission. These cease abruptly once intromission occurs. The marked deflections at the end of the recording trace are caused by the male as he dismounts after ejaculation. **B:** Note that the amplitude of pelvic thrusting is variable but the rate at which thrusts occur remains constant. (Adapted and redrawn from Contreras and Beyer, 1979.)

artiodactyls, they include the giraffe and okapi (Family Giraffidae), deer (Cervidae), the pronghorn (Antilocapridae), goats, sheep, cattle, bison, wildebeest, gazelles, antelopes and numerous other members of the Family Bovidae, as well as the tiny musk deer (Moschidae). Very little has been published concerning mating behaviour in the Moschidae, but mounts last for only a few seconds in these animals. A pattern no. 16 classification is likely, but currently uncertain. The presence of the same copulatory pattern in the five closely related families listed above indicates that it would probably have been present in their common ancestor. The chevrotains, or mouse deer, of the Family Tragulidae represent a sister group, and it is noteworthy that their copulatory pattern differs markedly, as it involves a prolonged intromission (e.g. 15–20 minutes in *Moschiola indica*: Parvathy *et al.*, 2014) and pelvic thrusting (in *Tragulus napa*: Ralls *et al.*, 1975). Other, more distantly related artiodactyl lineages such as pigs and camelids also exhibit divergent mating patterns (e.g. nos. 3 and 11), as is discussed below.

The phylogenetic position of the Family Hippopotamidae, as a sister group to the cetaceans (whales, dolphins and porpoises) within the Cetartiodactyla was noted in Chapter 2. The hippopotamus often mates in the water, and video recordings indicate that copulation involves a single, prolonged intromission without pelvic thrusting (pattern no. 15). Intromission lasted for almost 7 minutes in one recording that I was able to study in detail; mating took place in shallow water and both partners were able to breathe regularly. I have been unable find any information about the sexual behaviour of hippos when they leave the water. Both sexes move inland to graze at night, and it is likely that alternative nocturnal mating tactics might occur, particularly where subordinate males are concerned. Thus, pattern no. 15 might not be the only form of copulation displayed by the larger of the two hippo species.

The pygmy hippopotamus (*Choeropsis liberiensis*) is often regarded as simply a smaller version of the larger hippo, but ecologically it exhibits some major differences. It is a creature of the rainforest, and spends much of its time away from water (Robinson *et al.*, 2017). Copulations (pattern no. 16) typically occur on land in captive pygmy hippos (Flack, personal communication). Intromission is comparatively brief, as it lasts for about 25 seconds. The smaller of the two hippo species thus exhibits the same type of copulatory pattern as the bovids discussed above. Indeed, pattern no. 16 also occurs in cetaceans; at least, this is the case for members of the Odontoceti for which I could obtain data (the boto: *Inia geoffrensis*; harbour porpoise: *Phocoena phocoena*; dusky dolphin: *Lagenorhynchus obscurus* and the largest of the dolphins: *Orca orca*). It is also likely to be true of several other species, including the North Atlantic right whale (*Eubalaena glacialis*) for which only a partial classification of the copulatory pattern is currently available (see Appendix 1). It is possible that the mating patterns of hippos and cetaceans are homologous. Unusual features of vaginal morphology also link hippos with the cetaceans, as is discussed in Part III of this book.

Turning now to the Order Carnivora, copulatory pattern no. 16 occurs in all species of the Family Felidae for which there is sufficient information. Thus, a single brief intromission, without the occurrence of pelvic thrusting or a copulatory lock, is seen in tigers, lions and jaguars, as well as in the cheetah, and in smaller felids, such as ocelots, caracals and domestic cats. The emergence of pattern no. 16 in felids and in the cetartiodactyls discussed above undoubtedly results from markedly different selective pressures during their evolution. Thus, rapid copulation in ungulates such as deer, antelopes and wildebeest may be adaptive because it reduces the risk of being killed by predators. Any wildebeest that engaged in prolonged matings could easily fall prey to lions or hyenas. Cetaceans might have inherited the no. 16 copulatory pattern from amphibious ancestors, but whatever its origin, the evolution of the no. 16 pattern may have proven advantageous to aquatic animals, such as dolphins and whales. Copulations occur ventro-ventrally in cetaceans, and it has been noted that the female partner often occupies the upper position, with the male underneath her. This may allow the female better access to the surface of the water in order to breathe and also allow her to curtail intromission (e.g. in spinner dolphins: Johnson and Norris, 1994; dusky dolphins: Orbach et al., 2014). Male cetaceans have much less control over copulatory durations than in most mammals, so that the ability to intromit and ejaculate rapidly has undergone positive selection. Finally, there is the problem faced by all marine cetaceans of excluding the entry of sea water into the female's lower genital tract during mating, as contamination of the ejaculate by seawater can damage sperm. Rapid matings may be adaptive in this context; anatomical specializations of the reproductive organs may also reduce such risks during copulation, as is discussed in Chapter 8.

Mating in felids is complex; much more so than can be appreciated by considering masculine copulatory patterns in isolation. Most felids are non-gregarious, and the sexes rarely interact directly except when females become receptive. Aggressive tendencies have to be overcome at such times, as both sexes are capable of inflicting serious injuries upon prospective partners. Males commonly bite the skin on the nape of the neck of the female (the 'neck grip') to subdue her during copulation. Sexually receptive females exhibit several responses (tail deviation, treading and rump elevation) when mounted, and experiments using domestic cats have shown that at least two of them (tail deviation and treading) are mediated by effects of oestrogen at the spinal level (Hart, 1971). Females of a number of species also exhibit post-copulatory rolling and rubbing responses (Lanier and Dewsbury, 1976; Mellen, 1993). These responses may be elicited from intact domestic cats (but not in spinally transected females) by vaginal stimulation using a glass rod.

Felids, like some other carnivores, are induced ovulators (Bakker and Baum, 2000; Kauffman and Rissman, 2006). Thus, the act of mating triggers ovulation in species such as the domestic cat, and the puma, whereas in ruminants and cetaceans that exhibit the same no. 16 mating pattern, ovulation occurs spontaneously. Induced ovulation can have important consequences for male reproductive success in at least some taxa. Thus, Soulsbury (2010) has shown that males are better able to monopolize paternity of litters in species that are induced ovulators, as compared with spontaneous ovulators. The evolution of induced ovulation is discussed in Chapter 9.

The last group of mammals requiring consideration in relation to the prevalence of pattern no. 16 is the Order Lagomorpha. The lagomorphs are represented by two families: the rabbits and hares (Leporidae) and the pikas (Ochotonidae). As far as

I have been able to determine, rabbits and hares all copulate very rapidly. In the black-tailed jackrabbit (*Lepus californicus*), for example, mating lasts for less than 3 seconds. The male makes a single deep thrust to attain intromission and ejaculation, followed by a 'backward leap' as he dismounts (Lechleitner, 1958). In pygmy rabbits (*Brachylagus idahoensis*) mating is so rapid (<1 second) that is very difficult to verify whether an intromission has occurred (Scarlata *et al.*, 2012). In this species, aggressive interactions commonly occur post-mating, with the sexes wrestling, scratch-boxing and chasing each other.

Contreras and Beyer (1979) conducted a polygraphic analysis of events that occur during copulation in domesticated rabbits (*Oryctolagus cuniculus*). Their experiments reveal precisely what happens during this very rapid copulatory pattern (Figure 3.3). Experienced buck rabbits mount for an average of 2.61 seconds, during which time they may make up to 34 pelvic thrusts, prior to attaining intromission. The authors noted that the 'amplitude of pelvic oscillations usually decreased when the female displayed lordosis. This change was related to the process of orienting the penis towards the vaginal orifice'. Thus, the male's thrusting movements stimulate receptive (lordotic) responses by the female which, in turn, facilitate intromission. Thrusting then immediately ceases. Intromission lasts for less than 1 second (mean 722 ± 266 milliseconds), and after about 260 milliseconds the seminal vesicles begin to contract, as the male ejaculates. The mount is terminated by the male partner; he dismounts with an abrupt 'backward lunge'.

Rabbits are also induced ovulators (Bakker and Baum, 2000), and it has long been known that a variety of stimuli can cause ovulation (Fee and Parkes, 1930; Hammond and Marshall, 1925). Some pikas are also induced ovulators (Nakamura *et al.*, 1986; Suzuki 1984), but unfortunately no details of their copulatory patterns have been reported. Thus, we currently lack sufficient information to confirm that induced ovulation and a no. 16 copulatory pattern are homologous traits shared by the two extant families of lagomorphs.

Pattern Nos. 10, 11 and 12

Collectively, these three copulatory patterns are the most frequently encountered in mammals, as they occur in 55 per cent of all species for which classifications are available. Absence of a lock or tie between the sexes and the presence of pelvic thrusting characterize all these patterns. However, they differ as regards the number and duration of intromissions during mating. Multiple brief intromissions occur in pattern no. 10, whereas single intromissions occur in patterns 11 and 12 (intromission durations being prolonged in pattern no. 11 and brief in pattern no. 12: see Figure 3.1B).

Phylogenetically, these three patterns are also much more widespread than those considered thus far. In the marsupials, patterns 11 and 12 are well represented in the Diprotodontia, pattern no. 11 in the macropods and in wombats, and pattern no. 12 in the koala and the brush-tailed possum.

Pattern nos. 10, 11 or 12 are also represented in most groups of the placental mammals for which information exists (i.e. in 15 of 19 orders, as is shown in

Figure 3.4). Thus, all three patterns occur in the primates, carnivores and eulipotyph-lans. In the perissodactyls, pattern no. 11 is typical of both African and Asiatic rhinoceroses, and pattern no. 12 is found in equids and tapirs.

Interestingly, there are cases where more than one of these patterns is present in the same species. For example, among the primates, both patterns no. 10 and no. 12 have been recorded in one of the squirrel monkeys (*Saimiri sciureus*), in the chacma baboon (*Papio ursinus*) and the long-tailed macaque (*Macaca fascicularis*). Pattern

COPULATORY PATTERNS

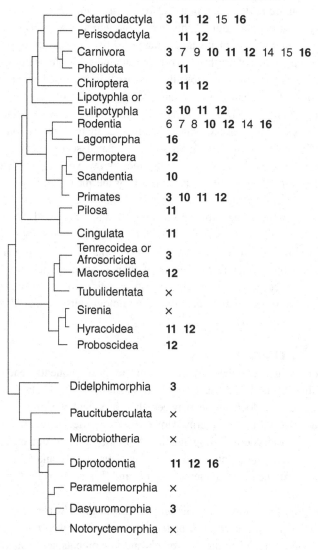

Cetartiodactyla	3 **11 12** 15 **16**
Perissodactyla	**11 12**
Carnivora	3 7 9 **10 11 12** 14 15 **16**
Pholidota	**11**
Chiroptera	3 **11 12**
Lipotyphla or Eulipotyphla	3 **10 11 12**
Rodentia	6 7 8 **10 12** 14 **16**
Lagomorpha	**16**
Dermoptera	**12**
Scandentia	**10**
Primates	3 **10 11 12**
Pilosa	**11**
Cingulata	**11**
Tenrecoidea or Afrosoricida	3
Macroscelidea	**12**
Tubulidentata	×
Sirenia	×
Hyracoidea	**11 12**
Proboscidea	**12**
Didelphimorphia	3
Paucituberculata	×
Microbiotheria	×
Diprotodontia	**11 12 16**
Peramelemorphia	×
Dasyuromorphia	3
Notoryctemorphia	×

Figure 3.4 Ordinal distribution of copulatory patterns in placental mammals and marsupials. The five most frequently occurring patterns (nos. **3, 10, 11, 12** and **16**) are shown in bold type. These patterns account for 92 per cent of all species classified so far.

no. 12 is the most frequent copulatory pattern observed in primates (Dixson, 2012). Transitions between patterns 12 and 10 might (in theory) occur in either direction, if males increase or decrease the number of intromissions that occur prior to ejaculation. That increases in the number of intromissions are more likely to occur under sexual selection will be discussed in the next chapter. On the other hand, gradual increases in the duration of intromission in a species with the no. 12 copulatory pattern might lead to the emergence of a no. 11 pattern. Again, it is likely that this transition has been favoured in some primate taxa by sexual selection. The widespread distribution of pattern nos. 10, 11 and 12 in placental mammals (Figure 3.4) may thus be partly due to effects of copulatory and post-copulatory sexual selection.

The Minor Patterns

Six masculine copulatory patterns (nos. 6, 7, 8, 9, 14 and 15) occur in only small numbers of taxa. Collectively, they are represented by 23 species, or less than 8 per cent of all species classified.

Pattern no. 6 has thus far been identified only in Molina's grass mouse (*Akodon molinae*). Yunes and Castro-Vazquez (1990) reported that males of this species make approximately 15 brief intromissions without pelvic thrusting, and exhibit a lock only during the final (ejaculatory) intromission of a series. The lock lasted for 1–6 seconds and the male was sometimes dragged along behind the female as she attempted to terminate the interaction by running from him. This peculiar pattern might occur, for example, if ejaculation is associated with a penile reflex (e.g. flaring of the glans penis) such as might cause a brief lock to occur. In another rodent species, the grasshopper mouse (*Ochrotomys torridus*), which exhibits a single brief intromission, ejaculation only occurs if a lock, lasting from 1 to 55 seconds, is established (see also pattern no. 8, below).

Pattern no. 7, in which copulation involves a prolonged single intromission with a lock and no pelvic thrusting has been recorded in the platypus (*Ornithorhynchus anatinus*), the Madagascan fossa (*Cryptoprocta ferox*) and the Australian hopping mouse (*Notomys alexis*). These three species mate under widely differing ecological conditions. The classification for the platypus is provisional (see Appendix 1), because some uncertainty surrounds whether a true lock is present. As we shall see in Chapter 5, the morphology of the penis gives few clues as to how a lock might become established in this species, but the answer may reside in certain features of the female's anatomy. The platypus mates in the water (Burrell, 1927; Temple-Smith, 1973), and it currently provides the only possible example of a prolonged lock occurring during aquatic copulation in a mammal. Hawkins and Battaglia (2009) noted that 'once intromission was achieved the female continued to drag the male as she swam and he stroked her laterally across her head and back'. Copulations lasted for up to 20 minutes. This 'dragging' of one sex by the other during extended matings was originally noted by Burrell (1927), but Hawkins and Battaglia add the interesting observation that it is the female that plays the active role in this respect.

Fossas mate in the trees, and when a female is in oestrus she attracts and copulates with multiple partners. These matings often involve aggression and loud vocalizations by both participants. Intromissions last for 9–119 minutes (Hawkins and Racey, 2009), and video recordings of wild fossas clearly show that the sexes sometimes have considerable difficulty separating at the end of copulation.

The Australian hopping mouse is a gregarious fossorial rodent and observations of captive groups indicate that receptive females sometimes mate with more than one male (Breed, 1990). Copulatory locks may last for a maximum of 9.2 minutes; the partners sometimes turn back to back, and the female may drag the male behind her during the lock.

Pattern no. 8 has been described only in a small number of species of mice belonging to the Family Cricetidae, although it probably occurs in further species of that group, for which partial classifications are listed in Appendix 1. It involves a single, relatively brief intromission, an absence of pelvic thrusting and the occurrence of a brief copulatory lock. Estep and Dewsbury (1976) made a study of this pattern using a laboratory colony of northern pygmy mice (*Baiomys taylori*). They predicted that this species might exhibit a copulatory lock on the basis of specializations of its penile morphology (a broad glans penis and large penile spines) and reductions in the size of certain of its accessory reproductive glands. In the event, a lock lasting between 21 and 43 seconds was identified, and the sexes sometimes turned back to back as they attempted to separate. The diverse specializations of reproductive anatomy that occur in mammals that exhibit such copulatory locks are discussed in detail in Chapter 5, which deals with penile morphology, and in Chapter 7, which considers the evolution and functions of the accessory reproductive glands.

Copulatory pattern no. 9 has been identified only in one species of carnivore, the masked palm civet (*Paguma larvata*). Jia *et al.* (2001) described this unusual pattern, which involves a series of prolonged intromissions (each lasting for 6.4 minutes on average) culminating in ejaculation. Deep pelvic thrusts occur, but there is no copulatory lock. Jia *et al.* noted that towards the end of the final mount in a series, the female emits a prolonged, loud vocalization, during which the male ceases thrusting and ejaculates. Intromission is then maintained during a post-ejaculatory 'pair-sit' which lasts for 66 seconds on average. A copulatory plug occurs in the masked palm civet, and interestingly its mass correlates positively with the duration of the female's loud vocalization. This might be an example of cryptic female choice operating at the copulatory level.

Pattern no. 14, which involves multiple brief intromissions, and the absence of a lock or pelvic thrusting, has been identified in some rodents and in one carnivore. Thus, with the exception of the dwarf mongoose (*Helogale parvula*), pattern no. 14 is confined to certain rodents belonging to the Cricetidae and Muridae. For example, it occurs in the laboratory rat (*Rattus norvegicus*), golden hamster (*Mesocricetus auratus*) and Mongolian gerbil (*Meriones unguiculatus*). These three species have been studied extensively by behavioural endocrinologists and reproductive biologists. Thus, a great deal is known about this copulatory pattern, and its relevance to understanding post-copulatory sexual selection, as females of all these species engage in multiple-partner matings.

Studies conducted using rats have shown that a cascade of reflexive responses shown by both sexes is required to ensure that the mount series proceeds successfully to culminate in ejaculation (Pfaff, 1980; Pfaff *et al.*, 1972, 1978). Thus, when a male rat mounts a receptive female, palpates her flanks with his forepaws and makes rapid pelvic thrusts prior to intromission, this stimulates her to exhibit lordosis. Her lordotic response, with rump and head raised and concave arching of the back, enables the male to perform the deep pelvic thrust required to achieve intromission. These events occur at lightning speed, so that specialized techniques were needed to capture them on film. Pfaff (1980) concluded that 'the female's lordosis reflex is a prerequisite for intromission by the male, rather than the reverse'.

The last of the six minor copulatory patterns to be considered (no. 15) consists of a single prolonged intromission without either a lock or pelvic thrusting. It has been identified in the larger of the two hippopotamus species, but not in the pygmy hippo, as was discussed above. The common ferret (*Mustela putorius*), in which intromission may last for up to 2 hours (Hammond and Walton, 1934), receives only a provisional classification, due to uncertainties about the absence of a lock or pelvic thrusts during mating. The remaining four species that exhibit this pattern are all pinnipeds belonging to the Family Phocidae. Thus, male elephant seals (*Mirounga angustirostris* and *M. leonina*), grey seals (*Halichoerus grypus*) and harbour seals (*Phoca vitulina*) cease making thrusting movements once intromission occurs. Nor is there any evidence of a lock, as the sexes are able to separate relatively easily. This must be advantageous during the aquatic copulations that occur in harbour seals and grey seals (Allen, 1985; Watkins, 1990).

Five copulatory patterns have not been considered so far because no species have yet been identified that exhibit any of them. Four of the patterns (nos. 1, 2, 4 and 5) include a copulatory lock; the fifth (no. 13) consists of multiple prolonged intromissions without a lock or pelvic thrusting. Given that the mating behaviour of most mammals still remains to be described, it is possible that examples of at least some of these patterns may come to light. It is unlikely, however, that any of them will prove to be widespread phylogenetically.

The Phylogenetic Distribution of Individual Copulatory Traits

Incomplete profiles of copulatory behaviour are available for 126 species, in addition to the 306 species with complete classifications that have been considered thus far. Here the data for all 432 species have been combined in order to examine how the presence or absence of the four individual traits might vary phylogenetically.

Copulatory Locks

A genital lock or tie between the sexes occurs in at least 42 species belonging to 9 orders of mammals (Table 3.1). This represents only 10 per cent of species, and less than half the orders of mammals included in Appendix 1.

Table 3.1 Mammals in which copulatory locks occur

Order	Family	Species
Monotremes		
Monotremata	Ornithorhynchidae	*Ornithorhynchus anatinus*?
Marsupials		
Dasyuromorphia	Dasyuridae	*Antechinus stuartii*
		A. agilis
Didelphimorphia	Marmosidae	*Monodelphis domestica*
Placentals		
Carnivora	Canidae	*Vulpes vulpes*
		Fennecus zerda
		Nyctereutes procyonides
		Speothos venaticus
		Canis mesomelas
		C. aureus; *C. simensis*; *C. latrans*;
		C. lupus; *C. familiaris*
		Lycaon pictus?
		Chrysocyon brachyurus
		Octocyon megalotis
		Cuon alpinus
	Hyaenidae	*Crocuta crocuta*
	Eupleridae	*Cryptoprocta ferox*
Chiroptera	Pteropodidae	*Pteropus livingstonii*
	Vespertilionidae	*Myotis nigricans*
Eulipotyphla	Soricidae	*Blarina brevicauda*
		Neomys fodiens
		Cryptotis parva
Rodentia	Cricetidae	*Neotoma albigulata**
		*N. floridana**
		*Ochrotomys nuttalli**
		*O. torridus**
		Onychomys leucogaster
		Ototylomys phyllotis
		*Akodon molinae**
		*Baiomys taylori**
		Tylomys nudicaudus
	Muridae	*Notomys alexis*
Primates	Daubentoniidae	*Daubentonia madagascariensis*
	Lorisidae	*Otolemur garnettii*
		O. crassicaudatus
		Galagoides demidoff
	Cercopithecidae	*Macaca arctoides*
Afrosoricida	Tenrecidae	*Geogale aurita*
		Setifer setosus

* Locks are of brief duration in these species; ? The case of the platypus is discussed in the text. *Lycaon pictus* is discussed in Chapter 5.

Clearly, this trait is not frequent or widespread among mammals, except in a few taxonomic groups such as the Family Canidae, which accounts for 14 species, members of the marsupial Family Dasyuridae and perhaps also among some groups of rodents. For example, Langtimm and Dewsbury (1991) conducted a cladistic analysis of copulatory patterns in 22 species of New World neotomine–peromyscine rodents and concluded that a mechanical tie between mating partners represents a primitive (plesiomorphic) trait, which has been lost in more derived species.

In the Order Eulipotyphla, several species of shrews are known to exhibit locks, but in some cases classifications of their copulatory patterns are currently incomplete (e.g. for *Neomys fodiens* and *Cryptotis parva*: see Appendix 1). It is likely that more examples of patterns that include a lock remain to be described among the Soricidae. In *B. brevicauda* (the northern short-tailed shrew), the copulatory pattern (no. 3) includes a lock that lasts for up to 25 minutes, with an average duration of 4.7 minutes (Pearson, 1944).

The canids are sufficiently well represented in the data set to justify the view that a lock during mating is a plesiomorphic trait for this family of the Carnivora, whose members also share a distinctive phallic morphology. Thus, canids, such as foxes, wolves and jackals, as well as the domestic dog, have a *bulbus glandis* at the base of the penis, which becomes tumescent and serves to lock the erect penis within the vagina once intromission is attained. Canids also possess an elongated baculum (*os penis*) that probably serves to strengthen the penis and protect the urethra from compression during prolonged matings.

For the majority of mammals in which locks occur, copulation involves a single prolonged intromission. This is the case in diverse species, such as the coyote (*Canis latrans*), fossa (*Cryptoprocta ferox*), greater hedgehog tenrec (*Setifer setosus*) and Garnett's galago (*Otolemur garnettii*). Prolonged intromission may facilitate the transfer of more spermatozoa and/or accessory glandular secretions to the female, and there is evidence that this is the case in domestic dogs. Isolated cases of taxa that exhibit mechanical ties and the diversity of their locking mechanisms indicate that this pattern has emerged independently in various lineages. An extreme example concerns the stump-tail macaque (*Macaca arctoides*), as it is the only member of its genus and indeed the only Old World monkey that exhibits a copulatory lock (Dixson, 2012, 2018).

With the possible exception of the platypus, no mammal that mates aquatically displays a copulatory lock. Being firmly tied together during mating could easily compromise the ability of aquatic mammals to surface and breathe, or place them at greater risk of attacks by predators. I have been unable to confirm whether a lock is absent in some amphibious mammals, such as the beaver, the yapok or the Pyrenean desman, due to the paucity of data on their copulatory patterns. A prolonged copulatory lock is present in the european water shrew (*Neomys fodiens*), but it is not known if these animals mate aquatically. It seems unlikely, given that individuals normally remain submerged for only 5–30 seconds while they are foraging (Nowak, 1999). The only detailed account of their copulatory behaviour that I have found (Köhler, 2012) includes photographs of captive animals mating on solid substrates.

Brief locks, that last for less than 60 seconds, occur in a number of small rodents belonging to the Family Cricetidae and it is likely that these differ qualitatively from the prolonged locks described above. For example, brief locks are closely coordinated with the occurrence of ejaculation, and appear to be less binding than prolonged locking patterns. Lock durations often appear to be determined by the female partners during such matings, rather than by males (e.g in *Akodon molinae*: Yunez and Castro-Vazquez, 1990; *Onychomys torridus*: Dewsbury and Jansen, 1972).

Pelvic Thrusting

Pelvic thrusting during intromission is exhibited by at least some species belonging to most orders of the Mammalia. Thus, it occurs in 238 (62 per cent) of the 384 species for which data are available concerning this trait. Among the monotremes, the male echidna makes vigorous thrusting movements for up to 60 minutes during some copulations (Wallage *et al.*, 2015). In marsupials, thrusting during intromission occurs in all but one species for which information exists (i.e. in the Diprotodontia, Dasyuromorphia and Didelphimorphia). Among the placental mammals, pelvic thrusting is widely represented, so that the Lagomorpha (rabbits and hares) is the only order in which this trait is completely absent. In the Cetartiodactyla, although ejaculation during a single brief copulatory thrust is the dominant pattern for the majority of its species, in several families (Suidae, Tayassuidae, Tragulidae and Camelidae) males engage in bouts of pelvic thrusting during intromission. This behaviour is also well represented among the carnivores (with the exception of the Felidae), rodents and bats, and is present in all species of the primates, perissodactyls, afrosoricidans and hyraxes for which copulatory patterns have been described.

Frey (1994) has pointed out that males of some testicond species, such as members of the Xenarthra, Cetacea and Sirenia, have a limited ability to flex the lumbar region of the spinal column when making pelvic thrusting movements. He noted that 'the construction of the trunk in the Testiconda (excepting the Hyracoidea) entirely or nearly entirely prevents sagittal bending. This is largely due to rigidity of the lumbar region or insufficient (dynamic) muscular control'. Males of many of these taxa have elongated penes, making it easier for them to attain intromission. This is the case, for example, in tapirs and in the African and Asian rhinoceros species. Males sometimes have some difficulty in manoeuvring the penis prior to intromission. Penile movements that assist bull elephants to attain intromission are controlled by the striated penile muscles.

It is probable that the capacity for males to make thrusting movements during copulation is an ancient trait that was present in the earliest mammals, and which has been incorporated into the majority of copulatory patterns displayed by the extant taxa. These include four of the five patterns most frequently displayed by mammals (nos. 3, 10, 11 and 12). Numerous variations in thrusting behaviour occur in different groups of mammals, however, so that classifying this as a single, uniform trait (as is the case in Figure 3.1) greatly over-simplifies matters. Diversity in the thrusting patterns displayed by mammals will be discussed in the next chapter, in relation to their possible involvement in sperm competition, copulatory courtship and cryptic female choice.

Multiple and Single Intromissions

Copulations that involve a series of mounts and intromissions have yet to be identified in any species belonging to the Monotremata, Afrotheria or Xenarthra. Among placental mammals, only some species belonging to the Superorders Laurasiatheria and Euarchontoglires exhibit multiple intromission copulatory patterns.

Seventy-seven species that exhibit multiple intromissions are included in Appendix 1, and most ($n = 50$) are rodents. Given that there are 29 families, and well over 2000 species, in the Order Rodentia, it is certain that many more examples have still to be documented. Of the remaining 27 species, 2 are marsupials (Genus *Perameles*), 8 are carnivores (all of which are members of the Feliformia), 1 is the shrew *Suncus murinus* (Order Eulipotyphla), 2 are treeshrews (Order Scandentia) and 14 are Old World and New World monkeys.

Individual intromissions during a multiple mount series are typically very brief; only the masked palm civet (*Paguma larvata*) is known to have long intromission times (pattern no. 9). Likewise, copulatory locks are lacking in all mammals that exhibit multiple intromissions, with the exception of Molina's grass mouse (*Akodon molinae*) in which a brief tie occurs only during the final, ejaculatory mount (pattern no. 6). The most frequently occurring pattern involves multiple brief intromissions with pelvic thrusting (pattern no. 10), with a small number of rodents also exhibiting pattern no. 14 (multiple brief intromissions with no pelvic thrusting).

In contrast to the situation outlined above, copulations that involve a single intromission occur in the vast majority of mammals, including monotremes and marsupials as well as most orders of the Placentalia. Thus, it appears that single intromissions probably represent the ancestral condition for mammals in general, as is also the case for pelvic thrusting during intromission (discussed in the previous section).

The number of mounts with intromission that constitute a multiple mounting series may vary considerably within the same species as well as between species. It has been shown experimentally, for example, that male rats can be conditioned to reduce the number of intromissions required to attain ejaculation. Silberberg and Adler (1974) conducted experiments in which male rats were allowed to make only seven intromissions during pair-tests with females. Most males initially failed to reach ejaculation under these conditions but when retested over the course of time, increasing numbers of them did so within the seven intromission criterion. By contrast, a control group of age-matched males that had unlimited access to female partners did not exhibit significant changes in numbers of intromissions. Silberberg and Adler noted that males in the experimental group had gradually extended the time that elapsed between intromissions. This was consistent with the results of earlier research by Larsson (1956) and Bermant (1964), who showed that by enforcing a fixed time interval between intromissions, male rats required fewer intromissions prior to ejaculation.

Observations of other species that have multiple intromission copulatory patterns confirm that intervals between intromissions vary between males and between pairings (e.g. in the green acouchi, *Myoprocta pratti*: Kleiman, 1971; Brazilian guinea pig, *Cavia aperea*: Rood, 1972). In Rood's study of Brazilian guinea pigs, some subordinate males ejaculated on the first intromission, whereas high-ranking males invariably completed a series of mounts. Such variations in copulatory behaviour may significantly affect the numbers of sperm that are transferred during mating, as is discussed in the next chapter.

Prolonged Intromission

There are 390 species represented in Appendix 1 for which intromission patterns are known; the majority of them (244 species or 62 per cent) exhibit brief intromission durations, whereas 146 species (38 per cent) maintain intromission for prolonged periods. The phylogenetic distribution of this latter group is listed in Table 3.2. Prolonged intromissions occur in at least some species of 41 families representing 118 genera of mammals.

Although this might appear to be an impressive total, in reality it is only a limited sample of mammalian diversity. Members of several orders of marsupials are not represented, as nothing is known about their mating behaviour. Among the placental mammals, pangolins (Pholidota), sloths (Pilosa) and armadillos (Cingulata) are poorly studied; only isolated examples are included in Table 3.2. For example, pangolins are

Table 3.2 Orders and families of mammals in which some species are known to exhibit prolonged intromission

Order	Families (no. of species with prolonged intromission)
Monotremata	Ornithorhynchidae (1), Tachyglossidae (1)
Diprotodontia	Macropodidae (6), Potoroidae (1), Vombatidae (2)
Dasyuromorphia	Dasyuridae (15)
Didelphimorphia	Marmosidae (4)
Cetartiodactyla	Camelidae (5), Hippopotamidae (1), Suidae (1), Tragulidae (2)
Perissodactyla	Rhinocerotidae (4)
Carnivora	Canidae (14), Eupleridae (1), Herpestidae (1), Hyaenidae (4), Mustelidae (22), Otariidae (4), Phocidae (6), Procyonidae (4), Ursidae (4), Viverridae (1)
Pholidota	Manidae (1)
Chiroptera	Pteropodidae (3), Vespertilionidae (4)
Eulipotyphla	Erinaceidae (2), Soricidae (2)
Rodentia	Heteromyidae (1), Muridae (1)
Scandentia	Tupaiidae (1)
Primates	Cebidae (5), Cercopithecidae (1), Cheirogaleidae (1), Daubentoniidae (1), Hominidae (2), Lorisidae (7)
Pilosa	Bradypodidae (1), Megalonychidae (1)
Cingulata	Chlamyphoridae (1)
Afrosoricida	Tenrecidae (6)
Hyracoidea	Procaviidae (1)

represented by a single species (*Manis javanica*) in which a pattern no. 11 type of copulation occurs. Many more cases of prolonged intromission must also exist among the rodents and bats, given the very large numbers of species in both these orders. However, the absence of some groups of mammals in Table 3.2 is indicative of the genuine lack of prolonged intromissions in certain lineages. None of the rabbits and hares (Lagomorpha) or elephants (Proboscidea) prolongs copulation, for example, and I think it unlikely that any of the manatees or the dugong (Sirenia) will be found to do so. Most of the even-toed ungulates (Cetartiodactyla) also mate quite rapidly. It is reasonable to ask why this should be the case, and this leads us to a discussion of the effects of natural selection, and of ecological factors that might influence mating durations in various taxa. The possible effects of sexual selection on mating durations are dealt with in the next chapter.

Ecological Factors That May Influence Copulatory Behaviour

Carnivorous Versus Herbivorous Modes of Life

In her monograph on *The Carnivores*, Ewer (1973) advanced the view that the act of mating, by its very nature, often places mammals at risk:

Vigilance and ability to take quick avoiding action are reduced and the pair are more than usually vulnerable to attack. It may therefore be advantageous for coupling to be of brief duration. This consideration, however, weighs much less heavily on predators than on prey species and one may therefore expect to find that carnivore matings may be relatively prolonged as compared with those of the species that constitute their prey.

An objective test of this hypothesis is possible by making statistical comparisons of intromission durations between carnivores versus herbivores. For the placental mammals, sufficient information is available (Appendix 2) to compare genera belonging to the Order Carnivora with herbivorous members of the terrestrial Cetartiodactyla. Intromission durations are indeed significantly longer among the carnivores (Figure 3.5A). The longest intromission times occur in the Caniformia, and especially in the various canids and mustelids. However, when considered individually, all three groups of the Carnivora (Caniformia, Feliformia and Pinnipedia) have longer intromission durations than the terrestrial cetartiodactyls ($P < 0.001$ in each case).

It is also possible to make a similar comparison between two orders of the marsupials: the herbivorous Diprotodontia and the Dasyuromorphia, which includes the Tasmanian devil, the native cats or quolls, and a number of smaller predatory taxa. Intromission durations tend to be prolonged among marsupials, as is the case in some diprotodonts; for example, in the eastern grey kangaroo (50 minutes: Sharman *et al.*, 1966) or the hairy-nosed wombat (64 minutes: Hogan *et al.*, 2010). However, intromissions are much more prolonged among the carnivorous dasyurids, lasting for 6 hours on average in the Tasmanian devil (Eisenberg *et al.*, 1975), and for up to 11 hours in the fat-tailed dunnart (Ewer, 1968). Hence the carnivorous marsupials

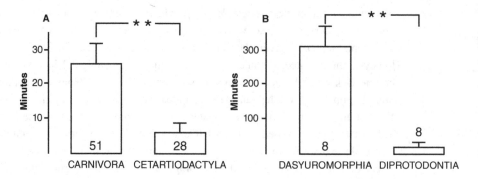

Figure 3.5 Intromission durations are longer in carnivorous mammals than in herbivores. **A:** Placentalia: Carnivora vs terrestrial Cetartiodactyla. **B:** Marsupialia: Dasyuromorphia vs Diprontodontia. **P < 0.001. Numbers of genera included in analyses are shown at the base of each histogram.

mate for considerably longer on average (307.5 ± 53.9 min) than the diprotodonts (11.8 ± 7.7 min: Figure 3.5B).

Copulation in Subterranean Mammals

Poor homeless wanderers in the roads and woods … delivered to all the perils of heaven and earth! I lie here in a room secured on every side

Franz Kafka, *The Burrow*

In his story, Kafka never reveals the identity of the solitary mammal that continually frets about the security of its burrow, and the reader is left to wonder if it ever interacts with others of its own kind. In reality, we know very little about how most of the subterranean mammals conduct their sexual lives. For example, the copulatory behaviour of marsupial moles (Order Notoryctemorphia), the moles of the Family Talpidae (Order Eulipotyphla) and the bizarre chrysochlorids or 'golden moles' of the Superorder Afrotheria has yet to be described. However, among the rodents there are significant numbers of burrowing species, some of which have been studied in detail. Copulatory patterns for 15 representatives of 7 families of such rodents are included in Table 3.3.

Some ground squirrels, such as *Spermophilus columbianus*, may mate above ground as well as in their burrows. One possible advantage favouring subterranean mating might be that it mitigates the risk of being killed by predators, such as ravens, hawks and falcons. However, competition between male Columbian ground squirrels for access to females is intense, so that mating below ground might be an alternative strategy to avoid interference by conspecifics. Manno *et al.* (2008) examined these questions by observing free-ranging Columbian ground squirrels during their annual mating season in Canada. They found that males living near the edge of the population occurred at lower densities but were at greater risk from predators. These males

Table 3.3 Copulatory patterns and intromission durations in fossorial rodents

Family	Species	Copulatory pattern no.	Intro. duration (min)	Source
Sciuridae*	*Xerus inauris*	12	0.42	Waterman, 1998
	Spermophilus richardsonii	12	3–4	Davis, 1982
			2.5	Denniston, 1957
	S. columbianus	12	–	–
	S. tridecemlineatus	12	0.42	McCarley, 1966 Wistrand, 1974
	S. beldingi	12	–	Sherman and Morton, 1979
Octodontidae	*Octodontomys gliroides*	12	0.83	Kleiman, 1974
	Octodon sp.	10**	0.17	Kleiman, 1974
Ctenomyidae	*Ctenomys pearsoni*	10	–	Kleiman 1974
	C. talarum	10	–	Fanjul and Zenuto, 2008
Geomyidae	*Thomomys talpoides*	10?	0.42	Andersen, 1978
				Schramm, 1961
Spalacidae	*Spalax ehrenbergi*	10	0.17? 0.54	Nevo, 1969 Gazit and Terkel, 2000
Heterocephalidae	*Heterocephalus glaber*	12	0.57	Sherman *et al.*, 1991
Bathergidae	*Heliophobius argenteocinereus*	12	0.33	Sumbera *et al.*, 1988
	Georychus capensis	10	<1	Bennett and Jarvis, 1988
	Cryptomys hottentotus	10	0.06	Hickman, 1982

* Copulations in some Sciurid species may occur above or below ground.
** Pattern no. 10 comprises a series of intromissions; the average intromission duration is listed here.

copulated above ground more frequently, however, whereas males situated in central areas were subject to heavy competition for access to receptive females and were significantly more likely to copulate in burrows. Avoiding interference with copulations rather than avoiding predators favours subterranean matings in this species. Much earlier, Hoogland (1995) had reached the same conclusion regarding subterranean matings in the black-tailed prairie dog (*Cynomys ludovicianus*). Copulation rarely occurs above ground in this species, but in three cases recorded by Hoogland, several brief mounts preceded a more prolonged (7–15 min) mount, which, he suggested, might be indicative of ejaculation. Unfortunately there is insufficient information to classify the copulatory pattern of this species with certainty. If it does involve a prolonged mount series, then this may have contributed to the requirement for males to mate underground, in order to avoid interference by rivals.

In the deserts of Southern Africa, female Cape ground squirrels (*Xerus inauris*) enter oestrus at unpredictable intervals throughout the year. Female relatives make their burrows close to one another, and these scattered 'burrow clusters' are visited by members of all-male groups whenever a female comes into oestrus. At such times the operational sex ratio (i.e. the ratio of potentially sexually active males to sexually receptive females) averages 10:1 (Waterman, 1998). Under these conditions multiple partner copulations are frequent and matings are often disrupted by rival males. Waterman was able to show that disruption was frequently avoided by couples entering burrows for the brief period required to achieve a copulation. Dominant males were more likely to employ this tactic, and they had significantly greater mating success than others.

Rodents that live exclusively underground face very different conditions from those described above. Theirs is a totally subterranean existence, in which potential partners must meet, and mate, in the darkness of closely confined burrows. An excellent example of how courtship and copulation has evolved under such conditions is provided by the blind mole-rat (*Spalax ehrenbergi*). This species is found throughout the Middle East; it is non-gregarious and territorial. The sexes occupy individual burrows, and neighbouring animals communicate by drumming their heads on the burrow walls and by sensing the vibrations so produced. Mutual avoidance is the rule, but during the annual mating season, females construct 'elaborate breeding mounds' in which copulation is thought to occur (Nevo, 1969).

Sexual behaviour has only been observed in captive blind mole-rats and even then with some difficulty, as they are highly aggressive to one another. Gazit and Terkel (2000) maintained mole-rats in an experimental burrow system, which allowed individuals freedom to remove a soil barrier and to interact directly during the mating season. Such encounters involved initial aggressive 'teeth-baring' displays and intense sniffing, which gave way to a lengthy courtship (mutual nibbling and head-pushing). By this stage, the male had widened the burrow to form a 'copulation hollow' and he attempted to manoeuvre the female into position for mating. This involved a series of 4–7 brief mounts with intromission and pelvic thrusting, during which the female made high-pitched vocalizations. Once mating was completed, the male promptly filled in the copulation burrow, and within 15–30 minutes both animals had renewed the soil barrier, and returned to their solitary lives.

Not all mole-rat species are non-gregarious; the most notable example of social grouping concerns the naked mole-rat (*Heterocephalus glaber*), which forms the largest groups of any fossorial mammal. They contain between 25 and 295 individuals of both sexes (Sherman *et al.*, 1991). Naked mole-rats are eusocial; only one adult female in the colony is fertile, and she initiates copulations with a select few of the many adult males that are present. When the breeding female is sexually receptive she invites mating by emitting trilling calls, exhibiting lordosis and backing towards any of her breeding partners that she encounters in the burrow system. Males have difficulty in mating with the (much larger) female, and copulations are brief, consisting of a single intromission with pelvic thrusting (pattern no. 12). The female only remains receptive for between 2 and 24 hours, and she copulates multiple times during this period. However, males do not compete for access to her, and courtship and mating appear to be under female control (Sherman *et al.*, 1991).

The burrowing species discussed here, along with others included in Table 3.3, employ just two masculine copulatory patterns (nos. 10 or 12). These fall within the group of five patterns which collectively occur in 92 per cent of all species listed in Appendix 1. Thus, it is likely that their presence in the various rodents shown in Table 3.3 is due to phylogenetic factors and not solely to their fossorial modes of life. However, it is interesting that patterns 10 and 12 are both brief types of copulation. Briefest of all is pattern no. 12, because only a single intromission is required to attain ejaculation. The ground squirrel species listed in Table 3.3 all display this pattern. These squirrels often mate when outside their burrows; the risk of interference by other males is always present, as is their vulnerability to predators. Thus it may be significant that certain major copulatory patterns that involve lengthy periods of intromission (e.g. pattern nos. 3 and 11) do not occur in these rodents.

Spiny Species: Effects of Body Armour

Convergent evolution has resulted in some members of four orders of mammals developing protective coverings of spines. Species as diverse as the echidna (Monotremata), hedgehogs (Eulipotyphla), porcupines and spiny rats (Rodentia) and tenrecs (Afrosoricida) all share spiny adaptations that help to deter potential predators. These are nocturnal animals and most of them are non-gregarious, so that they rarely associate except in order to reproduce. The question that naturally arises is how males deal with the barrier to mating imposed by the female's spines. The answer is that pre-copulatory communication is complex and involves both partners, as the following examples show.

During their studies of courtship and copulation in free-ranging echidnas (*Tachyglossus aculeatus*), Rissmiller and McKelvey (2000) noted that an unreceptive female responded to courtship attempts 'by digging in and erecting her spines, which caused the males to retreat'. However, when sexually receptive, she responded 'by lying flat on the ground with her spines in a relaxed position'. Males then jostled with each other, seeking to position themselves beside the immobile female and to to dig a furrow under her, in order to make it easier to gain intromission. The successful male 'continued digging until his tail was placed under the female's tail, cloaca on cloaca'.

The male crested porcupine (*Histrix cristata*) exhibits an unusual pattern of pre-copulatory behaviour, which Felicioli *et al.* (1997) have termed 'nose–quill'. The male uses his nose to gently touch and lift the specialized white quills on each side of the female's tail. These quills are highly sensitive to tactile stimuli; touching them normally evokes an aggressive response. However, a sexually receptive female responds by raising the quills on her back, arching her tail forwards to expose the anogenital region, and backing actively towards the male as he mounts.

North American porcupines (*Erithizon dorsatum*) also undergo marked changes in their behaviour during the period that precedes mating. Shadle (1946) noted that 'when the female is ready to mate, any stimulation of the hairs at the base of the tail and genital area results in raising of the tail, baring of the genitals, and actively seeking greater contact with any object which touches the labia'. The male repeatedly approaches the female, vocalizes and sniffs her body and genitalia. An unusual display also occurs, during which the male stands upright and 'begins to discharge urine in frequent, short spurts which in less than a minute may thoroughly wet the female. The quills of both animals are relaxed and kept flattened, as the female presents to the male, and backs towards him with her tail raised'. He stands upright, with the forepaws held well clear of her body. The male's hindlimbs and tail form a tripod, which supports him during mating (Shadle *et al.*, 1946).

The masculine copulatory patterns displayed by mammals that have protective spines are not in themselves unusual. The available information (Table 3.4) indicates that four of the five most frequent mammalian patterns are represented (nos. 3, 10, 11 and 12). These patterns are exhibited by other members of the same orders to which the spiny species belong. For example, prolonged intromission, such as occurs in the greater hedgehog tenrec (*Setifer setosus*), is also typical of tenrecs which lack spines, as is the case in the large-eared tenrec (*Geogale aurita*: Stephenson, 1993). By contrast, the porcupines included in Table 3.4 (i.e. *Hystrix* spp. and *Erethizon dorsatum*) exhibit quite brief intromissions (pattern nos. 10 and 12), as is the case for many other hystrichomorph rodents (e.g. green acouchi, *Myoprocta pratti*: no. 10; *Chinchilla lanigera*: no. 12).

Table 3.4 Copulatory patterns and intromission durations in spiny mammals

Order	Species	Copulatory pattern no.	Intro. duration (min)	Source
Monotremata	*Tachyglossus aculeatus*	?	30–180	Rissmiller and McKelvey, 2000
Eulipotyphla	*Atelerix albiventris*	11?	–	AFD
	A. algirus	11	5.5	AFD
Rodentia	*Proechimys semispinosus*	11	>5	Maliniak and Eisenberg, 1971
	Histrix cristata	10	0.14	Felicioli *et al.*, 1997
	H. africaeaustralis	12	2.5	Morris and Van Aarde, 1985
	H. indica	–	2	Tohmé and Tohmé, 1980
	Erethizon dorsatum	10?	0.27	AFD
			2–4	Shadle, 1946
Afrosoricida	*Tenrec ecaudatus*	–	4.5–12	Eisenberg, 1975
			21	Stephenson, 1993
	Setifer setosus	3	120	Paduschka, 1974
			>28	Eisenberg, 1975
	Hemicentetes nigriceps	–	10–21	Eisenberg, 1975
	Echinops telfairi	–	16–18+	Eisenberg, 1975, 1981

AFD: Author's observations, from filmed records.

A fifth copulatory pattern that occurs frequently in some mammals (no. 16) has not been identified in any of the spiny taxa. This is not surprising, given that this type of copulation requires the male to make a single rapid copulatory thrust, with intromission lasting for only a few seconds. It would be exceedingly difficult for male echidnas, hedgehogs, porcupines or tenrecs to behave in this way, given the care required to avoid the female's armoury of spines. The anatomical constraints posed by the female's spines may also have driven the convergent evolution of elongated penes in many of these species.

Aquatic and Terrestrial Copulations

Aquatic or amphibious species are to be found in eight orders of mammals: the Monotremata (platypus), Didelphimorphia (yapok), Cetartiodactyla (whales, dolphins and porpoises), Carnivora (pinnipeds and otters), Eulipotyphla (water shrews), Rodentia (capybaras, coypu and beavers), Afrosoricida (otter shrews) and Sirenia (manatees and dugong).

All of these taxa are the descendants of terrestrial precursors, and it is interesting that, in some cases, their masculine copulatory patterns closely resemble those of their current terrestrial relatives, making it likely that they are plesiomorphic traits. The cetaceans provide an example of this phenomenon. Most information concerns various dolphins and porpoises, all of which copulate rapidly by making a single intromission, without pelvic thrusts (pattern no. 16). For example, dusky dolphins take 1–17 seconds to complete intromission (mean = 4.9 s: Orbach et al., 2014). Cetacean biologists stationed on the Golden Gate Bridge in San Francisco Bay were able to look down on harbour porpoises (*Phocoena phocoena*) and to observe males as they rose from the depths, copulated with females near the surface of the water, and departed, all in less than 2 seconds (Keener et al., 2018). Further examples of cetacean intromission durations are included in Appendix 2; even the largest of the dolphins (*Orcinus orca*) maintains intromission for only about 30 seconds.

The copulatory pattern (no. 16) exhibited by dolphins and porpoises is essentially the same as that which occurs in many terrestrial cetartiodactyls, such as sheep, cattle, deer, giraffes and pigmy hippos. It may represent an ancient trait which was present among those ancestral cetaceans which first appear in the fossil record of the Eocene, some 50 million years ago. Brief patterns of copulation might have proven advantageous to such early aquatic forms, as they developed the ability to mate underwater. Prevention of salt water from entering the female's reproductive tract during mating may also have undergone positive selection; prolonged copulations, or multiple intromission patterns, could increase such risks.

Another likely influence of phylogeny upon the evolution of copulatory patterns concerns two groups of amphibious carnivores, the otters and the pinnipeds. The otters belong to the Family Mustelidae, which also includes weasels, martens, badgers and the wolverine. All the terrestrial mustelids for which I have been able to obtain sufficient information exhibit prolonged copulations involving a single intromission with pelvic thrusting (pattern no. 11). This is the case, for example, in the American mink (*Mustela vison*), in which intromission lasts up to 180 min (Enders, 1952); the black-footed ferret, *Mustela nigripes* (28–263 min: Williams *et al.*, 1991); the wolverine, *Gulo gulo* (12–56 min: Magoun and Volkenburg, 1983); and the striped skunk, *Mephitis mephitis* (5–20 min: Wright, 1931).

Otters may mate in the water or on land, and their copulatory patterns are the same as those of other mustelids. Copulatory pattern no. 11 occurs, for example, in the European river otter (*Lutra lutra*), Canadian river otter (*Lontra canadensis*) and oriental short-clawed otter (*Aonyx cinerea*). In such cases, aquatic conditions do not appear to present an obstacle to prolonged matings. Thus, captive giant otters (*Pteronura brasiliensis*) mate in the water for between 5 and 110 minutes (Londoño and Muñaz, 2006). The sea otter (*Enhydra lutris*), which can spend its whole life in the water, also mates for prolonged periods (>14 min: Kenyon, 1969).

Many seals and sea lions are capable of copulating either on land or (in polar regions) on the ice (Figure 3.6). Elephant seals (Genus *Mirounga*), for instance, come onshore to give birth and to mate. At such times, massive bulls compete to monopolize mating access to groups ('harems') of the much smaller females, and copulations involve a single prolonged intromission, without pelvic thrusting (pattern no. 15). Receptive females part their flippers and elevate the perineum, thus facilitating the male's attempts to gain intromission (Le Boeuf, 1972).

By contrast, Weddell seals (*Leptonychotes weddelli*) mate underwater. After female Weddell seals have given birth in the Antarctic, they stay on the ice in small groups.

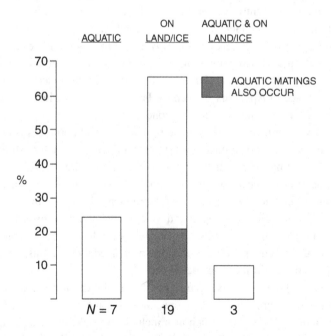

Figure 3.6 Aquatic vs terrestrial copulations in 29 species of pinnipeds. Data are percentages (the number of species is given at the foot of each histogram). 'Terrestrial' matings include those that occur on the ice. (Based on data in Riedman, 1990.)

Here they share an opening ('breathing hole') in the ice, which provides them with access to the water to hunt for food. Males do not monopolize harems under these conditions; instead, they establish underwater territories ('maritories') near the breathing holes used by females (Riedman, 1990). Male Weddell seals are somewhat smaller than the females, and they are agile swimmers. Copulations have rarely been observed, but they are quite long (>5 min: Cline *et al.*, 1971). The copulatory pattern, although only partially described, is likely to involve a single prolonged intromission, but it is not known whether males make thrusting movements.

The grey seal (*Halichoerus grypus*) has been observed mating on land, on ice and in the water. On Sable Island in Nova Scotia, Boness and James (1979) observed grey seal copulations that lasted for between 5 and 55 minutes (mean = 20 min). Watkins (1990) was able to record three aquatic copulations that occurred away from the terrestrial breeding grounds, in the Shetland Islands. They lasted for 8, 12 and 30 minutes (mean = 20 min). He noted that 'apart from pelvic flexions that were seen as evidence of intromission after mounting, pelvic movements by the male were irregular and of low intensity'. The copulatory pattern is thus classified as no. 15 for this species (a prolonged single intromission without pelvic thrusting or a genital lock).

Pinnipeds may have difficulty in making pelvic thrusts, especially when mating on land or on ice, due to the limitations imposed by the anatomy of their lower limbs (flippers) and pelvic girdle. This is particularly the case in members of the Phocidae (including the elephant seals and grey seal described above) because they are unable to turn their hind flippers under their bodies when moving about on ice or on land. All that is needed to transition from pattern no. 11 to pattern no. 15, seen in various phocids, is for pelvic thrusting to cease. Pattern no. 11 may be the ancestral copulatory pattern among pinnipeds. Aside from the reduction of pelvic thrusting, copulation in pinnipeds resembles that of mustelids and bears (Family Ursidae), which are their closest phylogenetic relatives in the Suborder Caniformia (Higdon *et al.*, 2007; Wyss and Flynn, 1993). Prolonged patterns of copulation and the possession of of an elongated penile bone (baculum) are also traits that the pinnipeds share with other members of the Caniformia, including the canids, as well as ursids and mustelids (Dixson, 1995c).

Effects of Body Size and Other Anatomical Constraints

Body mass influences many aspects of mammalian physiology and behaviour, so it might also be expected to affect patterns of copulatory behaviour. Stallmann and Harcourt (2006) reported that there is a negative correlation between body weight and the duration of copulation in mammals. They reasoned that smaller mammals 'may find the sustained maneuvering and body positioning of copulation easier than do large mammals'. Their sample comprised 113 species (85 genera) of marsupials and placental mammals. 'Copulation duration' was defined as the time from onset of the first intromission to the termination of mating once ejaculation had occurred. Problematic in this analysis was the inclusion of taxa in which mating involves a multiple intromission (MI) series (e.g. copulatory pattern nos. 10 and 14), because Stallmann and Harcourt's measure of copulation duration necessarily included all the intervals of non-genital contact between mounts, as well as the MI durations. Given that a larger data set for intromission durations is now available (see Appendix 2), I repeated the analysis, using only those taxa in which ejaculation occurs during a single intromission. The data set contained 217 species representing 170 genera and 19 orders of the monotremes, marsupials and placental mammals. This analysis confirmed Stallmann and Harcourt's findings; there is a negative correlation between intromission duration and body mass in mammals ($n = 170$; $r_s = -0.2083$; $P = 0.006$; two-tailed test).

The negative correlation between body size and intromission duration is not without exceptions, and it should not be taken to imply that a simple cause and effect relationship exists between the two variables. Indeed, some very large mammals, such as the various rhinoceros species, camels, grizzly bears and other ursids, mate for extended periods. Conversely, brief single intromission copulations occur in many small rodents, and in small-bodied diurnal monkeys such as the marmosets and tamarins. The differences in intromission durations between carnivorous and herbivorous mammals discussed earlier in this chapter did not take account of possible phylogenetic effects of body weight. However, differences in body weight between the samples of diprotodonts and dasyurids, or between the terrestrial artiodactyls and carnivores, represented in Figure 3.5 are not statistically significant. It appears likely, therefore, that carnivorous mammals copulate for longer periods of time than the herbivores that they prey upon.

Copulatory Postures

In the majority of mammals, copulation takes place with the male mounted upon the female in a dorsoventral position. Although dorsoventral postures are likely to represent the ancestral condition for therians, some interesting phylogenetic variations on this basic theme occur among the extant marsupials and placental mammals.

Prolonged dorsoventral copulations occur in many marsupials, during which males attempt to restrain females (Figures 3.7A–C). It is likely, but in most cases unproven, that prolonged copulations may serve to transfer larger numbers of spermatozoa to females. In the grey short-tailed opossum (*Monodelphis domestica*), for example, the male clasps the female around the waist, as well as using his feet to grasp her ankles. The animals usually lie on their right sides, as is also the case in the mouse opossum (*Marmosa robinsoni*). In this species, the male hangs by his prehensile tail during extended copulations (intromission lasts for 15–70 min: Trupin and Fadem, 1982). Lengthy matings also occur in many macropods, as in the red kangaroo (*Macropus rufus*: Figure 3.7C). The much larger male wraps his arms round the female's waist to restrain her during copulations that may last for 20 minutes. A different type of dorsoventral pattern is exemplified by the long-nosed bandicoot (*Perameles nasuta*). Mating involves a series of very brief (2–4 s) intromissions, during which the male remains upright and does not contact the female with his forepaws (Figure 3.7D).

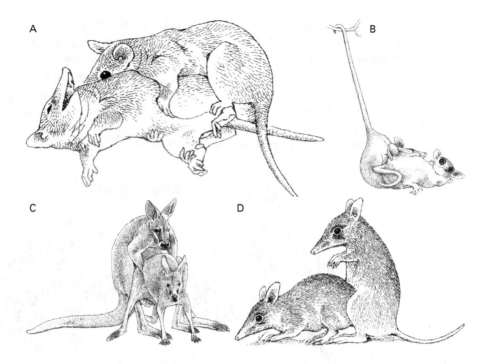

Figure 3.7 Examples of copulatory postures in marsupials. **A:** Grey short-tailed opossum: *Monodelphis domestica*. **B:** Mouse opossum: *Marmosa robinsoni*. **C:** Red kangaroo: *Macropus rufus*. **D:** Long-nosed bandicoot: *Perameles nasuta*. (From Tyndale-Biscoe and Renfree, 1987.)

Some examples of the dorsoventral copulatory postures displayed by various placental mammals are shown in Figure 3.8. Among the carnivores, members of the Family Felidae all exhibit brief copulations during which the male makes rhythmic 'treading' movements with his hind feet and grips the skin of the female's neck in his jaws (Figure 3.8A). Such 'neck-grips' occur in several other groups of mammals; their role in copulatory courtship is discussed in Chapter 8. Cats are induced ovulators, and males copulate repeatedly in order to provide sufficient tactile stimulation to trigger ovulation.

The copulatory posture typical of many artiodactyls is shown in Figure 3.8B. The bontebok (*Damaliscus pygargus*) mounts for only a few seconds, just long enough to deliver a single ejaculatory thrust and to dismount. A few artiodactyls mate for extended periods, most notably members of the Family Camelidae, in all of which both sexes crouch down on the ground during copulation. In the dromedary, for example (Figure 3.8C), intromission lasts for between 5 and 14.5 minutes. Multiple ejaculations occur throughout a single intromission (as observed during semen collections by artificial vagina: Al-Eknah *et al.*, 2001). This is significant in view of the fact that the semen of camelids contains an ovulation induction factor, as is discussed in Chapter 9.

A dorsolateral variant of the usual copulatory posture is seen in members of the Order Pholidota, such as the Sunda pangolin (*Manis javanica*: Figure 3.8D). The scaly armour and skeletal structure of these animals limits the male's ability to intromit and and to make pelvic thrusting movements during prolonged copulations.

The final example of unusual dorsoventral copulatory postures in placental mammals concerns some lorisiform primates, such as the slender loris (*Loris tardigradus*: Figure 3.8E). The male mounts the female in the usual way, but both partners are suspended in an inverted position beneath a branch. During copulation the male

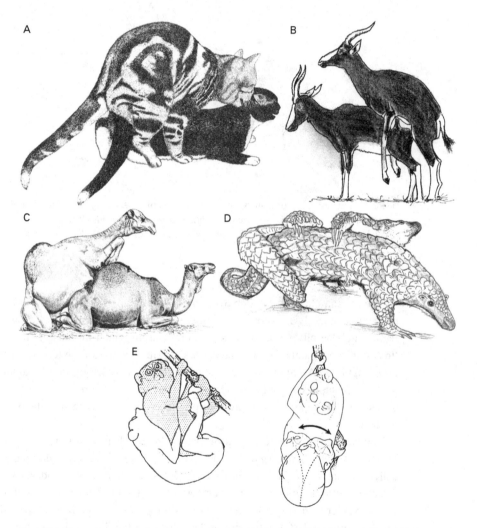

Figure 3.8 Examples of copulatory postures in placental mammals. **A:** Domestic cat (*Felis catus*). **B:** Bontebok (*Damaliscus pygargus*). **C:** Dromedary (*Camelus dromedarius*). **D:** Sunda pangolin (*Manis javanica*). **E:** Slender loris (*Loris tardigradus*). (**A**, From Herbert, 1972; **B**, author's drawing; **C**, from Short, 1984; **D**, author's drawing from a photograph in Zhang *et al.*, 2020; **E**, from Dixson, 2012, after Schulze and Meier, 1995.)

strokes the female's back by making side-to-side head movements, as is also shown in Figure 3.8E. Similar inverted copulatory postures also occur in the slow lorises of Asia and their African relatives, the potto and angwantibo. This posture was probably present in the stem forms from which the extant species are derived (Dixson, 2012). These slow-moving nocturnal primates are cryptic in their habits; the inverted copulatory posture may help to conceal them during their prolonged copulations.

Ventro-ventral copulations are rare in most groups of mammals. For example, only one rodent, the African four-striped mouse, has been reported to mate in this position (Dufour *et al.*, 2015). However, the anatomical specializations of cetaceans (whales, dolphins and porpoises) and sirenians (manatees and dugong) limit their ability to mate other than in a ventro-ventral or ventro-lateral position (Figures 3.9A,B). Females have much greater control over the duration of copulation in these taxa, as males are unable to restrain them. In many cases, the male partner approaches the female from below and remains below her during intromission. The female may thus surface to breathe, or terminate copulation more easily. Few of the largest whale species have been observed in the act of mating, the northern right whale (*Eubalaena glacialis*) being an exception. Both ventro-ventral and ventro-lateral matings by multiple partners have been recorded for this species (Mate *et al.*, 2005). A remarkable early record of mating in sperm whales is due to Captain James

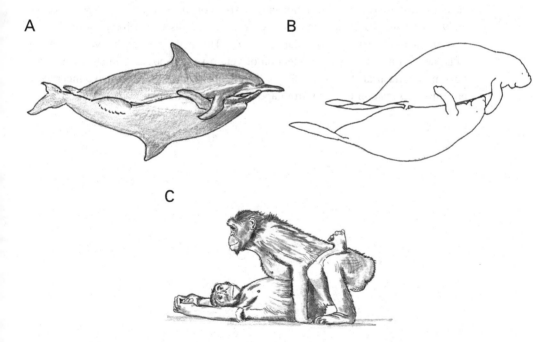

Figure 3.9 Ventro-ventral copulatory postures. **A:** Dolphins (*Stenella longirostris*). The male is underneath the female (redrawn and modified from Johnson and Norris, 1994). **B:** West Indian manatees (*Trichechus manatus*) (redrawn from Hartmann, 1979). **C:** Bonobo (*Pan paniscus*) (from Dixson, 2009, drawn from a photograph by Professor Frans de Waal).

Colnett, who visited the Galapagos Islands in 1793 as part of a British expedition in search of new whaling grounds. Philbrick (2000) records that Colnett and his crew 'witnessed something almost never seen by man: sperm whales copulating – the bull swimming upside down and beneath the female'.

Among the primates, face-to-face copulatory postures, as well as dorsoventral matings, have been described in some of the smaller apes (gibbons and siamangs) as well as in the great apes (orang-utans, bonobos and gorillas) and humans (Dixson, 2009, 2012). Figure 3.9C shows an example of ventro-ventral mating in the bonobo (*Pan paniscus*); the chimpanzee (*P. troglodytes*), however, copulates only in a dorso-ventral position.

The occurrence of ventro-ventral mating postures in the great apes, as well as in human beings, almost certainly represents homology, rather than being due to independent evolution of the trait. There may be several reasons why ancestral apes developed this mode of copulation. First, the increased brain development and intelligence of apes may be associated with a reduced reliance upon the stereotypical, dorsoventral copulatory patterns that occur in monkeys (Bingham, 1928). Second, ventro-ventral matings may serve to to facilitate continued (proceptive) eye contact between the partners, and thus constitute a form of copulatory courtship. Finally, the propensity for apes and humans to engage in ventro-ventral copulation may have been facilitated by the evolution of anatomical specializations of the shoulder joints, rib cage and forelimbs for locomotion and suspension in arboreal ancestors (Dixson, 2009). Apes that habitually hang or swing by their arms whilst foraging might also suspend themselves in this way during mating. This is the case in the orang-utan, for example, and may explain the retention of ventro-ventral postures in apes which are now more terrestrial (bonobos and gorillas). Humans may therefore have inherited a propensity to mate in this way from ape-like (australopithecine) precursors.

4 Copulatory Interactions and Sexual Selection

The last chapter considered the act of mating primarily from the perspective of male mammals, and discussed the effects of phylogeny and modes of life upon masculine patterns of copulatory behaviour. By contrast, this chapter addresses the interplay between the sexes that occurs during copulation. In many mammals, females mate with multiple partners during the fertile period. Under these conditions, the stage is set for sexual selection, via cryptic female choice, as well as sperm competition, to influence the fate of gametes that are deposited in the female reproductive tract by rival males. Thus, in what follows, the behaviour and physiological responses of both sexes will be discussed in relation to events that take place during and after copulation. Figure 4.1 shows, in diagrammatic form, relationships between sperm competition and cryptic female choice. On the left-hand side of the diagram, sperm from several males are depicted as 'competitors in a race', as they vie to to gain access to an ovum. The female's reproductive tract is a 'level playing field' in which this contest takes place. The right-hand side of the diagram introduces a note of reality into this androcentric vision. Sperm do not have direct access to ova; the vagina, cervix, uterus, uterotubal junction and oviduct all present challenges to the survival and onward progression of spermatozoa. The female's reproductive anatomy and physiology play crucial roles in transporting sperm, and also in controlling the temporary storage of gametes. Thus, although vast numbers of spermatozoa are released at ejaculation, few of them ever gain proximity to an ovum.

Caveats Concerning the Classification of Mating Systems

The likelihood that female mammals will engage in multiple-partner matings is dependent upon many factors, not the least of which is the nature of the mating system in which sexual interactions occur. The classification of mating systems has been detailed in a number of authoritative texts on animal behaviour (e.g. Alcock, 2013; Clutton-Brock, 2016; Davies *et al.*, 2012). Thus, it is not necessary to repeat this information. Rather, my purpose here is to discuss possible correlations between the various types of mammalian mating systems and likely occurrences of sperm competition and cryptic female choice. It is also necessary to point out some pitfalls that can arise when using current classification schemes.

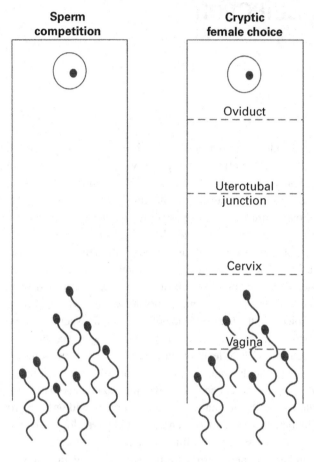

Figure 4.1 A schematic representation of sperm competition and cryptic female choice in mammals. As well as competition between the gametes of rival males for access to a given set of ova, the female's reproductive anatomy and physiology determine the fate of spermatozoa. (From Dixson, 2009.)

Figure 4.2 shows the patterns of copulatory interactions that characterize five major types of mammalian mating systems: monogamy, polygyny, polyandry, multimale–multifemale and dispersed. The members of dispersed mating systems are non-gregarious, but their individual home ranges or territories often overlap to varying degrees and multiple-partner matings occur. This is the case, for example, in many nocturnal marsupials, prosimians and rodents. The same is true of some mammals that form multimale–multifemale groups, such as many dolphins, macaques and chimpanzees. The members of such dispersed and multimale–multifemale mating systems are polygynandrous. They are thus much more likely to display reproductive adaptations

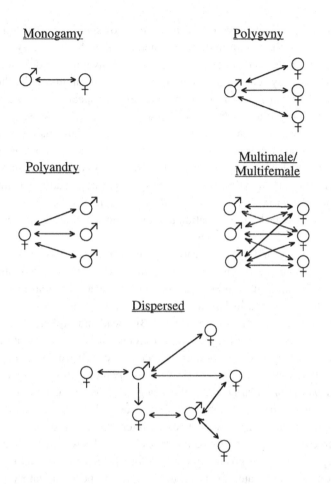

Figure 4.2 Copulatory interactions that characterize five major types of mammalian mating systems. (After Dixson, 2012.)

that result from copulatory and post-copulatory sexual selection than are mammals that have monogamous or polygynous mating systems.

A polygynous mating system is one in which a single male copulates with a number of females; several subtypes of polygyny have been described. The most robust of these, in terms of a single male controlling access to females, is female defence polygyny. In such a system a male defends a number of females, as for instance in many species of deer and pinnipeds, in some equids and in many of the Old World anthropoid primates, including hamadryas baboons and gorillas. Problems arise, however, when multimale–multifemale groups are classified as being polygynous on the basis that dominant males may establish priority of access to females. Their sexual relationships are often transitory, however, and other males may successfully employ alternative mating tactics to copulate with the same females. In multimale–multifemale groups of rhesus monkeys, for example, males have very large testes, indicative of the occurrence of sperm competition. Female rhesus monkeys also mate with multiple partners, so that the mating system might just as accurately be classified as being polyandrous. Polygyny is a delusion in such cases. In fact, mating systems of this type are often polygynandrous, and they differ markedly from the mating systems of highly polygynous species such as the gorilla, in which sperm competition is minimal (Dixson, 1998a, 2012). Waterman (2007) has identified exactly the same problem in classifying rodent mating systems as polygynous when, in numerous cases, both sexes engage in multiple-partner matings. Many authors also employ the term 'promiscuous' to describe mating systems in which both males and females mate with multiple partners. I advise against using the word promiscuous in this context. To do so encourages the notion that polygynandrous mammals lack discrimination in their choices of mating partners. This is not the case.

With the discovery of DNA fingerprinting by Jeffreys *et al.* (1985) it became possible to determine the parentage of offspring and to test theories about how mating systems function. It soon became apparent, for example, that in many avian species, hitherto considered to be monogamous, extra-pair matings accounted for significant numbers of the offspring produced (Birkhead and Møller, 1992). Studies of mammals have also revealed significant differences between behavioural assessments of mating success and genetic data on paternity of offspring (e.g. in primates: *Lemur catta*: Pereira and Weiss, 1991; *Macaca mulatta*: Widdig *et al.*, 2004; *Erythrocebus patas*: Ohsawa *et al.*, 1993; *Pongo abelii*: Utami Atmoko and Van Hooff, 2004; *Pan troglodytes*: Wroblewski *et al.*, 2009). It is exceedingly difficult to obtain a complete picture of the web of sexual interactions that occurs between the members of free-ranging groups. Covert matings by females with subordinate males, or extra-group males, often go unobserved. Another contributory factor is that in polygynandrous species, paternity is influenced by the post-copulatory processes that take place in the female reproductive tract, via sperm competition and/or cryptic female choice. The 'genetic mating system' often differs from the observed 'sexual mating system'.

How Common are Multiple-partner Matings by Female Mammals?

More than 30 years ago, Møller and Birkhead (1989) conducted a literature search to identify those mammalian species in which females mate with multiple males during a single period of sexual receptivity. They were able to locate information for 210 species, the majority of which were placental mammals. In 56 of these species females 'usually' or 'sometimes' engaged in multi-partner copulations. Nowadays, much more information is available, and it supports Møller and Birkhead's prediction that multiple-partner matings by females, and post-copulatory sexual selection, would prove to be widespread among mammals. The following brief review includes more recent information on the monotremes and marsupials, as well as the placental mammals.

Monotremes

Much of the evidence pertaining to multiple-partner matings by female monotremes is indirect, but it is compelling nonetheless. The presence of very large testes, in relation to body weight, in male platypuses and in short-beaked and long-beaked echidnas (Rose *et al.*, 1997; Taggart *et al.*, 1998) is indicative of sexual selection via sperm competition. This conclusion is supported by the observation that males produce specialized sperm 'bundles' (Johnston *et al.*, 2007; Jones *et al.*, 2004), the functions of which are discussed in Chapter 6.

Unfortunately, there is no direct information concerning the presence or absence of multiple-partner matings in the platypus, or in the long-beaked echidna species. However, field and laboratory studies of sexual behaviour in the short-beaked echidna (*Tachyglossus aculeatus*) have produced some important insights. In Tasmania, where colder conditions prevail, short-beaked echidnas form aggregations and hibernate for several months each year. Males sometimes mate repeatedly with females that are still torpid. Morrow and Nicol (2009) ascribe this tactic to the effects of 'extreme competition between promiscuous males'. Elsewhere in Australia, echidnas engage in prolonged periods of courtship, during which males line up to form 'trains' that follow a single female. Rissmiller (1999) records that 'Courtship lasts from one to six weeks and different males may join or drop out of the train ... mating can occur at any time of the day or night.' Despite past assumptions that only a single male is successful in mating under these conditions (Rissmiller and McKelvey, 2000), and that 'sperm competition is unlikely' (Taggart *et al.*, 1998), the fact is that the number of mating partners accepted by each female is not known. In captivity, female echidnas may sometimes remain receptive for a series of nights (3, 4 and 7 nights in several females observed by Wallage *et al.*, 2015). It is probable that, under natural conditions, female echidnas mate with multiple partners.

Marsupials

Most marsupial species are nocturnal; some, including the larger macropods, are crepuscular and just one species (the numbat: *Myrmecobius fasciatus*) is exclusively diurnal (Lee and Cockburn, 1985). The rarity of diurnal taxa among the marsupials is interesting in light of theories that link the evolution of diurnality in mammals to increases in brain development (Jerison, 1973; Eisenberg, 1981), as well as greater body size, gregariousness and behavioural complexity (Charles-Dominique, 1977).

Certainly, many marsupials are non-gregarious, and they often form dispersed social and mating systems in which individual home ranges overlap those of conspecifics. Polygynandrous matings may often occur under such conditions, as the following examples show.

The honey possum (*Tarsipes rostratus*) has a dispersed mating system in which 86 per cent of the population does not survive beyond its first year. Females may raise four litters of 2–3 young during this time, most of which are sired by more than one male (Bryant, 2004; Wooller *et al.*, 2000). Multiple-partner matings are thus known to occur (although they have not been observed directly). Residuals of testes weight are very large in honey possums (+0.74), as is consistent with high levels of sperm competition (Rose *et al.*, 1997).

Greater bilbies (*Macrotis lagotis*) have a dispersed social system, consisting of large individual ranges. Miller *et al.* (2010b) conducted a 5-year study of bilbies living in a 10-hectare enclosure. During each year, all offspring were sired by approximately 41 per cent of the males in this captive population; most fathered a single infant, and 30 per cent sired two or three infants. Miller *et al.* suggest that males adopt a 'roving strategy' in search of receptive females, but in the absence of data on copulatory behaviour, or multiple paternity of litters (litters may contain two infants), it is still unclear whether post-copulatory sexual selection occurs in this species.

Feathertail gliders (*Acrobates pygmaeus*) are mouse-sized, arboreal marsupials which sleep huddled together in small groups during the daylight hours. Fieldwork by Parrott *et al.* (2005) has shown that multiple paternity of litters occurs in these gliders; six of eight litters studied were sired by two or three males. Large relative testes sizes occur in this species (residuals of testes weight = +0.32; Rose *et al.*, 1997).

Multiple-partner matings occur in *Antechinus* species, such as *A. stuartii* (Hollely *et al.*, 2006), *A. agilis* (Kraaijeveld-Smit *et al.*, 2002) and *A. minimus* (Sale *et al.*, 2013). Multiple paternity of litters has been confirmed by fieldwork on all three species. In the case of *A. stuartii*, Hollely *et al.* found that 92 per cent of females mated with multiple partners, and that up to four sires were represented in each litter. Larger males (which also had the largest testes) had most reproductive success. As was noted in Chapter 2, *Antechinus* species are notable for their semelparous mating systems, in which all males in the population die following an intense and highly competitive period of multiple-partner copulations. Semelparity occurs in some other dasyurid marsupials (Tyndale-Biscoe, 2005), including the dibbler (*Parantechinus apicalis*), members of the genus *Phascogale*, the little red kaluta (*Dasykaluta rosamondae*) and the northern quoll (*Dasyurus hallacatus*). Among the South American marsupials, some opossums (Family Didelphidae) also have a semelparous mating system. Such is the case in the Brazilian slender opossum (*Marmosops paulensis*), in which both sexes exhibit post-reproductive mortality (Leiner *et al.*, 2008).

The macropods include the rat kangaroos (0.5–3.5 kg) which are non-gregarious and nocturnal, and the wallabies and kangaroos, the largest of which (the red kangaroo: *Macropus rufus*) may weigh over 80 kg. The rat kangaroos have dispersed mating systems in which multiple-partner matings are likely to occur, although their cryptic nocturnal behaviour has hampered attempts to establish the details of their sexual interactions (e.g. long-nosed potoroo, *Potorous tridactylus*: Long, 2001; rufous bettong, *Aepyprymnus rufescens*: Frederick and Johnson, 1996).

Among the wallabies, the tammar (*Macropus eugenii*) is the most extensively studied species, with regard to its reproductive physiology and sexual behaviour. Tammars exhibit a postpartum oestrus, and mating may take place an hour after females give birth. Rudd (1994) observed 'mating chases' involving several males, during which females copulated with multiple partners. Hynes *et al.* (2005) studied six captive groups of tammars, containing a total of 23 males and 50 females. Females 'usually mated with more than one male' in these groups, and male dominance rank provided 'only a moderate predictor of paternity'. Alpha males sired 50 per cent of offspring, beta males 35 per cent and lower-ranking sires accounted for the remaining 15 per cent of infants. It should be noted here that tammars do not normally live in groups; a system of overlapping individual home ranges is the norm, and sperm competition is likely to be more pronounced under such conditions.

The largest of the macropods, such as the eastern grey kangaroo (*Macropus giganteus*) and the red kangaroo (*M rufus*), aggregate to form labile groups ('mobs'). The adults are sexually dimorphic; males are far larger than the females and they have longer, more muscular arms, which are employed during sparring contests for access to mates (Jarman, 1983). Tyndale-Biscoe and Renfree (1987) discuss the behaviour of alpha males which compete to monopolize access to each female that enters oestrus, but subsequently allow other males to mate. Sperm competition is liable to occur under such conditions. They note, however, that only a brief window of time is available for fertilization to take place, as the ovum quickly becomes coated in a 'mucolemma' which prevents sperm from reaching the zona pellucida. Ova are most likely fertilized at the top of the oviduct in marsupials, rather than at the junction of the ampulla and isthmus, as is generally the case in placental mammals (Tyndale-Biscoe, 2005). Thus, the advantage to an alpha male may lie in ensuring that his spermatozoa enter the oviduct before the gametes of other males. Alpha males in three populations of eastern grey kangaroos studied by Rioux-Paquette *et al.* (2015) sired 54 per cent of the offspring, which is very similar to the reproductive success of alpha male tammars recorded by Hynes *et al.* (2005). In neither of these species have experiments determined whether a first male mating advantage might occur in relation to sperm competition. The mating systems of these macropods are most accurately defined as being multimale–multifemale (polygynandrous), rather than being strictly polygynous.

Placental Mammals

The placental mammals and marsupials share a nocturnal ancestry. However, in contrast to the marsupials, most of the 19 orders of placental mammals include diurnal as well as nocturnal taxa. There are exceptions, such as the bats (Chiroptera), colugos (Dermoptera) and shrews, and hedgehogs of the Order Eulipotyphla, all of which retain the plesiomorphic nocturnal condition. The extraordinary anatomical, eco-logical and behavioural diversity displayed by placental mammals was discussed in Chapter 2. Polygynandrous mating systems, large relative testes sizes and other traits indicative of the occurrence of post-copulatory sexual selection have been docu-mented for many members of the Cetartiodactyla, Carnivora, Chiroptera, Eulipotyphla, Rodentia, Lagomorpha and Primates. Some examples are discussed below. Polygynandry probably also occurs in manatees (Sirenia), in which mating groups of males congregate around a female that is receptive and compete for copulations (Florida manatee: O'Shea *et al.*, 1995). The limited information available for the Pilosa indicates that polygynandry may also occur in some sloths (e.g. in

Hoffmann's two-toed sloth, *Choelepus hoffmanni*: Peery and Pauli, 2012). However, there are still some orders, such as the Cingulata, Pholidota, Dermoptera and Tubilidentata, for which there is no information concerning the presence or absence of polygynandry.

In the Hyracoidea, both the bush hyrax (*Heterohyrax brucei*) and the rock hyrax (*Procavia johnstoni*) are considered to be polygynous (Hoeck *et al.*, 1982). Dominant males monopolize access to small groups of females, although peripheral males also attempt copulations during the mating season. To my knowledge, no paternity studies have been reported for any of the hyraxes. Polygyny also occurs in some perissodactyls, as for example in plains and mountain zebras (Estes, 1991). In the white rhinoceros, a dominant male mate-guards individual oestrous females that occupy adjacent home ranges (Owen-Smith, 1975). However, multiple-partner matings by females have been recorded in the black rhinoceros (Estes, 1991). Very little is known about the mating systems of any of the tapir species. Elephants (Order Proboscidea) are polygynous; individual mature bulls in breeding condition ('musth') adopt a roving strategy, visiting groups of females and controlling access to sexually receptive individuals (e.g. in the African elephant, *Loxodonta africana*: Hollister-Smith *et al.*, 2007).

Species belonging to two orders of placental mammals, the treeshrews (Scadentia) and elephant shrews (Macroscelidea), are usually considered to be monogamous. However, fieldwork on paternity in the large treeshrew (*Tupaia tana*) has revealed that 50 per cent of 22 offspring tested were the result of extra-pair copulations (Munshi-South, 2007). That 'social monogamy' does not necessarily equate to sexual monogamy is also indicated by the results of studies of paternity in alpine marmots (Goossens *et al.*, 1998), fat-tailed dwarf lemurs (Fietz *et al.*, 2000) and fork-marked lemurs (Schülke *et al.*, 2004). To my knowledge, no genetic studies have examined paternity in elephant shrews, and doubts remain as to whether they are monogamous.

Returning to a discussion of those orders of placental mammals in which polygynandrous taxa are well represented, I shall focus here on the primates, rodents, bats and cetartiodactyls. Collectively, these four orders comprise a huge variety of arboreal, terrestrial, volant and aquatic species with diverse mating systems.

Among the nocturnal primates many species have non-gregarious social systems and a dispersed type of mating system, in which individual males occupy home ranges that overlap those of a number of female conspecifics. Examples include the galagos, pottos, lorises, the aye-aye and various mouse lemur species (Dixson, 2012). Fieldwork has shown that females mate with multiple partners in mouse lemurs (*Microcebus murinus*: Eberle and Kappeler, 2004), lesser galagos (*Galago moholi*: Pullen *et al.*, 2000) and lorises (*Loris lydekkerianus*: Nekaris, 2003). In addition, the presence of very large testes in many nocturnal taxa is consistent with occurrences of multiple-partner matings and sperm competition (Dixson, 1995a; Kappeler, 1997).

Multimale–multifemale social groups, in which both sexes are known to copulate with numbers of partners, occur throughout the Order Primates (Dixson, 2012); such polygynandrous species include the ring-tailed lemur (*Lemur catta*: Koyama, 1988), sifaka (*Propithecus verreauxi*: Richard, 1976), Southern muriqui (*Brachyteles arachnoides*: Milton, 1985), brown capuchin (*Cebus apella*: Janson, 1984), tala-poin monkey (*Miopithecus talapoin*: Rowell and Dixson, 1975), yellow baboon (*Papio cynocephalus*) and mandrill (*Mandrillus sphinx*: Dixson, 2015b), as well as the various macaque species (e.g. *Macaca mulatta*: Manson, 1992). Among the apes, only the chimpanzee and bonobo exhibit a fusion–fission type of social organization, in which communities consist of changeable subgroups and females mate with numbers of males during the fertile period (Goodall, 1986; Kano, 1992). As an example, Goodall (1986) relates how during her studies of chimpanzees at Gombe she:

watched one party as it arrived at a new food source; the attractive female climbed into the tree along with eight bristling males, each of which copulated with her in quick succession in a period of five minutes.

Polygynandrous mating systems are also well represented among rodents. Waterman (2007) examined occurrences of multiple-partner matings by females of 95 species, representing 39 genera of rodents. She found that in 50 per cent of these taxa receptive females commonly mate with multiple partners. As examples, in the Family Sciuridae, female Columbian ground squirrels mate with four males on average (Murie, 1995), and females with an average of six males in California ground squirrels (Boellsstorff *et al.*, 1994).

Multiple paternity of litters is also common among squirrels; thus, 78 per cent of litters have multiple sires in Belding's ground squirrels (Hanken and Sherman, 1981), and in Gunnison's prairie dogs 61 per cent of infants are sired by 'extra-territory males' (Travis *et al.*, 1996). Waterman (2007) cites many other examples of multiple-partner matings by female rodents of the Families Heteromyidae (e.g. kangaroo rats: Genus *Dipodomys*) and Muridae (e.g. in many voles of the Genera *Microtus* and *Clethrionomys*, and mice of the Genus *Peromyscus*). Multiple-partner matings also occur in some cavies, including the greater guinea pig (*Cavia magna*) and the yellow-toothed cavy (*Galea musteloides*). In the latter species, multiple paternity of litters exceeds 80 per cent. In mate-choice experiments, Hohoff *et al.* (2003) found that female yellow-toothed cavies actively seek multiple partners and that 'both sperm competition and direct female choice seem to be important for increased offspring viability'.

Evidence concerning the prevalence of multiple-partner matings by female bats derives largely from studies of relative testes sizes and likely occurrences of sperm competition in various families of the Chiroptera, as well as information about long-term storage of sperm by females of some taxa. These topics are covered in Chapters 6 and 8 as part of more detailed discussions of sperm competition and cryptic female choice, so that only a brief account is provided here.

A positive correlation between relative testes size and social group sizes of bats at their roosting sites was reported by Hosken (1997), based upon his comparative studies of 31 species, representing 20 genera. Subsequently, Wilkinson and McCracken (2003) were able to assemble a larger data set (104 species) and to show that bats which form multimale–multifemale roosting assemblages have significantly greater relative testes sizes than those species which form single male–multifemale assemblages, or which roost in male–female pairs. Three of the 10 families included in this study exhibited larger than expected testes mass: the Vespertilionidae, Rhinopomatidae and Pteropodidae. Multimale–multifemale roosting assemblages of bats are thus likely to represent polygynandrous mating systems.

In many vespertilionid and some rhinolophid bats, sperm are stored for long periods in the female reproductive tract (examples are provided in Table 8.5). In at least one case, it is known that the sperm of up to five different males are represented at the storage site (in the common noctule bat, *Nyctalus noctula*: Gebhard, 1995). Direct observations of multiple-partner matings by female bats are few in number, but they reportedly occur in the Mexican free-tailed bat, *Tadarida brasiliensis*; the black mastiff bat, *Molossus ater* and the pale spear-nosed bat, *Phyllostomus discolor* (Wilkinson and McCracken, 2003).

Behavioural and anatomical evidence also indicates that multiple-partner matings and post-copulatory sexual selection have played significant roles in the evolution of reproduction in some members of the Cetartiodactyla. Examples of multiple-partner matings and multiple paternities of litters in even-toed ungulates are shown in Table 4.1. Polygynandry has also been documented in some whales, dolphins and porpoises (Connor *et al.*, 2000; Gowans *et al.*, 2008; Mate *et al.*, 2005). Post-copulatory sexual selection is likely to occur in taxa where males have very large testes in relation to body weight (Brownell and Ralls, 1986; Connor *et al.*, 2000; Dines *et al.*, 2015). An extreme example is provided by the northern right whale (*Eubalaena glacialis*) in which the testes weigh one metric ton and females have been observed

Table 4.1 Some examples of terrestrial artiodactyls in which multiple-partner matings (MM) and multiple paternity (MP) of litters are known to occur

Family: Species			Source
Tayassuidae: *Pecari tajacu* Collared peccary	MM	MP	Cooper *et al.*, 2011
Suidae *Sus scrofa* Domestic pig/wild boar	MM	MP	Delgado *et al.*, 2008; Spencer *et al.*, 2005
Bovidae: *Ovis canadensis* Bighorn sheep	MM	–	Hogg, 1988
Bovidae: *Ovis aries* Soay sheep	MM	–	Coltman *et al.*, 1999
Antilocapridae: *Antilocapra americana* Pronghorn	MM	MP	Byers *et al.*, 1994; Carling *et al.*, 2003
Cervidae: *Capreolus capreolus* Roe deer	MM	MP	Vanpé *et al.*, 2009
Cervidae *Odocoileus virginianus* White-tailed deer	MM	MP	De Young *et al.*, 2002

copulating with multiple partners (Mate *et al.*, 2005). Sperm competition in cetaceans is discussed in Chapter 6, and data on their relative testes sizes are provided in Table 6.1.

Copulatory Patterns, Sperm Competition and Cryptic Female Choice

Table 4.2 lists a number of ways in which copulatory and associated patterns of behaviour might affect reproductive success via sperm competition or cryptic female choice. A solid background of research on copulatory patterns and sperm competition in primates and rodents provides a suitable entry point to discussions of the Mammalia as a whole. I shall begin by considering the impact of sexual selection upon patterns of copulation in the prosimians, monkeys and apes.

Primates

Of the four copulatory patterns that occur among male primates, the most widespread is pattern number 12, in which there is no genital lock and a single brief intromission with pelvic thrusting culminates in ejaculation. This pattern is present across the mating spectrum, from species that are monogamous (e.g. owl monkeys and gibbons) or polygynous (e.g. proboscis monkeys and gorillas) to polygynandrous species, such

Table 4.2 Copulatory and associated mechanisms that may improve reproductive success via sperm competition, or cryptic female choice

---

Sperm competition
1. Increase sperm numbers in the ejaculate:
    Copulate multiple times
    Prolong copulation and transfer more sperm
2. Remove plugs of previous males and then:
    Deposit a copulatory plug
3. Deposit ejaculate(s) closer to ova:
    Adaptations for intracervical or intrauterine insemination
4. Stimulate and maintain the female's immobile, receptive posture
5. Stimulate physiological responses by the female that:
    Induce ovulation
    Enhance sperm transport
    Shorten the receptive period

Cryptic female choice
    Remate with another male(s)
    Prevent intromission
    Terminate copulation prior to ejaculation
    Fail to transport/store sperm
    Remove/dislodge copulatory plug
    Eject sperm/semen post-copulation
    Fail to ovulate

---

as talapoins, mandrills, Barbary macaques and chimpanzees. Polygynandrous primates that exhibit this pattern also have very large testes in relation to body weight and copulate at high frequencies. They exemplify the first sperm competition strategy listed in Table 4.2, which is to increase sperm numbers transferred to females by copulating multiple times. It is the ability to ejaculate frequently that has undergone selection, rather than the basic structure of the copulatory pattern. As examples, male Barbary macaques may copulate an average of 2.28 times/hour, male mandrills 0.85/h and chimpanzees 0.52/h, as compared to 0.07/h in owl monkeys, or 0.005/h in gibbons (Dixson, 1995b, 2012).

Another strategy that males may adopt to increase the numbers of sperm transferred to females is to copulate for longer periods of time. Members of 13 primate genera exhibit such prolonged single intromissions (pattern nos. 3 and 11); examples of the species concerned are included in Table 4.3. The great majority of them are polygynandrous and have large testes in relation to body weight. Bouts of pelvic thrusting take place at intervals during extended matings, and it is suspected (but unproven) that males may ejaculate multiple times, as for example in Garnett's greater galago (*Otolemur garnettii*). In this species intromission may last for over 4 hours (Eaton *et al.*, 1973). Extended matings might, of course, fulfil other functions such as allowing the male to mate guard a female; this may be particularly important in prosimians in which females are sexually receptive for limited periods of time. In *O. garnettii*, prolonged intromissions shorten the duration of the female's receptivity and reduce the time available for her to engage in multiple-partner matings (Dixson, 2012). It is also possible that during prolonged intromissions the glans penis serves to maintain semen in contact with the female's os cervix, thus facilitating sperm transport into the cervical canal and uterus.

Natural selection as well as sexual selection may have influenced the evolution of prolonged copulatory patterns in mammals, as was discussed in Chapter 3. Like many other mammals, prosimians such as galagos, lorises and pottos are nocturnal. Given that they occupy individual home ranges rather than forming social groups, prolonged matings may be adaptive in transferring the maximum number of sperm during a single encounter. The cryptic habits of these small, arboreal, nocturnal primates may also render them less likely to be attacked during extended periods of copulation. Among the diurnal primates, only a few of the larger arboreal New World monkeys engage in prolonged copulations (e.g. spider monkeys, woolly monkeys and muriquis: Table 4.3).

The last of the four copulatory patterns that occurs in primates (pattern no. 10) consists of a series of brief intromissions, each of which is accompanied by pelvic thrusting. There is no genital lock. This pattern has been described in several genera of the New World monkeys, as well as in various macaques and baboons (Table 4.3). Again, it is much more prevalent among species that have multimale–multifemale (polygynandrous) mating systems. Two exceptions to this rule are known; the golden lion tamarin (*Leontopithecus rosalia*) and the Hamadryas baboon (*Papio hamadryas*). Hamadryas baboons live in multilevel societies containing many polygynous one

Table 4.3 Copulatory patterns which occur in primates. Genital lock (GL), Prolonged intromission (PI); Brief intromission (BI) and Pelvic thrusting (PT)

Pattern no. 3	Pattern no. 10	Pattern no. 11	Pattern no. 12
Possible GL: a single PI + PT	No GL: multiple BI + PT	No GL: a single PI + PT	No: GL: a single BI + PT
Otolemur garnettii	*Cacajao calvus*	*Microcebus murinus*	*Lemur catta*[†]
O. crassicaudatus	*Saimiri sciureus**	*Galago moholi*	*Varecia variegata*
Galagoides demidoff	*Leontopithecus rosalia*	*Loris tardigradus*	*Cheirogaleus major*
Daubentonia	*Piliocolobus badius*	*Arctocebus calabarensis*	*Tarsius bancanus*
madagascariensis	*Macaca silenus*	*Lagothrix lagotricha*	*Callithrix jacchus*
Macaca arctoides	*M. nemestrina*	*Ateles belzebuth*	*Saguinus oedipus*
	M. nigra	*A. geoffroyi*	*Cebuella pygmaea*
	M. maura	*A. fusciceps*	*Callimico goeldii*
	*M. fascicularis**	*Brachyteles arachnoides*	*Callicebus moloch*
	M. mulatta	*Pongo pygmaeus*	*Aotus lemurinus*
	M. fuscata		*Cebus nigrivittatus*
	*M. thibetana?**		*Alouatta palliata*
	*Papio ursinus**		*Nasalis larvatus*
	P. hamadryas		*Miopithecus talapoin*
			Erythrocebus patas
			Chlorocebus aethiops
			Mandrillus sphinx
			Lophocebus albigena
			Theropithecus gelada
			Papio anubis
			Macaca radiata
			M. sylvanus
			Hylobates lar
			Pan troglodytes
			P. paniscus
			Gorilla gorilla
			Homo sapiens

* Pattern no. 12 also occurs in these species. [†]Copulatory pattern no. 10 also occurs in *L. catta*. Modified from Dixson (2012).

male units (Kummer, 1984, 1990). Kummer considered that the ancestral condition for *P. hamadryas* was a multimale–multifemale mating system such as occurs in most members of the genus *Papio*. If correct, this could explain the persistence of an ancestral mode of copulation (pattern no. 10) in this species. The significance of a multiple intromission copulatory pattern in the golden lion tamarin is unknown.

Might selection for a multiple intromission copulatory pattern have been influenced by sperm competition, given that it is present mainly in polygynandrous monkeys that have large relative testes sizes? One possible function of multiple intromissions may be to dislodge and remove coagulated semen deposited by rival males (item no. 2 in Table 4.2). It is also possible that cohorts of spermatozoa are transported from the cauda epididymis into the vas deferens during each intromission of a series, resulting in the transfer of larger numbers of gametes during the final, ejaculatory mount. Although this hypothesis has been mooted several times (Bercovitch and Nürnberg, 1996; Dixson 2012, 2018), it has not been tested by experiment. Some relevant experiments have been carried out using rodents, however, and these are discussed in the next section.

Finally, multiple intromissions and pelvic thrusting movements may affect subsequent sperm transport. During the peri-ovulatory phase of the ovarian cycle, the composition of cervical mucus alters; it develops an elastic quality ('spinnbarkheit') and becomes more penetrable by sperm. The thrusting actions exerted during repeated intromissions may assist in drawing out the mucus into long threads, so that spermatozoa may move from the vagina into the cervical canal (Dixson, 2012). Further discussion of the role played by the cervical mucus in cryptic female choice of spermatozoa is included in Chapter 8.

Several species of primates that have a multiple intromission copulatory pattern include some males that ejaculate during a single intromission with pelvic thrusting (pattern no. 12). This is the case for the squirrel monkey (*Saimiri sciureus*), chacma baboon (*Papio ursinus*) and the long-tailed macaque (*Macaca fascicularis*). Hall and DeVore (1965) reported this difference between a troop of chacma baboons in the Cape region of South Africa and two troops observed in Kenya's Nairobi National Park. The South African baboons were multiple mounters (pattern no. 10) whereas males in the two Kenyan groups were single mounters (pattern no. 12).

Marked variability in copulatory patterns may also occur between closely related species as, for example, in the Genus *Macaca*. The single brief intromission pattern no. 12 occurs in *M. sylvanus*, *M. sinica*, *M. radiata* and *M. assamensis*, pattern no. 3 in *M. arctoides*, and the multiple intromission pattern no. 10 in the remaining species for which behavioural data are available, such as *M. silenus* and *M. mulatta* (Figure 4.3). It is probable that pattern no. 12 represents the ancestral condition for this genus (Eudy, 1980) given that it occurs in the Barbary macaque (*M. sylvanus*), which represents the most ancient macaque lineage (Delson, 1980). The copulatory pattern of the stump-tail macaque is clearly derived; it consists of a prolonged single intromission with pelvic thrusting and a partial tie or lock between the male and female genitalia. Presumably, the multiple intromission pattern of macaques also derives from a brief single intromission pattern of copulation such as exists in *M. sylvanus*.

Rodents

Dewsbury (1975a, 1988) and Langtimm and Dewsbury (1991) conducted detailed studies of muroid rodents to investigate the evolution and functions of their patterns of copulatory behaviour. Dewsbury (1975a) noted that the Superfamily Muroidea contains 'more than 200 genera that are distributed throughout the world and that are adapted to virtually every possible habitat'. His laboratory studies focused on 31

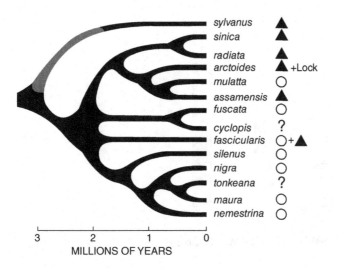

Figure 4.3 Phylogenetic distribution of copulatory patterns in the Genus *Macaca*.
▲ = Ejaculation occurs during a single mount, with pelvic thrusting. Note that *M. arctoides* exhibits a copulatory lock during the single intromission pattern. ○ = Copulation involves a series of intromissions with pelvic thrusting.

species, all of which were members of the Cricetidae and Muridae, and 32 per cent of them exhibited a multiple intromission copulatory pattern which lacked pelvic thrusts (pattern no. 14). A number of rodent species that have been extensively studied by reproductive biologists fall within this group, including the Norway rat (*Rattus novegicus*), golden hamster (*Mesocricetus auratus*) and Mongolian gerbil (*Meriones unguiculatus*). They display various anatomical and physiological adaptations indicative of post-copulatory sexual selection, some of which are discussed in later chapters. Thus, as in macaques, the evolution of multiple intromission copulatory patterns in rodents may be linked to sperm competition and cryptic female choice. Indeed, there is considerable evidence to support this hypothesis where the muroid rodents are concerned, as is illustrated by the following examples.

Unlike the female macaques and other primates described above, female muroid rodents such as rats and hamsters do not exhibit a spontaneous luteal phase during the ovarian cycle. Instead, copulatory stimulation is required to trigger a twice-daily surge of prolactin and the secretion of progesterone during pregnancy (Allen and Adler, 1985; Smith and Neill, 1976; Terkel and Sawyer, 1978). Female rats fail to become pregnant if males make too few pre-ejaculatory intromissions (Wilson *et al.*, 1965). Hence, cryptic female choice might favour some males over others via this mechanism. The male's multiple intromissions also affect the numbers of sperm transferred to the female at ejaculation. Adler and Toner (1986) conducted experiments where they switched the partners at different stages of an intromission series so that males and females experienced different numbers of pre-ejaculatory intromissions. Sperm counts in the female tract (vagina + uterus) increased in line with the numbers of pre-ejaculatory intromissions made by males, as is shown in Figure 4.4.

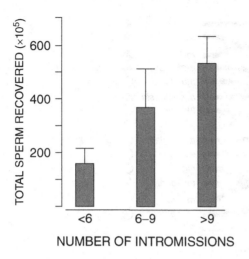

Figure 4.4 Numbers of sperm recovered from the reproductive tracts (vagina + uterus) of female rats after matings involving increasing numbers of intromissions by males. (Redrawn and modified from Adler and Toner, 1986.)

This result lends support to the hypothesis advanced previously: namely, that sperm may be transported from the cauda epididymis into the vas deferens during each pre-ejaculatory intromission, thus resulting in a higher sperm count. Where the rat is concerned, the efficiency of sperm transport is also affected by the male's behaviour throughout the mount series. His intromissions dislodge plugs deposited by previous males (Matthews and Adler, 1977). Tactile stimulation also facilitates the female's lordotic (sexually receptive) posture and assures that she remains immobile during ejaculation (Adler and Toner, 1986; Pfaff, 1980). A copulatory plug is thus deposited firmly against the cervix, which enhances sperm transport into the uterus (Matthews and Adler, 1977). Finally, it is important to consider that wild rats and mice live in small breeding units that contain a number of adults of both sexes and their offspring. Sexual interactions are much more complex and labile under such conditions; multiple-partner matings occur, and females exert more control over the timing ('pacing') of mounts and intromissions, and tend to create longer gaps between these events (McClintock, 1984; McClintock and Adler, 1978).

The information discussed above is consistent with the conclusion that mating patterns that include multiple brief intromissions (i.e. copulatory patterns nos. 10 and 14) have evolved under sexual selection in some primates and rodents. These two orders also account for 84 per cent of all mammalian species that are currently known to display these two patterns. Although Dewsbury's (1975a) comparative studies involved only 31 species of muroid rodents, 7 types of copulatory patterns were represented among this small sample of rodent diversity. Several of these patterns involved a genital lock during mating, and this was associated with thickening of the glans penis and the presence of large penile spines in males of the eight species concerned. Copulatory locks occur in some members of nine orders of mammals (see

Table 3.1). Sexual selection has produced a variety of genital specializations in such cases, as is discussed in Chapters 5 and 7. Dewsbury also noted that some of the voles included in his sample ovulate in response to copulatory stimulation. However, their copulatory patterns did not differ markedly from those of voles that are spontaneous ovulators. Chapter 9 deals with the evolution of mating-induced and spontaneous ovulation among mammals, and considers the role played by post-copulatory sexual selection during the evolution of induced ovulation.

Copulatory Courtship and Cryptic Female Choice

Comparative studies of insects and spiders have revealed that males of many species make rhythmic movements of their genitalia during mating and that in many cases these are likely to represent examples of 'copulatory courtship' that are subject to cryptic female choice (Eberhard, 1994). The same is true of some mammals in which the temporal patterning and duration of intravaginal thrusting varies tremendously between taxa. For example, among the dasyurid marsupials bouts of thrusting may occur with intervals in between, as for example in broad-footed marsupial mice (Genus *Antechinus*). In *A. stuartii*, copulation lasts for 5–12 hours (Woolley, 1966) and involves a genital lock. Active (pelvic thrusting) and quiescent phases of copulation have been described by Marlow (1961) as follows:

The onset of the active phase is heralded by a remarkable sinuous lateral wriggling of the tail of the male who then seizes the female's scruff in his jaws. He braces his hind feet against the female's rump and gives a single powerful coital thrust. Both animals roll over onto one side together and then resume their former position. This active phase lasts for about 10 seconds and alternates regularly with the quiescent stage which lasts for about 4 minutes.

Males of *A. agilis* exhibit bouts of thrusting (rather than single thrusts) lasting for 10–60 seconds, and incorporate 'side to side' movements of the pelvis into the thrusting pattern (Shimmin *et al.*, 2002). This occurs more frequently if the male is the first partner to mate with a female, and is more pronounced during the early stages of copulation.

Alternating between thrusting and quiescent phases has also been recorded during prolonged copulations in several other species of dasyurid marsupials (e.g. *Sminthopsis murina*: Fox and Whitford, 1982; *Ninguai* spp.: Fanning, 1982; *Planigale gilesi*: Whitford *et al.*, 1982; *Dasycercus cristicauda*: Sorenson, 1970 and *Dasyurus viverrinus*: Eisenberg, 1977; Godsell, 1983). Fanning (1982) noted that in several *Ninguai* species, pelvic thrusting continues during the quiescent phase of mating, but the thrusts are less frequent and deeper than during the active phase.

Further examples of the pelvic thrusting patterns exhibited by male mammals during prolonged copulations are listed in Table 4.4. Understanding the physiological significance of such behaviour will require much more detailed study in future. Prolonged intromission may allow males to transfer larger volumes of semen and/or spermatozoa to the female, as is known to be the case in the domestic dog (*Canis familiaris*). Intermittent bouts of thrusting in some taxa may be indicative of repeated

Table 4.4 Variations in patterns of pelvic thrusting (PT) during prolonged intromissions in mammals

Species	Copulatory behaviour	Source
Tachyglossus aculeatus	PT for up to 60 min during prolonged intromission	Wallage *et al.*, 2015
Macropus eugenii, M. giganteus, M. rufogriseus	Multiple ejaculations are thought to occur during prolonged intromission	Tyndale-Biscoe and Renfree, 1987
Monodelphis domestica	Intro = 4–7 min. PT in bouts with 'rest pauses'	Trupin and Fadem, 1982
Camelus bactrianus	Intro = 7.66 min. PT is 'intermittent'	Vyas *et al.*, 2015
Dicerorhinus sumatrensis	Intro = 5+ min. PT occurs intermittently in bouts	AFD
Rhinoceros unicornis	Intro = 30–60 min. Ejaculation is thought to occur at intervals	Laurie, 1982
Canis latrans	Lock = 15–20 min. PT occurs early, during lock formation	Bekoff and Diamond, 1976
Cuon alpinus	Lock = 14.7 min. PT slow and rhythmic until lock occurs	Paulraj *et al.*, 1992
Nasua narica	Intro = 60 min. PT bouts of 2–5 s with pauses of 1–5 s	Hass and Roback, 2000
Ailurus fulgens	Intro = 32.3 min. PT bouts of 8–79, mean = 39 thrusts	Roberts and Kessler, 1979
Mustela vison	Intro = up to 180 min. PT bouts are rapid, with periods of rest	Enders, 1952
Spilogale pygmaea	Intro = 18 min. PT in 7-s bursts	Teska *et al.*, 1981
Crocuta crocuta	Long mounts = 5 min. PT occurs early on during intro*	Szykman *et al.*, 2007
Arctocephalus forsteri	Intro = 6.56 min. PT more pronounced towards the end of the mount	Stirling, 1971
Myotis myotis	Several PT bouts occur, then pair remains suspended for 15–30 min	Zahn and Dippel, 1997
Atelerix algirus	Intro = 5.38 min. Slow PT bouts occur throughout the mount	AFD

AFD = author's observations using filmed records. *A post-copulatory pair-sit occurs.

ejaculations. Equally, they may serve to stimulate sperm transport within the female tract.

Eberhard (1996) reasoned that if copulatory thrusting serves as a form of courtship, then 'it should be relatively organized and stereotyped in at least some respects'. This is the case for both the Norway rat and the domestic rabbit. Both of these species exhibit very rapid, oscillating pelvic thrusts *prior to intromission*, and the duration and frequency of these thrusting movements is remarkably constant in both species (Contreras and Beyer, 1979; Morali and Beyer, 1992). One function of thrusting is to stimulate the receptive female to adopt the lordotic posture which, in turn, facilitates intromission by the male (see Figure 3.3, which shows polygraphic recordings of pelvic thrusting patterns in the rabbit). Where the rat is concerned, it has already been noted that the series of mounts and intromissions prior to ejaculation serves to trigger the secretion of progesterone required to support pregnancy. There are some rodents in which males continue to mount and intromit *after ejaculating*, so that females receive additional stimulation in the absence of further sperm being transferred. Such is the case in the cactus mouse (*Peromyscus eremicus*); prevention of post-ejaculatory intromissions (which are accompanied by pelvic thrusting in this species) resulted in 90 per cent of females failing to become pregnant, or pseudopregnant (Dewsbury and Estep, 1975). Data for the cactus mouse are included with those for nine other muroid rodents in Figure 4.5. This compares percentages of pregnancies that result from tests in which a single ejaculation occurs with those in which males ejaculate repeatedly during extended ('satiety') tests. In all but one species, higher percentages of pregnancies resulted from satiety tests.

The tendency for males of many species to copulate and ejaculate multiple times may relate to the courtship functions of copulation. As well as serving to increase sperm numbers transferred to the female, multiple matings may induce the surge of luteinizing hormone required to trigger ovulation (e.g. in rabbits and cats: see Chapter 9), induce the secretion of progesterone, as described for muroid rodents, or

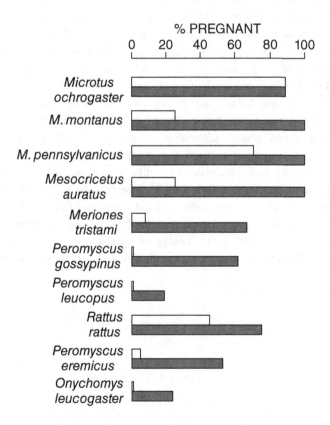

Figure 4.5 Percentages of females that become pregnant after receiving a single ejaculation (open bars) versus multiple ejaculations (during extended 'satiety' tests: closed bars) in 10 species of muroid rodents. (Redrawn and modified from Dewsbury, 1978.)

facilitate sperm transport within the female's reproductive tract. The prolonged matings and variable patterns of pelvic thrusting that occur in a variety of mammals (Table 4.4) may also include cases of copulatory courtship. Tactile stimulation during prolonged matings induces ovulation in mustelids, for example, whereas in camelids repeated ejaculations transfer an ovulation inducing factor in the male's semen. These examples, and others, are discussed in Chapter 9.

Although copulatory courtship is usually discussed primarily in terms of males courting females, females often strongly influence events that occur once genital contact has been established. Male courtship may not always succeed; thus, females may terminate matings before ejaculation occurs. Such behaviour has been observed during laboratory and field studies of a number of anthropoid primates (Dixson, 2012). In a few cases, females are known to contribute directly to copulatory thrusting movements. In the red uakari (*Cacajao calvus*), the female sometimes 'complements the male's pelvic thrusts with visible pelvic thrusts of her own' (Fontaine, 1981). Female mountain gorillas sometimes make thrusting movements during copulation and these tend to be slower and deeper than those made by the male. During copulations in which female orang-utans adopt a superior position on the male it is usual for the female to control pelvic thrusting movements (Nadler, 1988; Schurmann, 1982). Few detailed accounts exist concerning copulatory courtship in bats. However, Tan *et al.* (2009) have reported a possible case of such behaviour in short-nosed fruit bats (*Cynopterus sphinx*). Females of this species sometimes lick the base of the male's penis during mating, and the duration of copulation is increased as a result (Tan *et al.*, 2009). Why females behave in this way with some males but not others, and whether sperm transfer increases during longer copulations, is not known.

In addition to direct genital stimulation, cryptic female choice may include responses to other types of tactile stimulation provided by males during mating. In many invertebrates, for example, males may rub, lick or tap various parts of the female's body (Eberhard, 1991, 1994). Chapter 8 revisits the subject of copulatory courtship in greater detail, in order to discuss tactile and other forms of (non-genital) communication between the sexes. Cryptic female choice is also discussed in relation to events that take place during the passage of spermatozoa through the female reproductive tract, from the point at which ejaculation occurs to the site of fertilization in the oviduct.

Part III

The Evolution of Reproduction

Monotremata

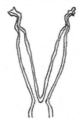

Marsupialia

Placentalia

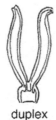

duplex

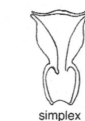

bicornuate   simplex

The Mammalian Uterus
Sharman, 1976

Part III
The Evolution of Reproduction

5 Phallic Structure and Function

In mammals, copulatory organs, especially male organs, are highly specialized and present very great diversity of structure, and there is equally great diversity in patterns of sexual behaviour, the functional significance of which is not always clear in our present state of knowledge.

Walton, 1960

When Arthur Walton wrote these words, which appeared in the third edition of *Marshall's Physiology of Reproduction*, he was unable to account for the evolutionary basis of phallic diversity in mammals, some examples of which are shown in Figure 5.1. Indeed, prior to the application of sexual selection theory to this problem (Eberhard, 1985, 1996; Parker, 1970), the presence of so much variability among male invertebrates, and among the vertebrates as a whole, had remained a mystery. The purpose of this chapter is to explore the various reasons for phallic morphological diversity, including the role that copulatory and post-copulatory sexual selection may have played in this context.

Phylogeny and Phallic Morphology

it is important to recognize at the outset that phylogenetic factors have played important roles in determining phallic structure. Possession of a phallus is an ancient trait, not just for the mammals but for most other amniotes. Thus, as is shown diagrammatically in Figure 5.2, males in virtually all the existing amniote lineages (i.e. squamate reptiles, turtles, crocodilians, some birds and all mammals) have a phallus. Notable exceptions to this rule are provided by the tuatara and also by more than 90 per cent of bird species (Sanger *et al.*, 2015).

The tuatara (*Sphenodon punctatus*) is an archaic, superficially lizard-like reptile which occurs only in New Zealand; it is the sole surviving representative of the Order Rhyncocephalia. Although the tuatara lacks a penis, Sanger *et al.* (2015) reported that, during embryonic life, the male passes through the earliest stages of phallic development, involving the growth of two external genital swellings. Development is halted at this initial stage, but Sanger *et al.* propose that forms ancestral to the tuatara would have displayed complete development of the phallus. Reduction and loss of the phallus is thus posited to have occurred in the tuatara, as is also the case for the great

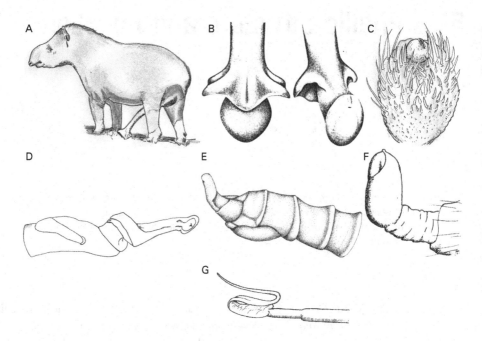

Figure 5.1 Examples of diverse penile morphologies in placental mammals. **A:** Brazilian tapir (*Tapirus terrestris*) to show the large lateral lobes on the erect glans penis (author's drawing). **B:** Glans penis of the Brazilian tapir; dorsal and ventral views (from Ottow, 1955). **C:** Hoary bat (*Lasiurus cinereus*) to show the greatly elongated spines on the glans penis (author's drawing, after Cryan *et al.*, 2012). **D:** Lesser mouse deer (*Tragulus javanicus*). (Redrawn from Vidyadaran *et al.*, 1999.) **E:** Chinese rock squirrel (*Sciurotamias davidianus*). (After Callahan and Davis, 1982.) **F:** Heart-nosed bat (*Cardioderma cor*). (After Matthews, 1942.) **G:** Northern short-tailed shrew (*Blarina brevicauda*). (After Pearson, 1944.)

majority of birds. A true (intromittent) phallus has been retained only in the Anseriformes (e.g. ducks, geese and swans) and the Struthioniformes (e.g. ostriches, cassowaries and kiwis: Montgomerie, 2010), whilst a rudimentary organ is present in the Galliformes (e.g. pheasants and quails: Montgomerie, 2010).

In amniotes other than the mammals, spermatozoa travel along an open groove in the phallus (the *sulcus spermaticus*) during copulation. However, in mammals (including the monotremes) an enclosed, penile canal fulfils this function. There are many other anatomical and physiological differences between the penes of the various amniote lineages. For example, in those birds in which a phallus is present, tumescence occurs via a lymphatic mechanism (Brennan and Prum, 2012), whereas in mammals it is controlled by the vascular system. Thus, given the current state of knowledge, the conclusion that the penes of extant reptiles, birds and mammals all originate from a single common ancestor (Gredler *et al.*, 2014; Sanger *et al.*, 2015) should be treated with caution.

Phylogenetic factors have greatly influenced the evolution of phallic structure among the various groups of mammals. A distinction is often made between the

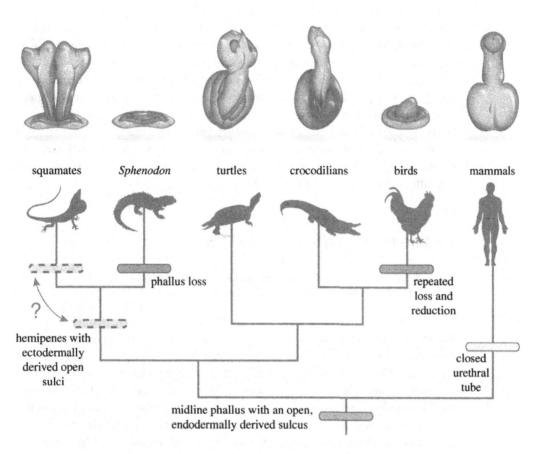

Figure 5.2 Phallic morphology and phylogenetic relationships among the extant amniotes. (After Sanger *et al.*, 2015.)

'fibroelastic' type of penis, which occurs in cetaceans and many ungulates (e.g. goats, sheep, cattle, deer and antelopes), and the 'vascular' penes that are more typical of the primates, carnivores, rodents and some others. In fact, a range of intermediate types occurs between these two extremes in the various mammalian lineages. It should be kept in mind that, in all mammals, penile erection depends to varying degrees upon vascular mechanisms that cause engorgement of the erectile tissues: the paired corpora cavernosa of the penile shaft and the corpus spongiosum which surrounds the urethra, and which also extends into the head of the penis (the glans, in certain cases). In a markedly fibroelastic type of penis, less erectile tissue is present in the distal shaft and head of the organ, most of the erectile capacity being concentrated at the root of the penis. In its non-erect state, the penis is withdrawn into the prepuce and held there, in a flexed position, by the action of paired retractor muscles. Such an arrangement occurs, for example, in cattle and sheep. During erection, blood enters the erectile bodies at the base of the penis, and the retractor muscles are relaxed; these two processes allow the organ to straighten out and to protrude from the prepuce. The situation in markedly vascular types of penes is quite different, as the *pars libera* of the non-erect organ is more flaccid and the corpora cavernosa and corpus spongiosum are more extensive. Erection thus entails greater increases in tumescence than in a fibroelastic penis.

Fundamental anatomical differences between fibroelastic penes as compared to highly vascular penes may have affected the evolution of certain other phallic traits. Penile spines, and bacula, for example, have evolved only in some mammals that have markedly vascular penes (e.g. among rodents, bats and primates, as examples). This has not been the case in mammalian lineages where fibroelastic morphologies predominate (e.g. among cetaceans and ungulates). Possible reasons for these phylogenetic differences are discussed later in this chapter.

The Evolution of Morphological Diversity

The study of genitalia probably represents the last major frontier of an old and very successful branch of biology: functional morphology.

William Eberhard

Taxonomists have long been aware that intromittent organs in many groups of animals vary tremendously in their morphology, even where closely related species are concerned. Thus, genitalic traits were originally studied because of their usefulness in classifying animals, rather than as a means of exploring their reproductive biology and its evolution. This may seem surprising, because intromittent organs clearly play a vital role in transferring spermatozoa to females. Yet, with so many other problems to claim their attention, most reproductive biologists did not assign a high priority to studies of intromittent organs, such as mammalian penes.

Given that the mammalian penis functions as a conduit for urine, as well as for semen, why should its morphology be so variable? Prior to the publication of William Eberhard's (1985) book entitled *Sexual Selection and Animal Genitalia*, a number of theories had been advanced to account for the evolution of such diversity. Alas, none of them was satisfactory. As an undergraduate student I was told that males of many invertebrate taxa have developed complex genitalia in order to mesh with complementary female structures that 'recognize' only the correct 'key' provided by members of the same species. It was thought that these arrangements helped to prevent hybridization, and functioned as *species isolating mechanisms*. One major objection to the 'lock-and-key' hypothesis is that selection should (and in fact does) favour mechanisms that allow animals to recognize prospective mating partners of their own species well before genital contact is attempted. Another objection is the absence of any anatomical evidence for lock-and-key meshing of the genitalia in so many invertebrate species (Eberhard, 1985). The same objections arise when attempts are made to apply the lock-and-key hypothesis to mammals. Penile complexity in many species of mammals is not necessarily matched by vaginal morphological complexity.

Ernst Mayr (1963) rejected the lock-and-key hypothesis and advanced an alternative 'pleiotropism hypothesis' to account for diversity in penile morphology.

This posited that variations, such as those shown in Figure 5.1, result from pleiotropic effects of genes in other systems that are favoured by natural selection. Mayr expressed his reasoning as follows:

The genitalic apparatus is a highly complicated structure, the pleiotropic by-product of very many genes of the species. Any change in the genetic contribution of the species may result in an incidental change in the structure of the genitalia.

According to this idea, pleiotropic effects are not subject to negative selection; providing, of course, that the penis continues to fulfil its basic functions effectively. Yet, even a cursory critique of this hypothesis raises the question: 'why should the penis be so burdened by pleiotropic effects, while other organs are not?' Given its essential role in reproduction we might expect that penile morphology would be 'especially likely to to be subject to selection' (Eberhard, 1985). It is also intriguing that males of many invertebrate species transfer their gametes to females by way of secondary structures, rather than via their primary genitalia. Examples of such secondary structures include the modified mouth parts (pedipalps) of male spiders and the specialized arm (hectocotylus) with which male cephalopods transfer their spermatophores to females (Figure 5.3). In such cases it is these secondary structures, rather than the primary genitalia, that have undergone species-specific morphological changes.

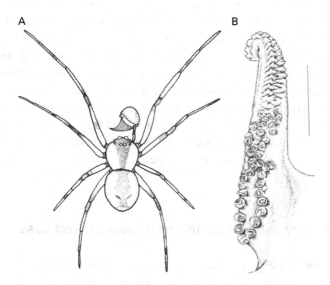

A   B

Figure 5.3 A: The spider *Tidarren fordum*. The male's greatly enlarged pedipalp is used to transfer sperm to the female. In this species the male sometimes removes one pedipalp; only one remains in this example. (After Chamberlin and Ivie, 1943.) **B:** The specialized arm (hectocotylus) of a male bottlenose squid (*Sepioloidea magna*). A series of flap-like structures occurs distally on the hectocotylus, which the male uses to transfer spermatophores during mating. (From Reid, 2009.)

The possibility that sexual selection might have influenced the evolution of penile morphology was not considered by Mayr. Indeed, his landmark volume on *Animal Species and Evolution* barely mentions the subject of sexual selection and, surprisingly, underestimates its importance:

Darwin had an inkling of the importance of reproductive success and discussed it in part under the heading of 'Sexual Selection.' Yet selection in favor of reproductive success has in many instances nothing to do with sexual selection. How much of Darwin's sexual selection falls under the heading of 'mere reproductive success' can be determined only after a complete reevaluation of his material. Mayr (1963)

The failure of existing theories to account for the evolution of complex genital morphologies led William Eberhard to seek alternative explanations. Comparative studies of invertebrate taxa led him to conclude that the male intromittent organ may sometimes function as an *internal courtship device*, encouraging the female to transport or store sperm within her reproductive tract (e.g. Eberhard, 1985, 1990, 1996). Thus, in those mating systems where females often copulate with multiple partners, possession of advantageous genitalic traits by certain males might result in them gaining a reproductive advantage via 'cryptic female choice' and not solely via inter-male (sperm) competition.

When mammals mate, spermatozoa must migrate (or be transported) from the vagina through the cervix, uterus and uterotubal junction before they reach the oviduct, where fertilization takes place. As we have seen in previous chapters, females of many mammalian species engage in multiple-partner matings. In such circumstances sperm competition takes place between the gametes of rival males for access to a given set of ova. However, at each stage of their journey to the oviduct, the sperm of rival males are also influenced by the female's reproductive anatomy and physiology. Such interactions affect their survival, motility and ability to penetrate the ovum. These hidden influences constitute cryptic female choices. In practice, sperm competition and cryptic female choice are not mutually exclusive; their effects become interwoven. The important insight arising from Eberhard's work is that some sperm may be favoured over others due to factors that are under *female control*. Thus, cryptic female choice, as well as sperm competition, may affect male reproductive success.

Penile Morphology and Primate Mating Systems: A Test Case

It is very remarkable, considering that the organs have the same rather limited functions to perform, how varied the male genitalia of primates are in their morphology.

Hill, 1972

A great deal is known about the genital morphology of primate species, thanks in no small measure to the painstaking work of comparative anatomists such as

W. C. Osman Hill. In his eight volumes on *The Primates: Comparative Anatomy and Taxonomy*, published between 1953 and 1974, Hill included detailed drawings and measurements of the external genitalia of many species of non-human primates. In 1985, when William Eberhard's book on *Sexual Selection and Animal Genitalia* was published, a colleague of mine who had been sent a copy for review passed it to me, as it fell outside of his own interests. I was intrigued by Eberhard's novel account of the part that sexual selection by female choice may have played in the evolution of invertebrate genitalia, and decided to test his ideas in a study of the primates. Hill's publications were to prove invaluable during this exercise.

Four traits were selected for study: penile length, length of the baculum (*os penis*), sizes of the keratinized penile spines on the distal region of the penis and complexity of the distal region in terms of its overall shape. Features such as distal penile complexity proved very difficult to quantify; thus, each character was rated on a five-point scale, in which 1 = least development and 5 = maximum development. Although open to subjective errors, this approach had a marked advantage, as it became possible to make numerical comparisons involving 130 species of primates.

Results of this initial study indicated that penile morphologies are most complex in those primate species in which females commonly mate with multiple males, rather than with a single partner during the fertile period (Dixson, 1987a). Thus, species that have polygynandrous mating systems tended to have longer penes, a more complex distal morphology, longer bacula and larger penile spines than polygynous or monogamous species. It is important to note that such correlations do not, by themselves, prove that there is a causative relationship between multiple-partner matings by females and the evolution of genitalic complexity in males. However, if it is the case that sexual selection is involved, then effects upon phallic morphology might be due to sperm competition, to cryptic female choice, or to the combined effects of both these types of sexual selection.

Lack of statistical control for phylogeny biased some results of the initial study, especially where the penile spines are concerned, as these structures are generally larger in prosimians than in monkeys and apes (Harcourt and Gardiner, 1994). Subsequent work (Dixson, 2009, 2012) has confirmed that ratings of penile length, distal complexity and baculum length are highest (scoring 4 or 5 on the five-point scale) for males of those genera where females mate with multiple partners (Figure 5.4).

The overall score for all four of the traits considered is 10 for *H. sapiens*, which is the same score as that assigned to monogamous and polygynous monkeys, such as *Callimico*, *Leontopithecus*, *Erythrocebus* and *Theropithecus*. Men have lower overall scores for penile complexity than 27 of the 48 genera included in the study. These findings do not support the view that sexual selection has influenced the evolution of human penile morphology, in contrast to a number of published accounts (e.g. Baker and Bellis, 1995; Gallup *et al.*, 2003; Smith, 1984).

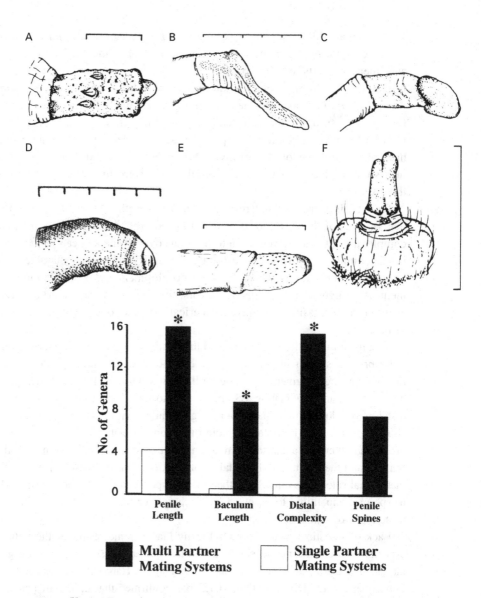

Figure 5.4 Upper: Examples of penile morphologies in primate species where females mate with multiple partners (polygynandry – **A**: *Eulemur fulvus*; **B**: *Macaca arctoides*), or with single partners (polygyny – **C**: *Erythrocebus patas*; **D**: *Gorilla gorilla*; monogamy – **E**: *Callithrix jacchus*; **F**: *Cebuella pygmaea*). Scales are in 1-cm divisions. (After Dixson, 2012.)
Lower: Penile morphologies are more complex in those primate genera where females mate with multiple partners than in genera where single partners are the norm.
*$P < 0.05$. (After Dixson, 2009.)

Pelvic Bones, Penes and Post-copulatory Sexual Selection in Cetaceans

> Thou didst, O lord, create the mighty whale,
> That wondrous monster of a mighty length;
> Vast his head and body, vast his tail,
> Beyond conception his unmeasured strength.
>
> Peleg Folger, Nantucket whaleman

The slaughter that resulted from commercial whaling produced one beneficial result. Biologists were sometimes able to gain access to fresh specimens in order to study their anatomy. Such observations, as well as those involving the carcasses of whales that had beached themselves or were washed ashore after their death, have provided much valuable information concerning their reproductive biology (e.g. Slijper, 1962, 1976). Indeed, for some cetaceans, such as the beaked whales of the Family Ziphiidae, virtually all our knowledge derives from studies of post-mortem material, as the living animals are only rarely glimpsed in the wild. Whales, dolphins and porpoises have fibroelastic penes, which are filiform at the tip and morphologically quite similar in the various taxa. An exception to this generalization concerns the Ganges River dolphin (*Platanista gangetica*) in which erectile side lobes occur on the penis. Unfortunately, this species is in danger of extinction, and nothing is known about its copulatory behaviour.

In all cetaceans, the non-erect penis is retracted within the abdomen where it forms an 'S'-shaped configuration. At its root, the penis and the ischiocavernosus muscles attach to the vestiges of the pelvis. Two small pelvic bones are present, and they are larger in adult males than in females (Figure 5.5). Dines *et al.* (2014) note that:

The ischiocavernosus muscles attach to the pelvis in all mammals, but cetacean pelvic bones are unique because they are no longer constrained by sacral and hindlimb attachments or by hindlimb locomotion, potentially freeing them to diverge according to penis morphology.

Comparative studies of 29 species (Dines, 2014; Dines *et al.*, 2014) have demonstrated that the sizes and shapes of these pelvic bones, as well as the length of the penis, are positively correlated with testes weights in cetaceans. Species with the largest testes (indicative of the occurrence of sperm competition) have the longest penes and largest pelvic bones in relation to their body sizes. For example, in the harbour porpoise (*Phocoena phocoena*), which is one of the species included in the Dines *et al.* (2014) study, the adult male's testes average 2.1 kg, or 4.1 per cent of adult male body weight. Fontaine and Barrette (1997) reasoned that the occurrence of such 'megatestes' in harbour porpoises indicates that their mating system involves multiple-partner matings by females and high levels of sperm competition. Recent observations of copulatory behaviour in this species support this conclusion (Keener *et al.*, 2018). Male harbour porpoises vie with one another to mate very rapidly with females, approaching them from below (always from the left side) and completing copulations in less than a second or two. The greatly elongated penis of the harbour porpoise is probably advantageous in this context (Figure 5.6).

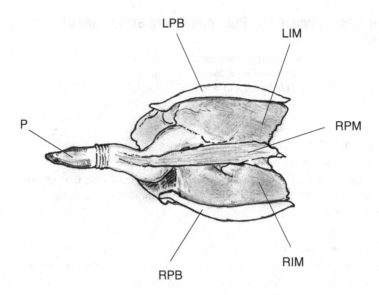

Figure 5.5 The penis, pelvic bones and associated muscles of the long-beaked common dolphin (*Delphinus capensis*). LIM and RIM, left and right ischiocavernosus muscles; LPB and RPB, left and right pelvic bones; P, penis; RPM, retractor penis muscle. Note the 'S'-shaped flexure of the penis. (Author's drawing from a photograph in Dines, 2014.)

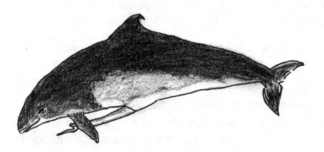

Figure 5.6 Adult male harbour porpoise (*Phocoena phocoena*) showing the length of the erect penis. (Author's drawing from photographs by Keener *et al.*, 2018 and Daniel Bianchetta.)

A second striking example is provided by the North Atlantic right whale (*Eubalaena glacialis*). In this species, aggregations of males assemble around a single receptive female and compete to mate with her. Male right whales have the largest testes of any mammal; their combined weight equals 1000 kg. Females mate with multiple partners, and a case has been reported where two males were observed mating simultaneously with the same female (Mate *et al.*, 2005). The great length and extreme mobility of the penis is adaptive in securing intromission under circumstances where the female sometimes rests at the surface with her ventral side uppermost.

Diverse Penile Morphologies in Marsupials

The penis fell next under my examination, the fabric of which appears not less
surprising than that you met with in the uterus of the female.

William Cowper, 1704

William Cowper wrote these words in 'A letter to Dr Edward Tyson. Giving an
account of the Anatomy of those Parts of a Male Opossum that differ from the
Female'. His account, which was published in 1704 in the *Philosophical
Transactions of the Royal Society*, contains a number of beautiful illustrations of the
reproductive anatomy of the male Virginia opossum (*Didelphis virginiana*). One of
them is shown here as Figure 5.7.

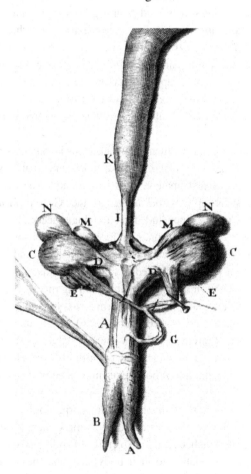

Figure 5.7 Part of William Cowper's dissection of the male reproductive tract of the Virginia
opossum (*Didelphis virginiana*). Note the bifurcated glans penis (A, B), the large prostate
gland (K), and the Cowper's (bulbourethral) glands (M, N), which he described as 'two
mucous bags on each side at the root of the penis, which empty themselves into the urethra'.
(From Cowper, 1704.)

In this species, as in many marsupials, the glans penis is divided longitudinally to form two distinct lobes. The urethra also undergoes bifurcation, so that it is represented by two furrows, one of which runs along the inner surface of each lobe of the glans. Marsupial taxa differ in the lengths of these urethral grooves; for example, in the Virginia opossum, they terminate at some distance from the distal ends of the forked glans, whereas in woolly opossums (*Caluromys*) they extend to their tips.

In addition to the positioning of the urethral grooves, many other penile traits exhibit taxonomic diversity in marsupials. Some striking examples which occur among South American opossums belonging to the Family Marmosidae have been described by Hershkovitz (1992). Figure 5.8 shows examples from four genera of the Marmosidae, three of which have the typical bifid glans penis, whereas the remaining example (*Marmosa mexicana*) has a non-bifid morphology. Hershkovitz noted the widespread occurrence of 'miniature spines' and 'spiral grooves and canals' on the surface of the glans, as well as 'lappets and other fleshy extrusions which may be erectile'. Thus, in Figure 5.8, *Gracilinanus agilis* has a ventral lappet on each lobe of the glans, *Micoureus cinereus* displays a pair of large lateral lappets and *M. mexicana* has two dorsal lappets and a single ventral lappet on its glans. In all cases, the glandes are clothed in keratinized spines, and their overall shapes differ markedly among the four genera. It is probable that, in the erect state, these differences would appear even more striking.

Hershkovitz observed that, during development, the glans penis is initially simple (i.e. 'single-headed') in very young specimens of these marsupials and that it gradually transitions to the bifid condition as they mature. This was found to be the case for *Gracilinanus agilis*, and also for species belonging to the Genera *Marmosops*, *Micoureus*, *Thylamys* and *Metachirus*. He concluded that the single-headed type of glans penis represents the primitive (plesiomorphic) condition for marsupials as a whole. Thus, some groups lack the bifid condition (e.g. the honey possums, kangaroos and wallabies).

The reasons for the evolution of the bifurcated glans penis in marsupials are not known. Cowper (1704) followed Tyson in suggesting that, during mating, the bilateral vaginae of the female might be better supplied with spermatozoa by a matching, bifid arrangement of the male genitalia (see also Biggers, 1966). This suggestion was rejected by Tyndale-Biscoe and Renfree (1987), on the basis that sperm travel up both lateral vaginae in the tammar wallaby, which has a non-bifid penis. However, the possibility that coevolution of the genitalia of both sexes may have occurred deserves further consideration.

A second example of the evolution of diverse penile morphologies among the marsupials concerns the Genus *Antechinus*, which contains more than 10 species of mouse-sized dasyurids, most of which occur in Australia (Tyndale-Biscoe, 2005). *Antechinus* males have large testes relative to their body size, and they amass very large stores of epididymal spermatozoa prior to the onset of the mating season (Taggart *et al.*, 1998). As discussed in Chapter 4, the majority of *Antechinus* species exhibit semelparity, a type of mating system in which all adult males die following a brief mating season that involves frequent and prolonged copulations (Braithwaite and Lee, 1979). Females mate with multiple partners and DNA-typing studies have

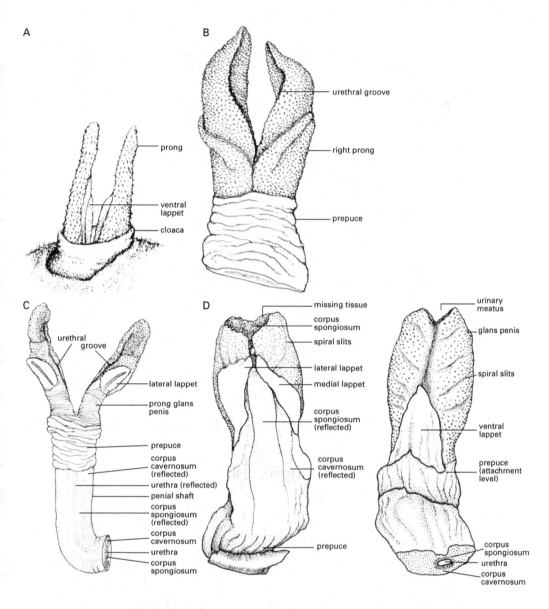

Figure 5.8 Morphology of the glans penis in South American marsupials belonging to four genera of the Family Marmosidae – **A:** *Gracilinanus agilis*; **B:** *Metachirus nudicaudatus*; **C:** *Micoureus cinereus*; **D:** *Marmosa mexicana* (left = dorsal and right = ventral view). (From Hershkovitz, 1992.)

confirmed that the resulting litters are often sired by more than one male (e.g in *Antechinus agilis*: Kraaijeveld-Smit *et al.*, 2002; *A. stuartii*: Holleley *et al.*, 2006; *A. minimus*: Sale *et al.*, 2013).

Figure 5.9 shows the great diversity of penile morphology that occurs in *Antechinus*, as revealed by Woolley's (1982) comparative studies of 12 Australian

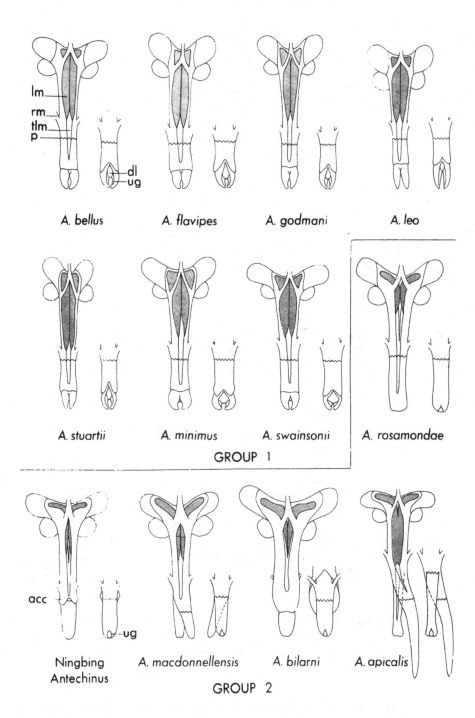

Figure 5.9 Interspecific variations of penile anatomy in marsupial mice of the Genus *Antechinus*. Ventral views are shown of the entire penis and dorsal views of the distal portion for each species. lm, levator muscle; tlm, tendons of levator muscles; rm, insertion of retractor muscle; p, level of attachment of preputial skin; dl, dorsal lobe; ug, urethral groove; acc, accessory structure. (From Woolley, 1982.)

species. Interspecific differences involve the shape of the tip of the penis, lengths of the urethral grooves, the morphology of medial dorsal lobe, the sizes of the *levator penis* muscles, and the extensions of the *corpus cavernosum* to form erectile accessory appendages (e.g. in *A. apicalis*). Woolley also distinguished between two groups of *Antechinus* species on the basis of the presence (Group 1) or absence (Group 2) of a bifid tip to the penis, and other traits shown in Figure 5.9.

These findings indicate that copulatory and post-copulatory sexual selection are likely to have played important roles during the evolution of the male genitalia in the Genus *Antechinus*. The data on penile morphology, relative testes sizes, multiple-partner matings and paternity of litters are consistent with this view. However, it must be acknowledged that they are correlational in nature and do not demonstrate caus-ation. The mechanisms by which sperm competition and (in particular) cryptic female choice might operate can only be inferred from such observations. For example, if the various phallic morphologies shown in Figure 5.9 do indeed operate as 'internal courtship devices' during the protracted copulations that occur in these marsupials, then detailed investigations are needed, in order to establish what takes place during and after copulation in both sexes. The morphological changes that occur during erection and the possible functions of the accessory appendages require investigation. In *A. agilis*, for example, Shimmin *et al.* (2002) observed that males make side-to-side pelvic thrusting movements, and knead and stroke the female's abdomen and hind-quarters during mating. They suggest that these behaviours 'may serve to improve the efficiency of sperm transport from the urogenital sinus to the sites of storage' (storage occurs in crypts in the isthmus of the oviduct).

Penile Morphology and Copulatory Locks in Diverse Taxa

The phylogenetic distribution of copulatory patterns that involve a mechanical 'lock' or 'tie' between the genitalia of the two sexes was discussed in Chapter 3. There, it was shown that at least 42 species representing 9 orders of mammals are currently known to exhibit these patterns (see Table 3.1). It was also concluded that copulatory locks have arisen independently a number of times in different mammalian lineages. This conclusion is strengthened when one considers the diverse anatomical special-izations that serve to bring about such locks in the various taxa, as the following examples show (Table 5.1 and Figure 5.10).

Among rodents of the Family Cricetidae, copulatory locks have been recorded in species belonging to a number of genera, including *Baiomys* and *Notomys*. Dewsbury predicted that a lock might occur in *Baiomys taylori*, on the basis of its penile morphology (this species has a relatively broad glans penis) as well as various features of the accessory reproductive glands. Confirmation of this prediction was obtained by conducting a series of pair-tests in the laboratory. Relatively few pairs mated under these conditions, but locks ranging from 21 to 43 seconds were recorded (Estep and Dewsbury, 1976). In *Notomys alexis* (the Australian hopping mouse) the glans penis differs markedly from that of *B. taylori*, being long and relatively narrow. However, it

Table 5.1 Copulatory locks (and possible locks) in mammals: anatomical specializations

*Platypus	The locking mechanism is unknown
Antechinus spp.	The locking mechanism is unknown
*Wild boar	Corkscrew-shaped distal penis engages with the cervix
Little brown bat	Accessory erectile tissue occurs behind prepuce of penis
Canids	Tumescence of *bulbus glandis* at base of glans penis
Fossa	Blocks of enlarged penile spines (on the penile shaft)
*Spotted hyena	Intromission occurs via the clitoral canal of the female. The exact mechanism by which the lock occurs is uncertain
Hopping mouse	Greatly enlarged penile spines (on the glans)
Greater galago	Robust penile spines (on the glans)
Stumptail macaque	Elongated, sagittate glans fits under the dorsal colliculus at the entrance to the vagina
Northern short-tailed shrew	The 'S'-shaped glans penis and its filiform tip are thought to engage with the coiled vagina

* These ambiguous examples are discussed in the text.

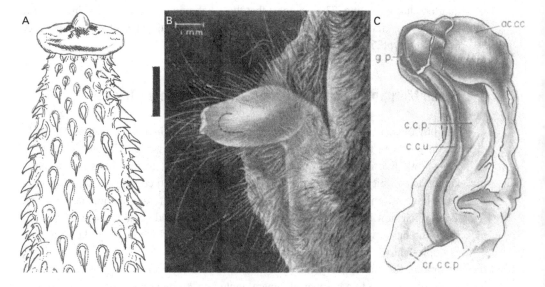

Figure 5.10 A: Glans penis of the Australian hopping mouse (*Notomys alexis*) to show the robust penile spines. Scale = 0.9 mm (author's drawing from a photograph by Professor Bill Breed). **B:** The distal end of the penis of the little brown bat (*Myotis lucifugus*). The position of the glans penis within the enlarged prepuce is indicated by the dashed line. (After Wimsatt and Kallen, 1952.) **C:** Dissection of the penis of *M. lucifugus*, to show the arrangement of the erectile tissues. ac.c.c., accessory cavernous body; c.c.p., corpora cavernosa penis; c.c.u., corpus cavernosum urethrae; cr.c.c.p., crura of corpora cavernosa penis; g.p., glans penis. (After Wimsatt and Kallen, 1952.)

is clothed in large, robust penile spines (Figure 5.10A), and these spines are thought to anchor the penis within the vagina (Breed, 1990; Dewsbury and Hodges, 1987).

Among the Chiroptera, copulations that involve a mechanical lock between the male and female genitalia have been described for a number of vespertillionid bats of the Genus *Myotis* (e.g. Wilson, 1971; Wimsatt, 1945). The anatomical basis of these locks has been studied in detail in the little brown bat (*Myotis lucifugus*) by Wimsatt and Kallen (1952). An accessory cavernous body lies behind and partly within the prepuce of the penis, and it surrounds the dorsal and lateral aspects of the penile shaft. This accessory cavernous body becomes greatly enlarged during copulation (Figures 5.10B,C). Enlargement only occurs after the male has ceased pelvic thrusting, when the pair remain locked together for an extended period. If they are disturbed and separated, then the accessory body is revealed in its fully swollen state. Wimsatt and Kallen (1952) cite one extreme case that occurred when a pair of bats was disturbed during hibernation:

One pair of bats was found *in coitu* in which both partners were hibernating and completely inactive. It is reasonable to assume that their copulatory embrace had already lasted, or might have lasted in the absence of human intervention, for days.

Turning to the Order Carnivora, foxes, wolves and dogs, of the Suborder Caniformia, exhibit tumescence of the proximal part of the glans penis (the *bulbus glandis*) once intromission has occurred, thus keeping the partners tied together. Figure 5.11 shows the marked changes that occur in the size and morphology of the glans penis of the domestic dog during erection. A baculum (os penis) is present in

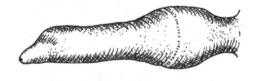

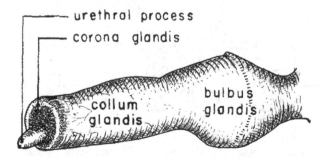

Figure 5.11 Domestic dog (*Canis familiaris*): morphology of the flaccid and erect glans penis. (Redrawn from Hart and Kitchell, 1965.)

canids, as is the case for the majority of carnivores. The bone is elongated and robust; it probably serves to strengthen the distal portion of the glans and to protect the urethra, as semen is gradually transferred to the female during the copulatory lock (Hart and Kitchell, 1966). The penis of the African wild dog (*Lycaon pictus*) also contains a prominent baculum (Figure 5.18D), deeply grooved along its ventral surface to surround the urethra. However, there is no distinct *bulbus glandis* and the erectile tissues are poorly developed in the glans (author's observations). Cade (1967) reported that a copulatory lock did not occur in captive members of this species. However, Frame *et al.* (1979) observed 'brief copulatory ties, up to 6 minutes in duration' during their studies of five packs of wild dogs in the Serengeti National Park. In the Madagascan fossa (Suborder Feliformia), by contrast, the lock is maintained by banks of enlarged penile spines on each side of the intra-preputial portion of the penile shaft (Figure 5.12).

The most unusual specializations of the external genitalia in carnivores, and among mammals in general, concern the spotted hyena (*Crocuta crocuta*). Matthews (1939) described in detail the reproductive anatomy of this species, in which the erectile clitoris of the female closely resembles the male organ (Figure 5.13) and there are two swellings on the female's perineum which are similar to the scrotal pouches of the male. Moreover, the female urogenital system opens to the exterior via the clitoris, rather than through the vagina. This bizarre arrangement led Matthews to comment wryly that 'from a consideration of the anatomy of the genitalia of the female spotted hyaena, copulation would appear to be a difficult feat'. Matters are assisted by the fact

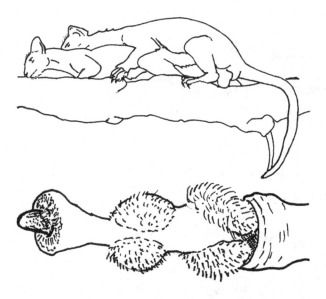

Figure 5.12 Upper: A pair of fossas (*Cryptoprocta ferox*) mating. (Author's drawing, from filmed records.) **Lower:** The penis of the fossa. Note the large banks of penile spines and the plunger-shaped glans with the tip of the baculum projecting at its distal end. (Author's drawing from a photograph in Hawkins *et al.*, 2002.)

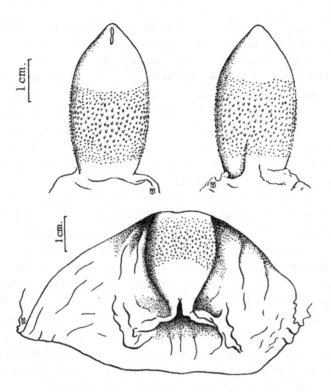

Figure 5.13 The external genitalia of the spotted hyena (*Crocuta crocuta*). **Upper:** Glans penis (dorsal and ventral views). **Lower:** Glans clitoridis of a parous female. The prepuce has been opened dorsally. (From Matthews, 1939.)

that in adulthood, and especially in parous females, the urogenital meatus of the glans clitoris is much enlarged and the prepuce is loose and slack (Figure 5.13). Sexually receptive females also withdraw the clitoris into the abdomen to facilitate intromission (Drea *et al.*, 2002). However, the mechanics of mating are certainly problematic for spotted hyenas, as this description, taken from a field study carried out in Kenya, shows:

the male mounted the female, and repeatedly attempted to achieve intromission. This task was apparently made extremely difficult by the female's peculiar genital morphology. The male had to squat down and under the female, so low that his rump was sometimes on the ground, to maneuver his erect penis into the female's flaccid phallus. (Szykman *et al.*, 2002)

Szykman *et al.* also noted that 'the extended time the male hyena spends in post-ejaculatory rest might function to facilitate sperm transfer, as does the copulatory lock in canids'. Neither these authors, nor Drea *et al.* (1999), who made careful observations of captive animals, specify whether a genital lock is present or absent in spotted hyenas. Dewsbury (1972) did not include it in his study, presumably because no information was available to him at that time. Given the very close fit that necessarily occurs between the genitalia of both sexes in the spotted hyena, I have provisionally classified its copulatory pattern as involving a lock (see Appendix 1).

A second ambiguous case concerns the domestic pig (*Sus scrofa*), in which the spiral tip of the boar's erect penis engages with the spiral folds and ridges lining the cervix of the sow. The close anatomical correspondence between penis and cervix may be important in preventing flowbacks of semen, as between 150 and 500 ml of fluid is transferred to the uterus during extended matings (review: Soede, 1993). However, although Dewsbury (1972) acknowledged that 'the boar thrusts until the glans penis becomes tightly lodged in the cervix', he was convinced on the basis of the published literature that there is no lock in this species.

Less problematic is the case of the platypus (*Ornithorhynchus anatinus*), in which one partner has been observed to swim along 'dragging' the other behind it during aquatic copulations (Burrell, 1927; Hawkins and Battaglia, 2009). Such behaviour indicates that a genital lock or tie occurs, but the anatomical basis of the connection is not known. Thus, the penis of the platypus lacks any obvious adaptations in this regard. The glans is bifid (the left lobe being larger than the right) and clothed in small spines (Temple-Smith and Grant, 2001). Might it be possible that the tie during copulation in the platypus is controlled primarily by the female? Enlargement of the left lobe of the glans penis correlates with the fact that only the left ovary is functional in the female. Temple-Smith and Grant (2001) suggest that the enlarged left lobe is specialized to contact and deposit sperm directly into the left uterus during copulation. This matter is discussed further in Chapter 8, which deals with the complex subject of coevolution of the male and female genitalia.

Urethral Processes and Related Structures

The opening of the urethra exhibits some unusual morphological specializations among mammals. For example, it may be situated at the apex of a vermiform appendage: the urethral process. Such extensions are found in many bovids, and they vary in size between the various taxa (Figure 5.14). In the domestic goat (*Capra aegagrus hircus*), histological studies have shown that the long, filiform urethral process contains an extension of the corpus spongiosum of the penis (Goshal and Bal, 1976). The urethral process is highly mobile, and Hafez (1968) speculated that it might rotate, so that semen is sprayed around the external opening of the cervix. In cattle, the entire terminal portion of the penis becomes coiled (Seidel and Foote, 1969). Ashdown and Smith (1969) describe the anatomical basis for this coiling response, and note that it effectively doubles the width of the intromittent organ, thus increasing its ability to impart tactile stimulation during ejaculation.

Other examples of mammals in which specialized structures occur include the yellow-spotted hyrax (*Heterohyrax brucei*), in which there is a urethral process (Glover and Sale, 1968). This vermiform appendage enlarges and becomes mobile during penile erection (author's observation). Among the monotremes, the echidna has a bifid glans penis, each half of which bears a pair of rosette-like structures.

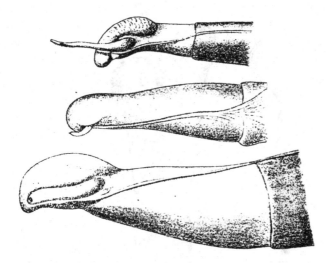

Figure 5.14. Examples of bovid penes, to show differences in the development of the urethral process, which arises from the left side of the glans. **Upper:** goat (*Capra aegagrus hircus*). **Middle:** yak (*Bos grunniens*). **Lower:** domestic cattle (*Bos taurus*). (From Ottow, 1955.)

Multiple branches of the urethra open on the surface of each rosette, via numerous tiny apertures 'similar to that of a showerhead' (Johnston *et al.*, 2007). Observations on a tame echidna made it possible to observe what occurs during penile erection. Only one pair of rosettes remains fully erect; the second pair gradually shrinks in size (Figure 5.15A). The pair of engorged rosettes is then rotated slightly, so that the arrangement is more symmetrical; Johnston *et al.* suggest that in this way the rosettes may be aligned with the paired uterine ostia during copulation. In the platypus the left side of the bilobed penis is larger, for the reasons discussed previously. At the apex of each lobe, surrounding the urethra, is a group of 'foliate papillae' (Temple-Smith and Grant, 2001). These are usually concealed from view but are extruded during penile erection. Lappets and papillae also surround the urethral meatus of the penis in some of the prosimian primates (Dixson, 2012). For example, three lappets occur in *Euoticus* (the needle-nailed galago) and smaller frills and lappets are present in pottos (*Perodicticus*) and lorises (*Nycticebus* and *Loris*). Even in such an extensively studied species as the laboratory mouse (*Mus musculus*) a novel phallic structure has only quite recently been described in detail. This is the 'male urogenital mating protuberance' (MUMP: Rodriguez *et al.*, 2011), a cartilaginous structure which is situated above the urinary meatus and extends beyond the tip of the glans penis.

Among hystricognath rodents, such as the New World porcupines, agoutis, tuco-tucos and cavies, there is a sac-like invagination, just below the urinary meatus at the distal end of the glans penis. This 'intromittent sac' is everted during penile erection to reveal a bulbous structure covered in penile spines and bearing two or more much larger spikes. An example is shown in Figure 5.16 of the remarkable morphological transition undergone by the penis of the Azara's agouti (*Dasyprocta azarae*) during

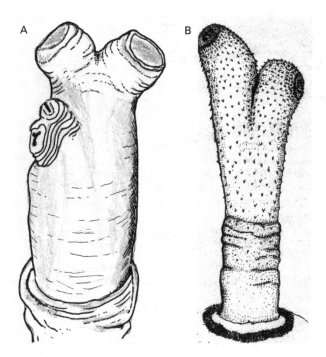

Figure 5.15 **A:** Ventral view of the erect penis of the echidna, to show unilateral enlargement of one pair of rosettes (author's drawing from a photograph in Johnston *et al.*, 2007). **B:** Dorsal view of the non-erect penis of the platypus showing the penile spines on the asymmetrical, bilobed glans (after Temple-Smith and Grant, 2001).

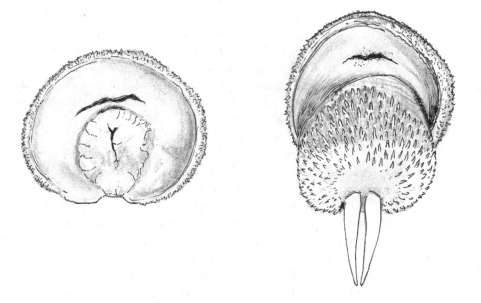

Figure 5.16 The tip of the glans penis of Azara's agouti (*Dasyprocta azarae*) when non-erect (left) and during erection (right) to show eversion of the intromittent sac and the very large penile spines. (Author's drawings, from photographs in Martinez *et al.*, 2013.)

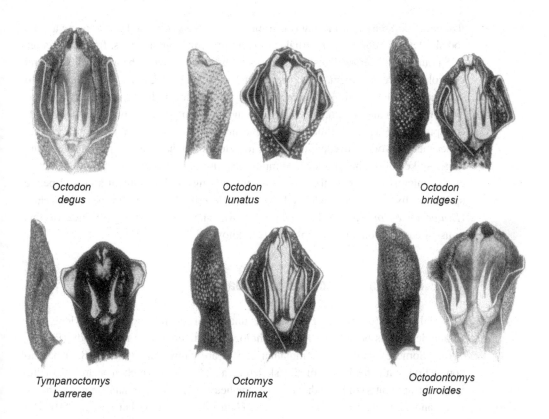

Octodon
degus

Octodon
lunatus

Octodon
bridgesi

Tympanoctomys
barrerae

Octomys
mimax

Octodontomys
gliroides

Figure 5.17 Morphological variability of the glans penis (lateral views) and intromittent sac in hystricognath rodents of the Family Octodontidae. (After Contreras *et al.*, 1993.)

erection. It is probable that the backward-pointing penile spines might grip or otherwise stimulate the walls of the vagina during copulation, whilst the pair of large spikes might probe deeper to contact the cervix.

Intromittent sacs, and the spines and spikes they contain, exhibit considerable taxonomic diversity among the Hystricognathi. Examples are shown in Figure 5.17 of the morphological variations displayed by species of the Family Octodontidae. The numbers and sizes of the large spikes contained in these sacs vary among the various taxa, and Contreras *et al.* (1993) also describe cases where the number of spikes varies within a single species.

The possible functions of these unusual penile structures have not received the experimental attention that they deserve. It has been suggested that they might be involved in some way with the short duration of oestrus and brief copulatory patterns in many hystrichognaths (Bignami and Beach, 1968; Kleiman, 1974), or that they might play some role in inducing ovulation (Weir, 1974). An intromittent sac is present in the domestic guinea pig (Cole, 1897) and guinea pigs might provide excellent subjects for research in this area. Thus, Goldfoot and Goy (1970) showed that either copulation or mechanical stimulation of the vagina and cervix using a glass rod shortens the duration of sexual receptivity in female guinea pigs, from an average of 5 hours to 1–2 hours. These inhibitory effects were shown to be under direct neural control and are not mediated by hormonal mechanisms. Uterine insemination and seminal coagulation within the uterine cavity also occur in the guinea pig and this, as Walton (1960) has commented, 'is convincing proof of the almost instantaneous transport of semen to the uterus by a spasmodic contraction of the vagina'. Further experimental work is needed, therefore, to determine what role the penile spines and larger spikes of the intromittent sac might play during copulation in the guinea pig. It is also interesting to note that structures resembling the intromittent sacs and penile spikes of hystricognath rodents have been described in the European hedgehog (*Erinaceus europaeus*: Akbari *et al.*, 2018). The functional significance of this unusual case of convergent evolution is unknown.

The Evolution and Functions of the Baculum

The penile bone (*os penis*), or baculum, is unusual in several respects. It has long been acknowledged as being the most morphologically diverse bone in the body (Romer, 1962). Some examples of mammalian bacula are shown in Figure 5.18. It has no connection with the bones of the skeleton, a distinction which it shares with the isolated fragment(s) of bone that occur in the hearts of some ruminants (e.g. the sheep: Frink and Merrick, 1974) and in the otter (*Lutra lutra*: Egerbacher *et al.*, 2000). The functional morphology of the baculum has given rise to considerable debate in the past, and continues to do so.

The baculum does not occur in the monotremes or the marsupials, being present only in some members of seven orders of the placental mammals (the Chiroptera, Rodentia, Eulipotyphla, Lagomorpha, Carnivora, Primates and Afrosoricida: Brindle and Opie, 2016; Schultz *et al.*, 2016). Prior to its discovery in the steppe pika (*Ochotona pusilla*: Erbajeva *et al.*, 2011) and the American pika (*O. princeps*: Weimann *et al.*, 2014), a baculum was thought to be lacking in lagomorphs. The bone is just 2.3 mm long in *O. princeps* and thus easily overlooked, so that other cases may exist of its presence in poorly studied taxa. The reorganization of the Order Insectivora described in Chapter 2 has also broadened our understanding of the phylogenetic distribution of the baculum. The lesser hedgehog tenrec (*Echinops telfairi*), which is now placed in the Order Afrosoricida, has been discovered to have a baculum (Riedelsheimer *et al.*, 2007), and among the insectivores (Order Eulipotyphla) the bone is present in some members of the Talpidae (e.g. in the European mole, *Talpa europaea*). Thus, over the course of time it has gradually become clear that the baculum must have arisen a number of times during the evolution of the placental mammals. Schultz *et al.* (2016) examined this question in detail, and concluded that the baculum has arisen a minimum of 9 times (including twice in the Order Primates), and that secondary loss has probably occurred at least 10 times.

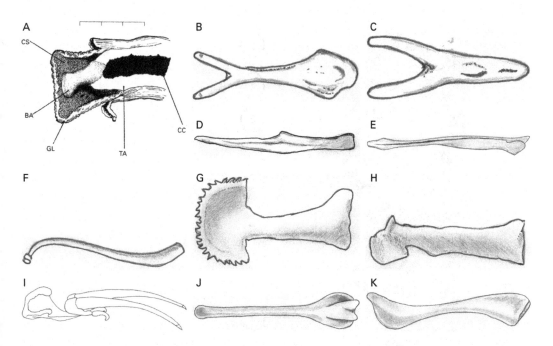

Figure 5.18 The mammalian baculum: some examples of morphological diversity. Primates – **A:** penis of the muriqui (*Brachyteles*) to show its internal structure. BA, baculum; CC, corpus callosum; CS, corpus spongiosum; GL, glans; TA, tunica albuginea. Scale is in 1-cm divisions. **B:** *Avahi laniger*; **C:** *Indri indri*; carnivores – **D:** *Lycaon pictus*; **E:** *Cryptoprocta ferox*; **F:** *Procyon lotor*; rodents – **G:** *Spermophilus annulatus*; **H:** *Sciurus alleni*; **I:** *Jerboa orientalis*; bats – **J:** *Lasionycteris noctivagans*; **K:** *Nicticeius humeralis*. (Author's drawings; **B–K** are not to scale.)

My own view remains that among the primates the baculum is likely to represent a plesiomorphic trait for the order as a whole. The bone is larger in most Old World monkeys than in New World monkeys, and it has undergone secondary reduction and loss in a number of genera (e.g. *Ateles*, *Chiropotes*, *Cacajao*, *Tarsius* and *Homo*). The African apes have very small bacula: just 6.9 mm long in the chimpanzee, 8.5 mm in the bonobo and 12.6 mm in a silverback gorilla (Dixson, 1987b, 2012, 2018).

It has been suggested that lack of homology might account for the morphological diversity and varied functions of the baculum among the various lineages of the placental mammals (Schultz *et al.*, 2016) . However, copulatory and post-copulatory sexual selection have also played important roles in both these respects, leading to similar adaptations across taxa, as is discussed in the following sections.

The baculum is situated in the distal region of the penis, its base being contiguous with the terminal part of the corpora cavernosa. Kelly (2000) notes that although the corpora cavernosa and baculum originate from the same mesenchymal mass during embryonic life in rats and mice, they then develop separately. Thus, strictly speaking, it is not correct to say that the baculum forms by ossification of the distal end of the corpus cavernosum. It is also important to acknowledge that bacular composition,

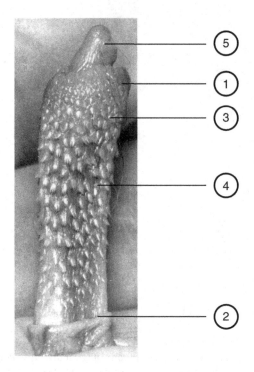

Figure 5.19 Glans penis of an adult greater galago *Otolemur garnettii*, to show the average age at which various testosterone-dependent morphological traits emerge during puberty. **1.** Prepuce begins to separate from the tip of the glans (199 days). **2.** Prepuce fully retractable (263 days). **3.** Penile spines first visible distally (228 days). **4.** Penile spines fully developed (296 days). **5.** Baculum reaches adult size and projects beyond tip of glans (344 days). (Author's unpublished data, based on a longitudinal study of puberty in eight galagos.)

including differences in osseous structure, as well as cartilaginous elements, vary among taxa (Brassey *et al.*, 2018; Schultz *et al.*, 2016).

Growth of the baculum is under androgenic control (e.g. Glucksmann *et al.*, 1976; Reddi and Prasad, 1967); the bone enlarges and increases in length during puberty, as the penis acquires its adult proportions (e.g. Dixson and Nevison, 1997; Fooden, 1975; Hutchinson *et al.*, 2015). Figure 5.19 provides provides an example of the time course of testosterone's effects during puberty upon the growth of the baculum, glans penis and penile spines of Garnett's greater galago.

There is an allometric relationship between body mass and the size of the baculum in mammals, as is shown in the upper part of Figure 5.20. Baculum length scales in a predictable way with body size, but there are marked variations in the relationship between the two variables, as indicated by the distances that various points fall either above, or below, the regression line. In adult males of those species which fall above the regression line, the baculum is longer than would be expected on the basis of body weight. Included among this group are some nocturnal primates such as galagos, mouse lemurs, lorises and the aye-aye, as well the stump-tail macaque

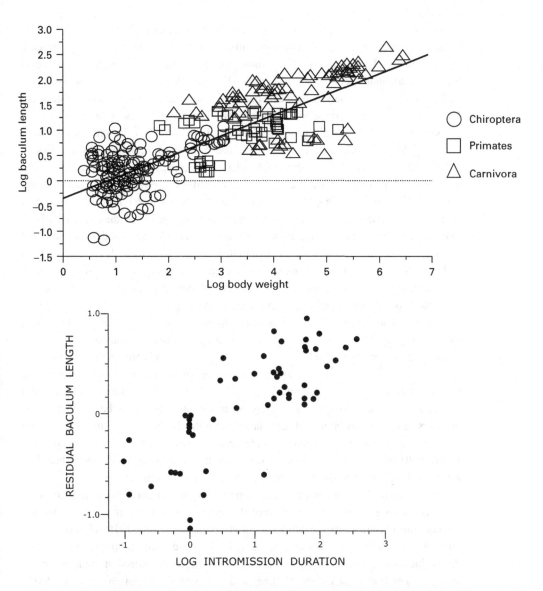

Figure 5.20 Upper: Double logarithmic plot of baculum length vs body weight for 315 species of carnivores, bats and primates. (From Dixson *et al.*, 2004b.) **Lower:** Relationship between residuals of baculum length and intromission duration in 23 species of primates ($r_s = 0.62$; $P < 0.002$) and 31 species of carnivores, including pinnipeds ($r_s = 0.663$; $P < 0.001$). (Based on data from Dixson, 2018; Dixson *et al.*, 2004b.)

(*Macaca arctoides*). All of these primates exhibit copulatory patterns which involve prolonged intromission (Dixson, 1987a, 1987b, 1989). Baculum length is thus significantly greater in those primates that exhibit copulatory pattern number 3 (which involves a single prolonged intromission, with pelvic thrusting and a lock) or number 11 (in which a lock is absent, pelvic thrusting occurs and intromission is prolonged).

Among the carnivores, there is also evidence that species with elongated bacula (in relation to body weight) maintain intromission for long periods. This is the case among the canids, but also in many mustelids, including otters, and in those bears for which adequate behavioural data exist (Dixson, 1995c). Larivière and Ferguson (2002) found no correlation between baculum length and intromission duration for North American carnivores but, as these authors state, this result 'may have been weakened by our data set' (which included only 18 species). Pinnipeds also have relatively large bacula and intromissions are prolonged in many cases (Dixson, 1995c). Data on copulatory behaviour are more complete for those pinnipeds that mate on land, or on the polar ice, given the difficulties of observing aquatic matings (as was discussed in Chapter 3). Thus, the copulatory behaviour of the walrus (*Odobenus rosmarus*) has never been observed in the wild, as these Arctic giants mate underwater. Yet at 54 cm, the walrus baculum is the longest, both absolutely and relative to body size, of any extant mammal. I venture to predict that copulations in walruses also involve long intromissions. Such predictions are also possible for other taxa, such as the mountain beaver (*Aplodonta rufa*). Nothing is known about about the copulatory behaviour of this primitive rodent species, which is rarely seen outside its burrow. The 30-mm baculum is much longer than expected for body weight (650–700 g), however, and indicative of a prolonged pattern of copulation.

In the earlier studies, cited above, those primates or carnivores in which intromission lasts for <3 minutes were classified as having 'short' intromissions, as compared to 'long' intromissions (>3 minutes) in the second group. The 3-minute cut-off point between these two groups was purely arbitrary; its advantage being that larger numbers of taxa could be included in data sets on this basis. The use of data on exact intromission durations is clearly preferable, however, and the lower part of Figure 5.20 shows that there is a positive correlation between residuals of baculum length and intromission durations in both the primates and carnivores.

From a biomechanical perspective, it appears that the baculum, in conjunction with the corpora cavernosa, forms a functional unit that strengthens the erect penis and protects the urethra during extended matings (Brassey *et al.*, 2018; Herdina *et al.*, 2015; Kelly, 2000). Brindle and Opie (2016), who conducted comparative studies on the evolution of the baculum, concluded that 'prolonged intromission predicts significantly longer bacula in extant primates and carnivores' and emphasized the likely importance of post-copulatory sexual selection in this context.

How, then, should one attempt to explain the presence of bacula in some orders of placental mammals but not others? If the baculum enhances reproductive success, why is it not universally present throughout the Placentalia? Given that bacula vary so greatly in shape and size, what selective forces might have resulted in such diversity of form and function? First, bacula occur primarily in those mammals that have vascular penes, as is the case for primates, carnivores, rodents and bats. In fibroelastic penes, such those of bovids and other ungulates, less erectile tissue is present in the distal shaft and head of the penis. Given that the corpora cavernosa and baculum form a 'functional unit', as described above, the presence of more erectile tissue in the shaft and head of vascular penes may have been pre-adaptive to initial development of a penile bone. Second, it seems logical to suggest that the baculum would have initially been a morphologically simple structure: a small rod of ossified or cartilaginous material that developed in close association with erectile tissue in the distal part of the penis. Such rudimentary structures are seen in some extant species, for example in the American pika (Weimann *et al.*, 2014) and the lesser hedgehog tenrec (Riedelsheimer *et al.*, 2007). Positive selection for enlargement and elaboration of the baculum may have occurred for biomechanical reasons, because (in combination with the corpora cavernosa) it strengthened and stiffened the erect penis (Kelly, 2000). Thus, sexual selection might have begun to influence the evolution of bacular morphology from an early stage. Individual variations between males in the size and shape of the bone would have led to subtle differences in erectile capacity, with resultant effects upon copulatory and reproductive success.

There is now experimental evidence for the effect of sexual selection on the baculum in a rodent species: the laboratory mouse (Simmons and Firman, 2014; Stockley *et al.*, 2013). Both these studies, one conducted in the UK and the other in Australia, showed that mice bred through multiple generations, under conditions that favoured post-copulatory sexual selection (females mated in quick succession with three males during a single oestrus), developed thicker bacula than controls maintained under conditions of enforced monogamy (Figure 5.21).

Mice do not exhibit a lock or prolonged intromission; their mating pattern comprises a series of brief intromissions with pelvic thrusting (pattern no. 10). This stimulates neuroendocrine responses in female mice that are required for the support of the corpus luteum during pregnancy. Thickening of the baculum may therefore enhance the effectiveness of stimulation transmitted to the vagina and cervix during copulation.

Several hypotheses have been advanced to account for elongation of the penile bone in some taxa. One possibility is that a long baculum might assist the male to gain intromission, especially in those species where sexual dimorphism is pronounced and

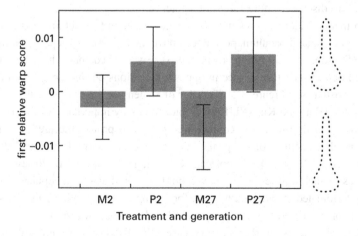

Figure 5.21 Baculum shape diverges at generations 2 and 27 under post-copulatory sexual selection in mice. M = Enforced monogamy; P = females mate with multiple partners. (After Simmons and Firman, 2014.)

males are much larger than their prospective mates (Long and Frank, 1968; Patterson and Thaeler, 1982). However, the results of comparative work on carnivores (Larivière and Ferguson, 2002), and biomechanical studies of bacular function (Brassey *et al.*, 2018) do not support this hypothesis.

Might tactile stimulation by the baculum during copulation be important in those mammals that are induced ovulators, as for example in mustelids (King, 1989) and badgers (Neal, 1986)? Baculum length is probably not related to the occurrence, or absence, of induced ovulation in carnivores (Larivière and Ferguson, 2002). Thus, members of the Family Felidae have small bacula, although some species are known to be induced ovulators. Conversely, the baculum is elongated in canids, yet females of most species are spontaneous ovulators. As far as is known, rabbits and hares (Order Lagomorpha) do not have bacula (although they are present in pikas), but induced ovulation occurs in this group. Spontaneous ovulation is the rule for members of the the Order Primates, including those species that have large bacula, such as stump-tail macaques and greater galagos.

Despite the negative correlational evidence cited above, it is important to bear in mind that the baculum has arisen multiple times during the evolution of placental mammals. Copulatory stimulation results in the secretion of pituitary hormones such as luteinizing hormone (LH), prolactin, or oxytocin by females belonging to certain domesticated species, but the vast majority of the world's mammals have not been sufficiently studied to rule out the possibility that induced ovulation might occur. Could it be the case, for instance, that in some spontaneously ovulating species, copulatory stimuli may advance the onset of the LH surge in otherwise 'spontaneously ovulating' females, rather than being an essential trigger, as in induced ovulators? In the laboratory rat, which is a spontaneous ovulator, copulatory stimuli have been reported to advance the timing of ovulation in just this way (Rodgers, 1971; Rodgers and Schwartz, 1973). Evolutionary relationships between induced and spontaneous ovulation are discussed more fully in Chapter 9.

Given that considerable pressure may be exerted upon the urethra during prolonged matings, an elongated baculum, positioned above the urethra, might protect it from such stresses (Dixson, 1987a, 1987b; Ewer, 1973). Ewer noted that when dogs mate for prolonged periods and turn to face in opposite directions during the tie, then the penis becomes twisted (see Figure 3.2). Transfer of semen continues during the lock in the domestic dog (Hart and Kitchell, 1966); hence the likely importance of the baculum, as it is grooved on its lower surface, and well-placed to protect the urethra during this process. Healed fractures of the penile bone have been reported in several carnivores (e.g. otter: Bland Sutton, 1905; polecat: Kierdorf, 1996; walrus: Bartosiewicz, 2000). The causes of such injuries are unknown, but they could arise if a copulatory lock was suddenly terminated. This could happen, for example, if the mating pair was surprised by a predator, or forced to separate by a rival male (Bartosiewicz, 2000).

Finally, it is interesting that, in some cases, the distal end of the baculum extends beyond the tip of the penis, with the urinary meatus opening onto its perineal surface, as for example in galagos, lorises and angwantibos (Dixson, 2012). This arrangement is likely to bring the tip of the baculum into contact with the os cervix during copulation, as was noted by Coe (1969) in the case of the South African rodent *Pedetes surdaster*. The cervix is the guardian of the uterus, serving to repel pathogens and to protect the developing offspring until the time for parturition arrives. For those mammals in which intravaginal ejaculation is the norm, the cervix also represents a major barrier that spermatozoa must traverse in order to gain access to the upper regions of the female reproductive tract. Adaptations of phallic morphology that assist in circumventing this barrier should prove advantageous to males, especially so in those species where females mate with multiple partners and post-copulatory sexual selection occurs. Placement of semen directly into the cervical canal might be advantageous, therefore, and the projecting baculum, being rounded at its tip in many cases, would be less likely to damage the cervix.

Some Observations Concerning Fossil Bacula

Fossil bacula are rarely discovered by palaeontologists, but some examples that have come to light are worth noting here. Most of them are from carnivores, including giant bear dogs, dire wolves and walruses (Table 5.2). However, a baculum belonging to a

Table 5.2 Examples of fossil bacula from carnivores

Indarctos arctoides (Abella *et al.*, 2013). Five bacula; Madrid basin/Spain, Late Miocene. Average baculum length 23.36 cm; body wt. 265.74 kg.
This was a large bear, similar in size to the European brown bear. The authors conclude that the long baculum is consistent with this bear having had a prolonged intromission type of copulatory pattern.

Amphicyon (Olsen, 1959) from the Miocene of Florida. Considered to be related to either canids or ursids. I measured the figure which has a scale. The baculum is 29.52 cm long, a rod-like bone with a groove on its ventral side, at the distal end.

Plesiogulo marshalli. A type of extinct wolverine (Harrison, 1981). Two bacula 18.4 and 18.2 cm long are described. Both bones are slightly bowed. A urethral groove is present distally.

Megalictis ferox. A giant early Miocene mustelid (Valenciano *et al.*, 2016). Harrison (1981) figures the partial baculum of *M. ferox* in her paper and, by comparison with the *Plesiogulo* specimens of known length, the *M. ferox* specimen (AMNH 12881) is 15.51 cm long.

Canis dirus. The dire wolf. Hartstone-Rose *et al.* (2015) record that for 137 presumptively mature specimens, baculum lengths (cm) = 15.9 ± 1.97 (mean $\pm$ SD) as compared to 10.9 ± 0.81 cm for 10 *C. lupus* specimens ($P < 0.001$). Dire wolf bacula are also thicker than those of extant wolves. A fractured, displaced and healed specimen is described by Hartstone-Rose *et al.* The authors attribute the rarity of such fractures to the robustness of the dire wolf baculum. Average body weight for adult male dire wolves is estimated at 60 kg (Anyonge and Roman, 2006).

Enaliarctos mealsi. An archaic pinniped (Berta and Ray, 1990), dating from the Late Oligocene or early Miocene. Baculum length = 21.7 cm. Estimated body weight = 73–88 kg. The baculum is 'slender and ventrally curved'. It displays some primitive traits consistent with an ursid ancestry, as well as derived pinniped characters.

Titanotaria orangensis. A tuskless walrus, from the Late Miocene of Orange County in California. Baculum = 34.2 cm long (Magallanes *et al.*, 2018).

member of an extinct group of primates (Adapidae) was discovered in 1979 by Von Koenigswald. Post-cranial remains of a medium-sized, lemur-like adapid were found in Eocene oil shale deposits at Messel, close to the German city of Darmstadt. A baculum 46 mm in length was present, and it was shown to be very large in relation to body size; thus, copulation involving prolonged intromission would, in all probability, have occurred in this extinct primate (Dixson, 1987a, 1987b).

The most complete collection of fossil bacula from a single species contains approximately 400 specimens. These are the bacula of dire wolves (*Canis dirus*) from the La Brea Tar Pits in California. They represent a range of developmental stages, from young specimens up to mature males (Hartstone-Rose *et al.*, 2015). Adult dire wolves had longer and thicker bacula than those of modern wolves (*Canis lupus*), and they were long in relation to body size, falling above the regression line in the double logarithmic plot of baculum weight vs body mass in mammals (Figure 5.20A). The same is also true for two other extinct carnivores included in Table 5.2 and for which body weight estimates are available: an archaic pinniped (*Enaliarctos mealsi*) and the bear *Indarctos arctoides*. The latter species was predicted, on the basis of its large relative baculum length, to have had a prolonged intromission type of copulatory pattern (Abella *et al.*, 2013). Possible correlations should be tested for the other carnivores listed in Table 5.2, as and when estimates of their body weights become available.

The Evolution and Functions of Penile Spines

Penile spines occur on the surface of the glans penis (and adjacent areas) of many placental mammals (e.g. rodents, carnivores, bats and primates), as well as some marsupials and in the platypus (Dixson, 2012; Orr and Brennan, 2016). They are keratinized, androgen-dependent structures; hence, they atrophy after castration and are restored by testosterone treatment (e.g. in the rat: Beach and Levinson, 1950; Phoenix *et al.*, 1976; hamster: Whitsett *et al.*, 1980; domestic cat: Aronson and Cooper, 1967; and in several primate species: Dixson, 1976; Dixson and Herbert, 1974; Herbert, 1974).

Penile spines may be divided into three broad morphological categories (Dixson, 2012): Type 1, single-pointed small structures; Type 2, much larger, robust, single-pointed spines; and Type 3, large, complex, multi-pointed structures. Examples of these spine-types are shown in Figure 5.15 (platypus: Type 1); Figure 5.10A (Australian hopping mouse: Type 2) and Figure 5.19 (Garnett's galago: Type 3). Exceptional cases also occur, such as the assemblages of very large single-pointed spines on the penile shaft of the fossa (*Cryptoprocta ferox*: Figure 5.12) and the peculiar, elongated, forwardly directed spines that encircle the glans of the hoary bat (*Lasiurus cinereus*: Figure 5.1C).

It is reasonable to assume that, *ab initio*, the earliest mammalian penile spines would probably have been small, Type 1 structures. Thus, I shall discuss the possible functions of these simple spines first, before considering the more complex types.

Simple, Type 1 spines probably arose because they enhance the sensory feedback required to attain intromission and ejaculation (Dixson, 2012, 2018). Beach and Levinson (1950) originally suggested that the penile spines of the laboratory rat (*Rattus norvegicus*) might function in this way, as their deflection during copulation would be expected to stimulate sensory receptors in the underlying dermis. An interesting suggestion made by Johnson *et al.* (1986), who were studying penile mechanoreceptors in the cat, is that 'perhaps a function of penile spines is to extend the receptive fields in a centrifugal direction, thus increasing contact with the vaginal walls'. This could well be the case, as spines change orientation to point up and outwards from the surface of the erect penis (e.g. in rats: Sachs *et al.*, 1983; marmosets: author's observation) and engage with the vaginal epithelium.

Beach and Levinson (1950) reported that the declines in sexual behaviour that occur after castration in rats might be due, in part, to atrophy of the penile spines. Subsequent experimental work has shown, however, that the behavioural deficits that emerge after castration in a wide range of mammals are mediated primarily at the level of the brain (e.g. Larsson, 1979; Sachs and Meisel, 1988). This does not mean that hormonal effects on penile spines and tactile sensitivity are negligible, merely that they are likely to be subtle. In this regard, it is interesting that selective removal of the penile spines from gonadally intact marmosets (by application of thioglycollate cream) results in an increased intromission latency and a greater duration of pelvic thrusting to attain ejaculation (Figure 5.22).

Penile spines are concave at the base and each contains a papilla of dermal tissue. This is made clearer in Figure 5.22A, which shows the glans penis of a marmoset before and after removal of spines. No histological information is available concerning the distribution of tactile receptors in the glans of the marmoset. Beach and Levinson (1950) thought that tactile receptors were situated in the dermal papillae immediately beneath the penile spines of rats, but Johnson and Halata (1991) showed that the dermal papillae are devoid of such structures. In the cat, by contrast, free nerve endings are present throughout the dermis of the glans penis, including dermal papillae beneath the large spines that are grouped at the proximal end of the glans (Cooper, 1972). Johnson *et al.* (1986) reported that rapidly adapting mechanoreceptors predominate in this spiny area of the glans in the domestic cat, whereas slowly adapting receptors are present in greater numbers in the distal glans, where they probably play an important role in facilitating intromission. For the vast majority of mammals, however, there is no anatomical or electrophysiological information concerning functional relationships between penile spines and sensory receptors; comparative investigations of this question would be most worthwhile.

At the beginning of this chapter it was noted that penile spines are more commonly present in those mammals that have vascular, rather than fibroelastic, penes. The reason for this difference may reside in the fact that penile spines require circulating testosterone for their growth and maintenance, and hence were more likely to arise in those taxa in where the penis is highly vascular and the corpus spongiosum well-developed.

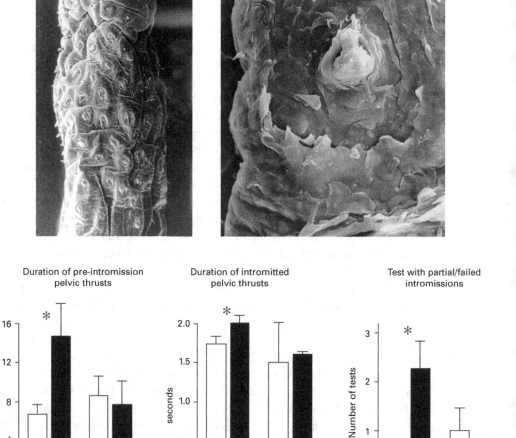

Figure 5.22 A: Scanning electron micrographs of the glans penis of the marmoset (*Callithrix jacchus*) before (left) and after (right) application of thioglycollate cream to remove the penile spines. The dermal papillae are exposed after removal of the spines. **B:** Effects of penile spine removal (Spine X) or a sham operation (Control) upon copulatory behaviour of male marmosets. Open bars = preoperative data; closed bars = postoperative data. *$P \leq 0.05$. (After Dixson, 1991, 2018.)

The role that penile spines might play in copulatory and post-copulatory sexual selection is still largely a matter for conjecture. There are at least four possible lines of enquiry, and these mainly concern the larger Type 2 and Type 3 spines. It should be stressed that these possible functions are not mutually exclusive.

1. Large spines may grip the walls of the vagina during prolonged copulations that involve a lock, or a partial lock, between the sexes. For example, Types 2 and 3 spines occur on the glans penis of a number of nocturnal prosimian primates which mate in this way (e.g. in *Otolemur*, *Galagoides* and *Microcebus*: Dixson, 2012). The very large Type 2 spines of the Australian hopping mouse (*Notomys alexis*: Figure 5.10A) are also thought to fulfil this function (Breed, 1990; Dewsbury and Hodges, 1987). The Madagascan fossa (*Cryptoprocta ferox*) has striking arrays of spines on the distal penile shaft (Figure 5.12). In the wild, female fossas may mate with 10 males during a single oestrus, and their copulations can last for 39 minutes (Luhrs and Kappeler, 2014).

In the cases described above, where the male's spines are potentially large enough to damage the vagina or cervix, conflicts between the sexes might result in antagonistic coevolution of their genitalia (Arnqvist and Rowe, 2005; Eberhard, 2004). For most species in which males have very large penile spines, it is clear that post-copulatory sexual selection of some kind has taken place; thus, they have large testes in relation to body weight, indicative of sperm competition. Unfortunately, for most of these species (the fossa being a prime example), the question of antagonistic coevolution is impossible to assess, as the structure of the vagina and cervix has not been reported.

A peculiar exception concerns the hopping mouse (*N. alexis*), as males of this Australian rodent have very small testes (equivalent to 0.15 per cent of body weight), yet there is evidence that genitalic coevolution has occurred in this species (Breed *et al.*, 2013). Thus, the vagina is muscular and narrow, blending with the cervical lumen, so that the fornices which usually occupy the vault of the vagina are absent. This arrangement is well adapted to receive the long, narrow glans penis and its enlarged spines, and thus to facilitate a copulatory lock. There is no copulatory plug (the male's seminal vesicles and coagulating glands are atrophic) and sperm are known to gain access to female's uterus 10–16 minutes after mating (Breed *et al.*, 2013). Doubts remain concerning the mating system of *N. alexis* in the wild, and of what role sexual selection may have played in the evolution of its genitalia, given its exceptionally small testes and apparent absence of sperm competition.

2. Spines may impart tactile stimulation to the female that facilitate sperm transport within her reproductive tract, that trigger ovulation, or shorten the duration of her receptive period. For example, copulation results in reductions in the duration of sexual receptivity in female mammals belonging to a variety of species, including spontaneous and induced ovulators (e.g. Huck and Lisk, 1986). The mechanisms underlying such effects are likely to be extremely complex, however, and may include factors such as the timing and duration of intromissions (e.g. in the golden hamster: see Huck *et al.*, 1987a, 1987b). Identifying what role (if any) is played by

the penile spines is very difficult, and has not yet been accomplished experimentally in any mammal. Some pertinent observations and possible lines of enquiry are discussed below.

The large penile 'spikes' and spines contained in the eversible intromittent sacs of hystricognath rodents (see Figures 5.16 and 5.17) may prove to be important in this respect. Copulation reduces the duration of sexual receptivity in female guinea pigs (Goldfoot and Goy, 1970) and semen rapidly enters the uterus during copulation in this species (Walton, 1960). The intromittent sac, positioned just below the urethral meatus, is everted during penile erection, bringing its spines into contact with the vagina and cervix. There is also the possibility that such copulatory stimulation might trigger or advance the timing of ovulation in some histricognaths (Weir, 1974).

Penile spines may also be involved in shortening the duration of sexual receptivity in some prosimian primate species in which large Type 2 or Type 3 spines are present. In *Otolemur garnettii*, for example, laboratory work has shown that the duration of female receptivity is reduced if prolonged copulations are allowed to run their full course, rather than separating the partners (Dixson, 2012). In *Lemur catta*, copulations are quite brief and females are receptive for up to 24 hours when pair-tested in the laboratory (Van Horn and Resko, 1977). However, in the wild, where females mate with multiple partners, receptivity is reduced to 4 hours on average (Koyama, 1988). Whether this is due to copulatory stimulation or to a post-mating effect of the copulatory plugs deposited by males of this species is not known.

Sexual selection might favour copulatory stimuli that reduce receptivity because this shortens the time available for rival males to mate with the same female. Stockley (2002) conducted a comparative study of receptivity durations and penile spine sizes in primates and reported a correlation between greater spinosity in males and shorter receptive periods in females. She noted that 'although caution is required in interpreting correlational evidence, these results indicate that penile spines might function to reduce sperm competition risk via a mechanism involving increased or exaggerated copulatory stimulation'.

Another example of a possible correlation between penile spinosity and post-copulatory sexual selection concerns African mole-rats of the Family Bathyergidae. Parag *et al.* (2006) examined the penile spines in five mole-rat species that differed in their social organizations and mating systems, as well as the presence or absence of induced ovulation. Spines were well developed in two polgynandrous, non-gregarious, seasonally breeding species that are induced ovulators (*Bathyergus suillus* and *Georychus capensis*). By contrast, spines were absent in two eusocial, spontaneous ovulators (*Heterocephalus glaber* and *Cryptomys damarensis*). The fifth species studied (*C. hottentotus natalensis*) lives in small colonies with 8–12 members, including a single breeding pair. It breeds seasonally and exhibits induced ovulation. Males of this mole-rat species have only small, rounded protrusions on the glans, rather than prominent spines. Whether a causative relationship might exist between spine sizes, induced ovulation and multiple-partner matings in mole-rats thus remains an open question.

3. Female mammals of many species exhibit behavioural responses during copulation that result directly from tactile stimulation of the vagina or cervix. The presence of penile spines might, in theory, increase the effectiveness of such tactile stimuli. In the rat, for example, the female's sexually receptive posture (lordosis) initially occurs in response to the male as he mounts, palpates her flanks and thrusts against her perineum (Pfaff, 1980). Once intromission occurs, however, lordosis duration is prolonged by penile stimulation of the vagina and cervix (Rodriquez-Sierra *et al.*, 1975). These female responses, which involve concave arching of the back with elevation of the rump and head, are largely reflexive in nature; removal of the cerebral cortex of the brain results in a more extreme and prolonged lordotic response (Beach, 1967).

There is currently no experimental evidence that penile spines affect the expression of lordosis in rodents, or the 'treading' behaviour of receptive female cats, and other behavioural reactions shown by female mammals. Vaginal and cervical stimulation during copulation in prosimian primates might possibly influence behaviour, given that lordosis occurs in some species (Dixson, 1983a, 1998a) and receptivity is under rigid control by ovarian hormones. In monkeys and apes, by contrast, reflexive lordotic postures and oestrus are absent. Female responses during copulation are much more varied than those exhibited by prosimians. In the marmoset *Callithrix jacchus*, for example, females struggle, shake their heads, open their mouths and attempt to terminate intromission. All these responses are blocked by local anaesthesia of the vagina and cervix (Dixson, 1986), whereas removal of penile spines has no apparent effect on the female's behaviour (Dixson, 1991). Only small Type 1 penile spines occur in the marmoset; no experiments have yet examined the effects of removing the much larger complex spines that occur in some prosimians, rodents, carnivores and bats.

4. It is possible that penile spines may assist in the removal of coagulated semen, or copulatory plugs, deposited by other males, thus reducing the risk of sperm competition. Removal of copulatory plugs manually has been observed in some species of tree shrews and monkeys (Parga *et al.*, 2006), but we are concerned here with removals that occur during the act of mating. The repeated intromissions made by male rats before ejaculation occurs serve multiple functions, one of them being to dislodge plugs left by previous matings (Wallach and Hart, 1983). During each intromission, a reflexive flaring of the glans penis occurs; spines in the concave distal portion of the glans, as well as on its sides, may then assist in breaking up and dislodging plugs (Figure 5.23). Then, during the final ejaculatory intromission, the male lodges his own plug tightly against the cervix.

Removal of copulatory plugs may be most likely to occur in mammals that have a multiple intromission pattern of copulation, and a multiple-partner mating system in which post-copulatory sexual selection occurs. In Chapter 3 it was noted that at least 75 species have multiple intromission copulatory patterns, and that many more examples have yet to be described. Most of the species classified thus far are rodents,

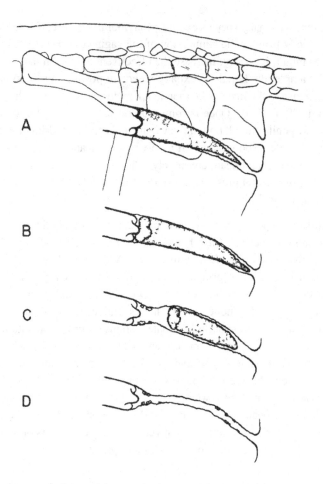

Figure 5.23 Sequential stages in the removal of a copulatory plug from the vagina of a female rat during a series of pre-ejaculatory intromissions (copulatory pattern no. 14). **A:** Prior to re-mating the plug adheres tightly to the cervix and vaginal walls. **B, C** and **D** show the gradual removal of the plug over the course of three or four intromissions. (After Wallach and Hart, 1983.)

but some are monkeys and carnivores. One member of the Eulipotyphla (*Suncus murinus*) also mates in this way. The ring-tailed lemur (*Lemur catta*) may also intromit several times and thus remove plugs from previous matings (Parga, 2003), although males of this species are also capable of ejaculating during a single intromission. Ring-tails have both large and small spines on the glans penis, but there is no direct evidence that they dislodge copulatory plugs. The same is true for one of the New World monkeys (*Cacajao rubicundus*) which has large Type 2 spines. Hershkovitz (1993) suggested that these function to dislodge semen during multiple intromissions. As always, such correlations are interesting, but they do not establish cause and effect. Experimental investigations of the possible functions of penile spines in mammals, other than rats, are badly needed.

With the exception of the marmoset studies discussed above (Figure 5.22), the only experimental work I know of that has measured the effects of removing penile spines is due to Friesen *et al.* (2014), who studied red-sided garter snakes (*Thamnophis sirtalis*). Ablation of the large Type 1 spine, which occurs at the base of each hemipenis in this species, resulted in males copulating for shorter periods and depositing smaller copulatory plugs. However, anaesthesia of the cloaca in female garter snakes resulted in longer copulations, 'suggesting that cloacal and vaginal contractions play a role in controlling copulation duration' (Friesen *et al.*, 2014).

The Evolution and Functions of the Striated Penile Muscles

The striated penile muscles are situated at the base of the penis. Depending upon the species concerned, their functions include facilitation of penile erection, the control of reflexive penile movements and the expulsion of semen during ejaculation. These muscles might therefore make important contributions to the role of the penis as an 'internal courtship device'. They could also be concerned in inter-male competition to displace rival ejaculates. Several penile muscles have been described; of especial interest to discussions of post-copulatory sexual selection are the ischiocavernosus and bulbocavernosus (sometimes called bulbospongiosus) muscles.

In placental mammals (Figure 5.24), the paired ischiocavernosus (IC) muscles arise from the ischia of the pelvic girdle and insert along the sides of the vascular erectile bodies (*corpora cavernosa*) of the penile shaft. Contractions of these muscles elevate the penis and assist the male in gaining intromission; indeed, if the IC muscles of the rat are removed, then males become 'virtually incapable of achieving penile insertion' (Sachs, 1982). In the whales and dolphins, the IC muscles attach to the small remnants of the ischial bones of the pelvis and control the penile movements that are required to attain intromission. As described earlier in this chapter, the pelvic bones are larger, and the penes are longer, in those cetaceans that engage in sperm competition (Dines *et al.*, 2014).

The IC muscles also facilitate penile erection in some mammals (e.g. in cattle and sheep: Watson, 1964; goat: Beckett *et al.*, 1972; horse: Beckett *et al.*, 1973; and dog: Hart and Kitchell, 1966; Purohit and Beckett, 1976). Figure 5.25 shows the rapid build up in pressure that occurs in the corpus cavernosum of the erect penis of the goat during copulation. IC muscle activity and corpus cavernosum pressure peak together, followed by a burst of activity by the bulbocavernosus (BC) muscles during ejaculation.

The BC muscles insert along the perineal surface of the proximal part of the penis, where they surround the corpus spongiosum and urethra (Figure 5.24C,D). Powerful contractions of these muscles occur during ejaculation. The BC muscles tend to be larger in primates that engage in sperm competition. This is the case, for example, in the muriqui (*Brachyteles*: Dixson *et al.*, 2004a) which has very large testes in relation to its body weight (Arakaki *et al.*, 2019) and a polygynandrous mating system. Preliminary studies of primates indicate that the BC muscles are larger in genera that

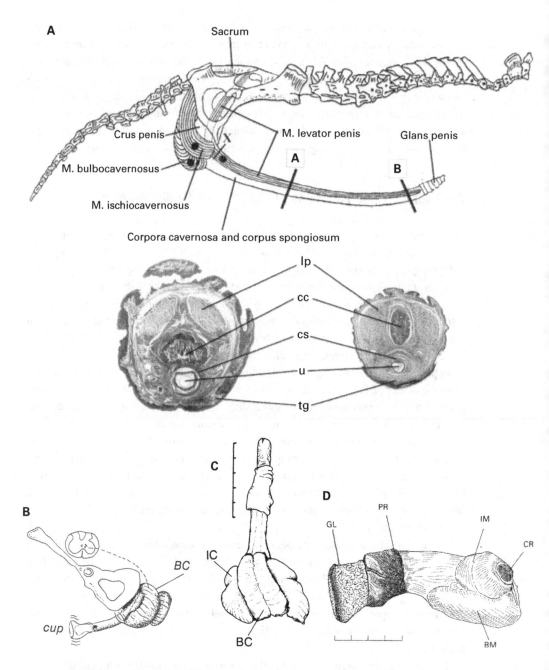

Figure 5.24 Examples of the anatomical arrangement of the penile muscles in placental mammals. **A:** Armadillo (*Chaetophractus villosus*). lp, levator penis muscles; cc, corpus cavernosum; cs, corpus spongiosum; u, urethra; tg, tegument. **B:** Rat (*Rattus norvegicus*). cup, the flaring response of the glans which is controlled by the bulbocavernosus muscles. **C:** Bornean orang-utan (*Pongo pygmaeus*). **D:** Muriqui (*Brachyteles* sp.). BC and BM, bulbocavernosus muscles; IC and IM, ischiocavernosus muscles; CR, crus penis; GL, glans; PR, prepuce. (**A** after Affanni *et al.*, 2001; **B** after Wallach and Hart, 1983; **C** after Dixson, 2012; **D** after Dixson *et al.*, 2004a.)

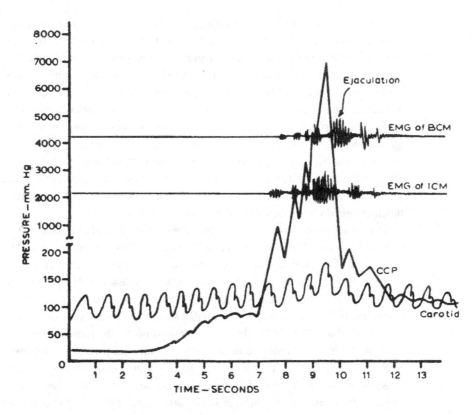

Figure 5.25 Cavernosal pressures and electromyograms (EMGs) associated with erection and ejaculation in the goat. CCP, corpus cavernosum; IC, ischiocavernosus muscles; BC, bulbocavernosus muscles. (After Beckett *et al.*, 1972.)

have multi-partner mating systems than in genera where single-partner matings by females predominate (Dixson, 2012). Quantitative studies of the weights of the BC muscles in mammals are required in order to establish whether there is a correlation between muscle mass and relative testes size. Unfortunately, accurate weights of the penile muscles are known for very few taxa.

As well as controlling ejaculation, the BC muscles can also cause changes in the distal morphology of the penis during copulation. In some groups of placental mammals (e.g. primates, bats, carnivores and rodents), the corpus spongiosum is enlarged at the distal end of the penis to form the glans. Rhythmic contractions of the BC muscles compress the corpus spongiosum in the proximal part of the penis so that blood is moved distally, causing the glans to swell and make pulsing movements. In the rat, these reflexive responses are called 'cups', and they are known to fulfil several functions. They break up and remove copulatory plugs deposited by other males (see Figure 5.23), they pack and seal the current male's plug firmly against the cervix and (via a series of non-ejaculatory intromissions) they trigger the increases in progesterone required to support pregnancy (Adler, 1978; Sachs, 1982).

Marked changes in penile morphology also occur during erection and ejaculation in some primates (Dixson, 2012). In capuchins (*Cebus*), for instance, the glans sometimes expands rapidly and repeatedly during penile erection, in a similar way to the reflexive cupping response seen in the rat. The glans pulsates during ejaculation in some species, presumably as a result of contractions of the BC muscles (e.g. in *Mandrillus sphinx* and *Miopithecus talapoin*). In the rhesus monkey, males sometimes show rapid 'flip' movements of the penis during the inter-mount intervals that precede ejaculation. These movements are probably caused by rhythmic contractions of the ischiocavernosus muscles (author's observations). In the woolly monkey (*Lagothrix lagotricha*) the glans is particularly prominent and plunger-shaped in erection, whilst in spider monkeys Campbell (2007) notes that the distal end of the penis becomes much enlarged and 'mushroom-shaped' during erection.

In contrast to the vascular penes discussed above, fibroelastic penes such as those that occur in ungulates do not include large amounts of spongiose erectile tissue in distal part of the organ. Many ungulates have a vermiform extension, the urethral process, at the tip of the penis, however, as was discussed earlier in this chapter (see Figure 5.14 for examples). Histological studies show that the urethral process contains an extension of the *corpus spongiosum* that surrounds the urethra (e.g. in the domestic goat: Goshal and Bal, 1976). Thus, contractions of the BC muscles might also influence tumescence and reflexive responses of the urethral process during copulation.

Scattered throughout the anatomical literature are descriptions of '*levator penis*' muscles in diverse species of mammals. It is unclear to what extent these muscles might be homologous structures. In some cases muscles that serve to retract and retain the flaccid penis within the body have also been described as *levator penis* muscles. Several examples are discussed here. Figure 5.24A shows the *levator penis* (LP) muscles of an armadillo (*Chaetophractus villosus*). These paired muscles arise from the sacrum, extend along the dorsal side of the elongated penis and insert close to its distal end (Affanni *et al.*, 2001). Electrical recordings show that the LP, BC and IC muscles are all active during the spontaneous erections that occur during slow-wave sleep in this species. After transection of the LP muscles, the flaccid penis cannot be retracted into its normal resting position beneath the skin of the lower abdomen. The exact role played by the LP muscles during mating remains uncertain.

Levator penis muscles have been described in African and Indian elephants (Schulte, 1937; Short *et al.*, 1967; Watson, 1872). Of these, Watson's (1872) account is most thorough, as he clearly describes the IC and BC muscles, as well as the pair of long, thick 'levatores penis' muscles situated on the dorsal side of the penis. Each muscle terminates in a tendon, and these fuse together and become firmly attached to the penis. Attaining intromission is a difficult process for bull elephants, given their huge size and the anatomy of the female genitalia. Short *et al.* (1967) proposed that the LP muscles may facilitate this process:

It is this muscle which probably accounts for the S-shaped flexure of the penis at erection. Presumably the male hooks the upwardly flexed tip of his penis into the ventrally situated vulva of the female, and she then retracts it caudally and dorsally, using the powerfully developed levator clitoris muscles. The male can then insert the full length of his penis into the female.

A final example of LP musculature concerns its representation in some members of the Order Primates. In the rhesus macaque, Wislocki (1933) described a separate, smaller, pair of levator muscles which clearly derive from the ischiocavenosus muscles and insert along the cranial border of the penis. These muscles, he suggested, function 'to elevate and straighten the pendulous end of the penis'. It is likely that similar LP muscles occur in many of the Old World monkeys (Hill, 1966), although information about their distribution and structure is still very limited. In the male ring-tailed lemur, Drea and Weil (2008) have described LP muscles which are not derived from a division of the ishiocavernosus muscles, and thus differ from the condition that occurs in the rhesus monkey. They point out that 'considering the varying origins of the muscles referred to as *levator penis* within primates, it seems unlikely that the structures are all homologous'.

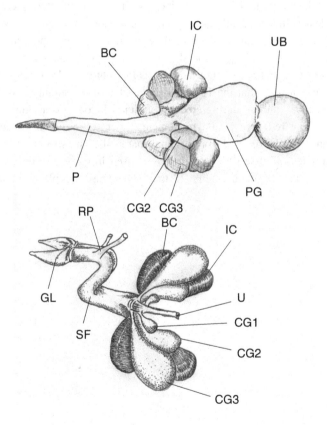

Figure 5.26 The male reproductive tracts of (**upper**) a western grey kangaroo (*Macropus fuliginosus*) and (**lower**) the brown four-eyed opossum (*Metachirus nudicaudatus*) to show the anatomical arrangement of the striated penile muscles. BC, bulbocavernosus muscle; IC, ischiocavernosus muscle; CG 1, 2, and 3, the three pairs of Cowper's (bulbourethral) glands. The third pair of glands is not visible in this dorsal view of the *M. fuliginosus* tract; GL, bifid glans penis; P, penis; PG, prostate gland; RP, retractor penis muscle; SF, sigmoid flexure of penis; U, urethra; UB, urinary bladder. (Author's drawings from Nogueira *et al.*, 1999 and Warburton *et al.*, 2019.)

This discussion of the anatomy and functions of the striated penile muscles has focused on the placental mammals. It is important, in concluding this chapter, to acknowledge that there are important differences between the IC and BC muscles of placental mammals and those of the marsupials. Figure 5.26 shows the arrangement of the penile muscles and associated organs in an Australian marsupial (the western grey kangaroo: *Macropus fuliginosus*) and a South American marsupial species (the brown four-eyed opossum: *Metachirus nudicaudatus*). The paired IC and BC muscles of both these species are globular in shape, however, and in contrast to the situation in placental mammals, the IC muscles do not arise from the pelvis and the BC muscles do not unite in the midline to surround the corpus spongiosum and urethra. Histological studies of the IC and BC muscles of the grey kangaroo (Warburton *et al.*, 2019) have shown that the IC and BC muscles of *M. fuliginosus* have a multipennate architecture, which probably increases their strength during contraction. Each IC muscle acts independently and surrounds one root of the corpus cavernosum. Each BC muscle likewise surrounds a single bulb of the corpus spongiosum. Both pairs of muscles are thus well-positioned to exert pressure on the cavernous bodies during penile erection and ejaculation, and this is thought to be their major function. Warburton *et al.* consider that the IC and BC muscles of marsupials thus 'function purely as mechanical pumps' during erection and ejaculation, and are unlikely to be involved in causing reflexive penile movements, such as those that occur during intromission and ejaculation in many placental mammals. The specializations of the IC and BC muscles discussed here might have arisen in early marsupials, or have been present in the therian ancestors of the marsupials and placental mammals (Warburton *et al.*, 2019).

6 The Testes and Spermatozoa

Evidence concerning occurrences of multiple-partner matings by female mammals was reviewed in Chapter 4. There, the conclusion reached was that sperm competition is widespread among extant members of the Monotremata, Marsupialia and Placentalia. Because sperm competition arises when the gametes of two or more males are situated in contention for access to a given set of ova, males that are able to produce and store larger numbers of sperm prior to mating may then gain a reproductive advantage via post-copulatory sexual selection. Greater sperm production may be achieved by increasing the mass of gamete-producing (seminiferous) tissue in the testes, or by increasing the rate of spermatogenesis. Evidence regarding both these mechanisms is discussed in this chapter. When sperm leave the testis, they pass via the excurrent ducts into the epididymis and are stored in its terminal region (cauda) prior to copulation. Transit times and numbers of sperm stored in the cauda are discussed here, as they may also be affected by post-copulatory sexual selection.

Aside from the production and storage of greater sperm numbers, post-copulatory sexual selection might also result in the evolution of traits that enhance the 'quality' of spermatozoa, such as their ability to move more rapidly or to survive for longer periods in the female reproductive tract. It is interesting that in artificial insemination experiments where equal volumes of semen, or equal numbers of spermatozoa, from two males are mixed together prior to insemination, one male may sire a disproportionate number of the resulting offspring (e.g. in rabbits: Beatty, 1960; cattle: Beatty *et al.*, 1969; mice: Edwards, 1955). Hence individual differences might exist between males in their sperm and/or semen quality. The question of motility and sperm competition is addressed here. However, where sperm survival is concerned, it is the female's reproductive anatomy and physiology that ultimately determines sperm survival. This subject is discussed in Chapter 8.

Mammalian testes not only vary tremendously in size relative to body mass, but also as regards their anatomical position in the body. In many species the testes are retained in the peritoneal cavity (the testicond condition), whereas in others they are housed outside the body in an external pouch, the scrotum. Much debate has concerned the factors that have resulted in testicular descent and the evolution of the scrotum in therian mammals. These debates are revisited in the final section of this chapter, in the light of some recent developments concerning the genetic basis of testicular descent.

Relative Testes Size and Sperm Competition

Measurements of testes size relative to body weight have proven useful as indirect measures of sperm competition occurrence in a variety of mammals, including the monotremes and marsupials (Paplinska *et al.*, 2010; Rose *et al.*, 1997; Taggart *et al.*, 1998); cetaceans (Brownell and Ralls, 1986; Connor *et al.*, 2000; Dines *et al.*, 2015); carnivores (Fitzpatrick *et al.*, 2012; Iossa *et al.*, 2008); rodents (Breed and Taylor, 2000; see also Kenagy and Trombulak, 1986); bats (Hosken, 1997; Wilkinson and McCracken, 2003) and primates (Harcourt *et al.*, 1981, 1995). Rather than attempting to review all of these studies, I have selected several examples from research on bats, primates, carnivores and cetaceans to illustrate the major findings.

Sperm Competition in Bats

Wilkinson and McCracken (2003) assembled data on testes weights and body weights for 104 species of bats. They pointed out that bats exhibit a very wide range of testes sizes, from as little as 0.12 per cent up to 8.4 per cent of adult body weight. A significant amount of this variation is probably due to interspecific differences in sperm competition. In some species, females store sperm for up to 6 months in the uterus, uterotubal junction or oviduct (see Table 8.5). In the common noctule bat (*Nyctalus noctula*), for example, sperm from up to five males may be stored by a single female in this manner (Gebhard, 1995).

Multiple-partner copulations are most likely to occur in bats that roost in multimale–multifemale assemblages and, as discussed in Chapter 4, they have much larger testes relative to weight than putatively polygynous or pair-living species (Figure 6.1A). Phylogenetic differences are also marked; 3 of the 10 families of bats in Wilkinson and McCracken's study have significantly larger testes than expected, given their body weights. Residuals of testes size have negative values in six of the seven remaining families (Figure 6.1B).

Wilkinson and McCracken did not find any effects of seasonal breeding upon relative testes sizes in the 72 species for which adequate information was available. However, within a single species, population differences did occur. Thus, a sixfold difference in testes weight was measured in males belonging to two populations of the common fruit bat (*Artibus jamaicensis*). This is interesting in view of the fact that many studies of relative testes sizes in mammals do not take account of potential differences between populations.

Sperm Competition in Primates

Large differences in testes weight, relative to body weight, in monkeys, apes and humans were first documented by Adolph Schultz in 1938, but at that time there was no functional explanation for them. The first comparative study of relative testes sizes and mating systems in the anthropoid primates was reported by Harcourt *et al.* (1981).

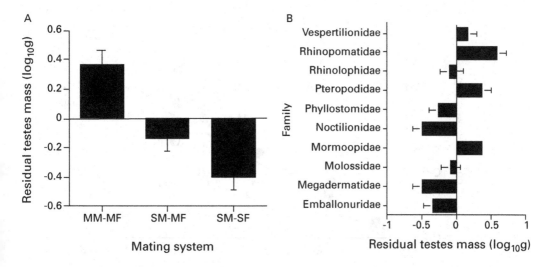

Figure 6.1 A: Residuals of testes mass (means + SEM) for bats that exhibit three types of roosting assemblages during mating periods. Multiple male–multiple female (MM-MF), single male–multiple female (SM-MF) and single male–single female (SM-SF). **B:** Residuals (means + SEM) of combined testes mass for 10 families of bats. (From Wilkinson and McCracken, 2003.)

Subsequently, Harcourt *et al.* (1995) included prosimians in an enlarged data set (37 genera and 58 species) which examined the possible effects of seasonal breeding, as well as mating systems, on relative testes sizes (Figure 6.2).

Taken together, these two reports clearly established that (independent of seasonality) relative testes sizes are largest in those primates that have multiple-partner mating systems, as is consistent with the occurrence of sperm competition. Examples of such species are represented by the closed circles in Figure 6.2. They include various macaques and baboons, as well as vervets, talapoin monkeys and chimpanzees. All but one of the closed circles fall above the regression line, indicating that the species concerned have larger testes than expected for their body weights. The same is true for the smaller-bodied nocturnal prosimians (galagos, mouse lemurs, dwarf lemurs and lorises) represented by the closed squares at the lower end of the regression line. These species have dispersed mating systems in which individuals occupy overlapping home ranges. Multiple-partner matings by females are also frequent in these cases, and males have larger testes than expected (Dixson, 1995a). By contrast, relative testes sizes are usually small in polygynous species, such as gorillas, proboscis monkeys and geladas, and in monogamous primates, such as owl monkeys and gibbons. The polygynous and monogamous species are represented by the open circles and squares, respectively, in Figure 6.2.

Given that the great apes are the closest phylogenetic relatives of *Homo sapiens*, comparative studies of their testes sizes might yield some insights concerning the question of human sperm competition. Results of a study that included data on more than 7000 men belonging to 14 human populations worldwide, as well as

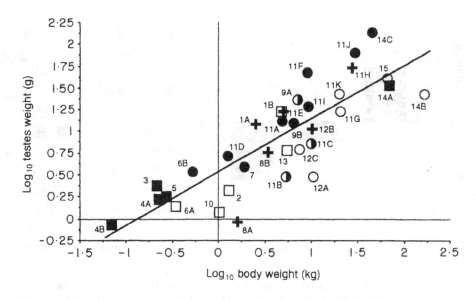

Figure 6.2 Testes weight (g) in relation to body weight (kg) in primates. Closed symbols = polygynandrous taxa (closed circles = multimale–multifemale mating systems; closed squares = dispersed mating systems). Open symbols = polygynous (circles) or monogamous (squares) taxa. Crosses denote taxa for which mating systems were unknown at the time this study was carried out. 1, Lemuridae (A, *Petterus* (*Eulemur*); B, *Varecia*); 2, Indriidae (*Avahi*); 3, Cheirogaleidae (*Cheirogaleus, Microcebus*); 4, Galagidae (A, *Galago*; B, *Galagoides*); 5, Lorisidae (*Loris*); 6, Callitrichidae (A, *Callithrix, Cebuella, Leontopithecus*; B, *Saguinus*); 7, Cebidae (*Cebus, Saimiri*); 8, Pithecinae (A, *Pithecia*; B, *Cacajao*); 9, Atelinae (A, *Alouatta*; B, *Ateles, Lagothrix*); 10, Aotinae (*Aotus*); 11, Cercopithecinae (A, *Cercopithecus aethiops*; B, *C. Ascanius*; C, *Erythrocebus*; D, *Miopithecus*; E, *Allenopithecus*; F, *Macaca*; G, *Theropithecus*; H, *Mandrillus*; I, *Cercocebus*; J, *Papio cynocephalus*; K, *P. hamadryas*); 12, Colobinae (A, *Colobus guereza*; B, *Colobus polykomos*; C, *Presbytis, Nasalis*); 13, Hylobatidae (*Hylobates*); 14, Pongidae (A, *Pongo*; B, *Gorilla*; C, *Pan*); 15, Hominidae (*Homo*). (From Harcourt *et al.*, 1995.)

measurements of all the great apes, are shown in Figure 6.3. Both the chimpanzee and bonobo have very large testes (averaging 149 and 168 g, respectively), as is consistent with their multiple-partner mating systems and high copulatory frequencies. I should mention that chimpanzees belonging to the eastern subspecies (*Pan troglodytes schweinfurthii*) may have larger testes than the values cited here for *P. t. troglodytes* (Professor Martin Muller, personal communication). In the gorilla, which has a polygynous mating system, massive silverbacks weighing more than 160 kg have extremely small testes (combined weight = 16.5 g in *Gorilla gorilla*, and 29 g in *G. beringei*). Human testes are not large in relation to body weight; they are much smaller than those of chimpanzees or bonobos, and resemble the condition found in both species of the orang-utan (Figure 6.3). Population and ethnic differences are pronounced in *H. sapiens*. Testes are smallest in some Asian populations (e.g. in China (Hong Kong), South Korea and Japan) and largest in men of European and

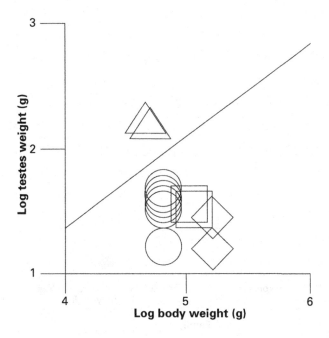

Figure 6.3 Relative testes sizes in the great apes and human populations worldwide. ◯ = *Homo*; ◇ = *Gorilla* (data for the western lowland gorilla are plotted separately and fall below the mountain gorilla on the graph); ☐ = *Pongo* (Sumatran and Bornean species are shown separately); △ = *Pan* (data for the bonobo and chimpanzee are plotted separately). (From Dixson, 2009.)

African descent (Dixson, 2009). Data for all 14 human populations fall below the regression line in Figure 6.3, which is consistent with an evolutionary history involving pair formation or polygyny. Sperm competition pressure would have been low under these conditions.

Sperm Competition in Terrestrial Carnivores

Data on relative testes sizes for 79 species of terrestrial carnivores are shown in Figure 6.4, which has been modified from the work of Iossa *et al.* (2008). An eighth family of Malagasy Carnivores, the Eupleridae, is not included in Figure 6.4, but it contains the fossa (*Cryptoprocta ferox*), which has large testes and a multiple-partner mating system (Luhrs and Kappeler, 2014).

Iossa *et al.* found that families belonging to the Caniformia, and especially the Canidae and Mustelidae, have larger testes than members of the Feliformia. The lowest relative testes sizes are found in the Felidae and Hyaenidae. They also reported that carnivores which have shorter mating seasons have larger testes in relation to their body weights, and that spontaneously ovulating species have larger testes than induced ovulators, indicative of more pronounced sperm competition in the former. Soulsbury (2010) subsequently reported that paternity representation in litters of

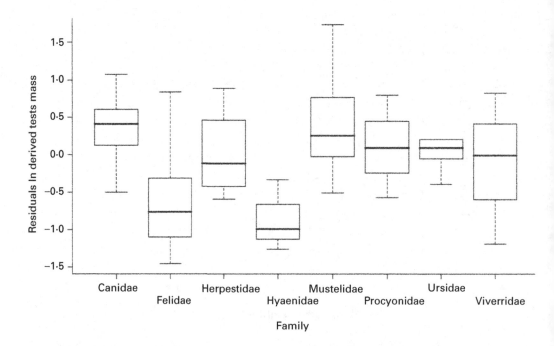

Figure 6.4 Relative testes sizes in eight families of terrestrial carnivores (Canidae, $n = 16$; Felidae, $n = 22$; Herpestidae, $n = 4$; Hyaenidae, $n = 3$; Mustelidae, $n = 23$; Procyonidae, $n = 3$; Ursidae, $n = 5$; Viverridae, $n = 3$). (From Iossa *et al.*, 2008.)

offspring varied depending upon the mode of ovulation, more than one male being likely to be represented in litters born to spontaneous ovulators. Sperm competition risk may be lower in induced ovulators, because the gametes of the first male to copulate with a female may have some priority of access to her ova (see Chapter 9 for discussions of post-copulatory sexual selection in induced ovulators).

Surprisingly, Iossa *et al.* (2008) did not find any correlation between relative testes sizes and mating systems in carnivores, probably because the importance of multiple-partner matings was underestimated for some taxa. In order to classify mating systems accurately, it is necessary to have a clear understanding of the networks of copulatory interactions that occur between individuals. This is more easily said than done, especially for animals in which alternative mating tactics and covert copulations can easily obscure reality. These factors have doubtless led to confusion where some carnivore mating systems are concerned, especially so in the case of the Canidae. The wolves, dogs and foxes have traditionally been considered as monogamous mammals. Kleiman (1977), for example, included 17 species of canids in her review of 'Monogamy in mammals' published in the *Quarterly Review of Biology*. However, Lawick and Lawick-Goodall (1971) recorded that the dominant female in a group of African hunting dogs mated with three males. Genetic studies have revealed that multiple paternity of litters occurs in some canids (red fox: Baker *et al.*, 2004; Arctic fox: Carmichael *et al.*, 2007; island fox: Roemer *et al.*, 2001). A combination of factors (spontaneous ovulation, short mating seasons and multiple-partner matings by some females) may thus explain the relatively large testes sizes of canids. This being so, it may also help to explain their complex penile morphologies, which were discussed in the last chapter. Elongated bacula and lengthy copulations involving a genital lock are not traits that one would expect to find in monogamous mammals. It is likely that sperm competition and complex male genitalia represent plesiomorphic traits for this family of the Carnivora.

Sperm Competition in Cetaceans

Every whale has its louse

T.H. Huxley

Huxley's barbed quip (concerning one of Darwin's detractors) was both witty and biologically accurate. For whale lice are species-specific; they transfer to a new member of their particular host species only when two whales make close physical contact, as occurs during copulation, for example. Measurements of genetic markers in *Cyamus boopis*, a louse which parasitizes the humpback whale, have provided new information about such contacts between members of the geographically disparate breeding stocks of humpbacks in the Southern Hemisphere (Isawa-Arai *et al.*, 2018). Yet, to my knowledge, no one has actually observed humpback whales in the act of mating. Indeed, the same is true for most of the other great whale species, an exception being the North Atlantic right whale (Mate *et al.*, 2005). However, in the absence of such direct evidence, it is possible to infer whether multiple-partner matings and sperm competition might occur in cetacean species by examining their relative testes sizes.

Dines *et al.* (2015) have analysed data on body mass and testes mass for 58 species of whales, dolphins and porpoises. Table 6.1 contains information on some of these species; the negative values in this table indicate that testes sizes are smaller than expected in relation to body size. The humpback whale has exceptionally small testes for its size, an indication of low sperm competition pressure during its evolution. Male humpback whales display by vocalizing ('singing') and there is intense competition for mating opportunities. Females are widely dispersed, however, and it appears unlikely that a male could monopolize more than one mate at a time (Clapham, 1996). Sperm whales also have relatively small testes, which accords with their roving males, female groups and pronounced male-biased sexual dimorphism (Whitehead, 2003). Yet it is among the beaked whales of the Genus *Mesoplodon* that relative testes sizes are smallest, as is the case for True's beaked whale and Perrin's beaked whale (Table 6.1). Some beaked whales are almost certainly polygynous, as their small groups usually contain a single adult male (Macleod and D'Amico, 2006). Males have a pair of enlarged, tusk-like teeth in the lower jaw (e.g. in the strap-toothed and spade-toothed beaked whales). Such weaponry is likely to

Table 6.1 Male body weight, testes weight and residuals of testes weight (RTW) for selected whales, dolphins and porpoises (Data are from Dines *et al.*, 2015)

Common name and Latin name	Body wt (kg)	Testes wt (kg)	RTW
Baleen whales			
Bowhead: *Balaena mysticetus*	71,470	423.6	+1.1
Sei: *Balaenoptera borealis*	17,977	23.26	−0.069
Blue: *B. musculus*	107,000	70.0	−0.065
Fin: *B. physalus*	62,500	58.3	0.014
Humpback: *Megaptera novaeangliae*	56,340	4.0?	−0.896
North Pacific right: *Eubalaena japonica*	78,499	972	+1.437
Toothed whales			
Sperm: *Physeter macrocephalus*	57,000	18.0	−0.341
Beluga: *Delphinapterus leucas*	1254	1.664	−0.353
Short-finned pilot: *Globicephala macrorhynchus*	3600	14.4	+0.298
Narwhal: *Monodon Monoceros*	2131	1.207	−0.561
True's beaked: *Mesoplodon myrus*	1020	0.327	−1.106
Perrin's beaked: *M. perrini*	1200	0.20	−1.07
Dolphins and porpoises			
Short-beaked common dolphin: *Delphinus delphis*	163	7.94	+0.871
Risso's dolphin: *Grampus griseus*	500	12.72	+0.748
Dusky dolphin: *Lagenorhynchus obscurus*	85	9.73	+1.107
Orca: *Orcinus orca*	10,488	46.2	+0.617
Harbour porpoise: *Phocoena phocoena*	61.2	3.814	+0.873
Dall's porpoise: *Phocoenoides dalli*	190.0	0.92	+0.042

be part of the trade-off that occurs between armaments and testes size in males of polygynous species (Dines *et al.*, 2015).

By contrast with the examples cited above, there are numerous cases of cetaceans that have very large testes in relation to their body weights. Examples listed in Table 6.1 include the bowhead whale of the high Arctic and the North Pacific right whale (*Eubalaena japonica*). In its close relative, the North Atlantic right whale (*E. glacialis*), as many as 40 males have been observed to gather around a single receptive female (Kraus *et al.*, 2007). Frasier *et al.* (2007), who conducted paternity studies of North Atlantic right whales, also advance the view that multiple-partner matings by females are likely to occur in this species.

Dolphins and porpoises include many species that have large testes in relation to their body weights; examples in Table 6.1 include the common dolphin, dusky and Risso's dolphins, and the harbour porpoise. Harbour porpoises also have exceptionally long penes and males employ specialized copulatory tactics (Keener *et al.*, 2018), as was discussed in Chapter 5. Many of the oceanic dolphins (Family Delphinidae) form large multimale–multifemale 'pods' and their mating systems are considered to be polygynandrous (Gowans *et al.*, 2008).

A Caveat Concerning the Compartments of the Testis

The testes contain both sperm-producing tissue (the seminiferous tubules) and inter-tubular elements, such as blood vessels, lymphatic sinusoids, connective tissue, nerves and endocrine tissue (the interstitial Leydig cells, which secrete testosterone). It is necessary, therefore, to consider the relative proportions of tubular and inter-tubular tissues in the testis, because cases could arise where large relative testes sizes are due to the proliferation of non-gamete-producing tissue. Interspecific variations in the percentages of tubular and inter-tubular tissue have been measured in some primates, for example, but it is unlikely that they seriously impact assessments of relative testes size in relation to sperm competition (Dixson, 2012). However, in certain groups of mammals, research has brought to light scattered examples of species in which the interstitial Leydig cells take up most of the inter-tubular spaces and constitute anywhere between 20 per cent and 60 per cent of the overall volume of the testis. Fawcett *et al.* (1973) found this condition to be present in the testes of the domestic pig (*Sus scrofa*), warthog (*Phacochoerus africanus*), zebra (*Equus quagga*), Virginia opossum (*Didelphis virginiana*) and naked mole-rat (*Heterocephaulus glaber*). Similar findings have been reported for the woodchuck (*Marmosa monax*: Christian *et al.*, 1972), as well as for an Australian murid rodent (*Leggadina delicatula*: Taylor and Horner, 1970) and a number of South American opossums belonging to the Didelphidae and Caenolestidae (Rodger, 1982).

An extreme example of this type of testicular organization occurs in the South American capybara (*Hydrochoerus hydrochairis*), which is the largest rodent species. Moreira *et al.* (1997) calculated the percentage of interstitial tissue in the testes of 80 adult capybaras and found that it accounted, on average, for 72 per cent of testes volume. Histological studies showed that large masses of interstitial tissue were interspersed with clusters of seminiferous tubules, as also occurs in some opossums (Rodger, 1982) and suiformes (Parkes, 1966). The functional significance of this proliferation of interstitial Leydig cells is not well understood. I mention it here because it indicates that, in exceptional cases, measurements of relative testes size do not provide a reliable indicator of sperm competition.

Sperm Production

As well as investing in a greater mass of seminiferous tissue in the testes, sperm production can also be boosted by increasing the rate of spermatogenesis. Does this occur in mammals that engage in sperm competition? Ramm and Stockley (2010) explored this question by examining the length of the seminiferous epithelium cycle (SEC) in 50 species representing 9 orders of mammals. They found that SEC length is negatively correlated with relative testes sizes in this sample of

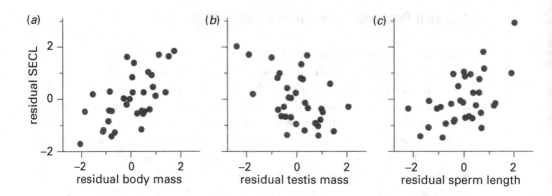

Figure 6.5 Correlations between **(a)** body mass, **(b)** testis mass and **(c)** sperm length and seminiferous epithelium cycle lengths (SECL) in mammals. (From Ramm and Stockley, 2010.)

mammals, which included three species discussed above (capybara, pig and brush-tail possum) that have excessive amounts of interstitial tissue in their testes. However, this is unlikely to have biased the results, given that it involved only 6 per cent of the species studied. Ramm and Stockley's findings are thus consistent with sperm competition selecting for shorter SEC lengths, and hence for faster rates of spermatogenesis (Figure 6.5). This is because the duration of spermatogenesis (i.e. the time taken by the seminiferous epithelium to produce spermatozoa) is equivalent to 4.5 SEC lengths. Also included in Figure 6.5 are two positive correlations: between SEC lengths and body mass, and SEC lengths and sperm length. Thus, larger mammals and those that have longer sperm tend to have slower rates of sperm production. Ramm and Stockley (2010) suggested that some trade-off may occur between sperm production (and hence sperm numbers) and sperm length in mammals: those species with the highest rates of production may tend to have smaller gametes. They did not discuss the significance of the correlation between SEC lengths and body size. However, body size affects many physiological processes in mammals, including heart rate and basal metabolic rate. Given the correlation between body mass and SEC lengths, vast creatures, such as bowhead and North Pacific right whales, which engage in sperm competition may have to invest even more in their testes sizes, given that rates of spermatogenesis are slower. Indeed, these whales both appear as outliers on log–log plots of testes weight versus body weight for cetaceans (Dines *et al.*, 2015).

Ramm and Stockley's findings also lead to the prediction that daily sperm production (DSP) should be negatively correlated with SEC lengths. Measurements of DSP (per gram of testicular parenchyma) exist for only a small number of placental mammals, as listed in Table 6.2. For this sample there is a negative correlation with SEC length ($r_s = -0.691$; $N = 10$; $P = 0.05$; two-tailed test).

Table 6.2 Daily sperm production (per gram of testicular parenchyma) and seminiferous epithelial cycle lengths (SECL) in placental mammals

Species	DSP (millions/g)	SECL (days)
Rabbit	25.0	10.70
Hamster	24.0	8.74
Rat	24.0	12.44
Rhesus macaque	23.0	10.50
Human	4.4	16.00
Pig	23.0	9.05
Sheep	21.0	10.40
Horse	16.0	12.20
Cattle	13.0	13.50
Cat	10.4	16.00

Data are from Amann (1981) and Ramm and Stockley (2010).

The Epididymis: Sperm Maturation and Storage

The epididymis is a highly convoluted, tightly packed, tubular duct which receives spermatozoa via the excurrent ducts of the testis. Sperm then pass gradually along the epididymis, from its initial segment (caput), through the middle segment (corpus) to the terminal segment (cauda), where they are stored prior to copulation. This is a considerable journey; for example, the epididymis is about 6 m long in the human male, and 50 m in the ram. As they pass through the initial and middle segments of the duct, sperm undergo important maturational changes involving the cell membrane and acrosome. Sperm also acquire their fertilizing ability during their passage through the epididymis; gametes in the initial segment are capable only of feeble movements, whereas those in the terminal segment are motile (Bedford, 2015; Bedford and Hoskins, 1990). However, spermatozoa also undergo significant changes once they enter the female reproductive tract; these will be described in Chapter 8, in relation to mechanisms of cryptic female choice.

Figure 6.6 shows anatomical relationships between the testis and epididymis in various mammals, including two testicond species (the echidna and the elephant shrew). In contrast to the therian mammals, monotremes lack a distinct middle segment of the epididymis, as is shown here for the echidna. In the elephant shrew, the epididymis is elongated and the terminal segment is situated at some distance from the testis. Possible reasons for this will be addressed later in this chapter, in relation to the question of testicular descent, and the evolution of the scrotum.

First, it is necessary to consider those factors that determine how many spermatozoa pass through the epididymis and become available for transfer to the female during copulation. How do the transit times of sperm through the epididymis vary among mammals? How large are the stores in the terminal segment, and how might they vary in relation to mating frequencies?

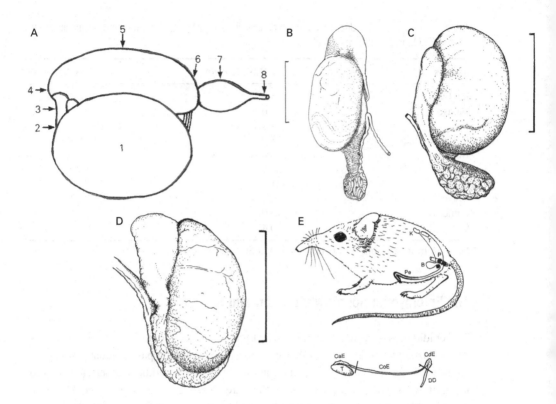

Figure 6.6 Epididymal morphology in mammals. **A:** Short-beaked echidna (*Tachyglossus aculeatus*). **1**, Testis; **2**, rete testis; **3**, ductuli efferentes; **4–6**, initial segment of epididymis; **7**, terminal segment of epididymis; **8**, vas deferens. **B:** Honey possum (*Tarsipes rostratus*). **C:** Mouse lemur (*Microcebus murinus*). **D:** Common marmoset (*Callithrix jacchus*). Scale = 1 cm in each case. **E:** Eastern rock elephant shrew (*Elephantulus myurus*) to show the position of the reproductive organs and divisions of the elongated epididymis. K, kidney; T, testis; B, urinary bladder; P, prostate; Pe, penis; CaE, caput epididymis; CoE, corpus epididymis; CdE, cauda epididymis; DD, ductus deferens.
(**A**, after Djakiew and Jones, 1983; **B**, author's drawing, after Cummins *et al.*, 1986; **C** and **D**, author's drawings and specimens; **E**, after Woodall, 1995.)

Measurements of transit times for spermatozoa through the epididymis are available for a small number of mammals. In the short-beaked echidna, the total transit time is 14.1 days (9.9 days via the initial segment and 4.2 days in the terminal segment: Djakiew, 1982). Transit times through the whole length of the epididymis have been recorded for the tammar wallaby (*Macropus eugenii*: 13 days) and the brush-tail possum (*Trichosurus vulpecula*: 11 days) by Setchell and Carrick (1973). Table 6.3 provides information on 12 placental species. Like Table 6.2, it includes a preponderance of domestic livestock and laboratory rodents, but also several primates, including data for the chimpanzee as well as the human male. Transit times through the whole epididymis range from 2 to 15.6 days (mean = 10.3 days). The shortest duration is for the chimpanzee (Smithwick *et al.*, 1996), and the longest is for the golden hamster.

Table 6.3 Sperm transit times through the epididymis in placental mammals

Species	Sperm transit times (days)		
	Whole epididymis	**Caput + corpus**	**Cauda**
Pig	14.0	5.00	9.00
Sheep	12.0	4.00	8.00
Cattle	14.0	5.00	9.00
Horse	11.7	3.80	7.90
Rabbit	11.1	3.50	7.60
Rat	8.4	3.40	5.00
Mouse	9.2	3.50	5.70
Hamster	15.6	2.00	13.6
Coyote	14.0	–	–
Rhesus macaque	10.5	4.90	5.60
Chimpanzee	2.0	–	–
Human	5.5	1.45	4.05

Data are from Orgebin-Crist and Olson (1984).

Although both these species have large relative testes sizes, they lie at opposite ends of the transit time continuum.

Sperm are transported through the initial and middle segments of the epididymis relatively quickly in placental mammals, in 3.5 days on average, and this is about half the time taken to move through the terminal segment (7.2 days: $N = 10$, $t = 3.8505$; $P < 0.01$). Movement through the terminal segment is also affected by copulatory behaviour, and transit times may be shortened by several days in sexually active males (Amann, 1981; França $et\ al.$, 2005).

Setting transit times aside, intuitively it seems most probable that sperm competition should select for mechanisms that result in greater numbers of mature gametes being stored in the terminal segment (cauda) of the epididymis. Rupert Amann (1981) assembled information on numbers of sperm in the epididymides of 10 species of placental mammals. The measurements involved males that were at 'sexual rest' (i.e. sexually inactive for some days prior to sampling). One finding was that between 54 per cent and 87 per cent (average = 66 per cent) of all extra-gonadal sperm reserves are stored in the cauda epididymis. Larger sperm stores might be expected to occur in polygynandrous species, given that females mate with multiple partners and males may also copulate frequently. Included in Amann's data set were several polygynandrous species (e.g. the domestic sheep, the rhesus monkey and the European rabbit). It is interesting to compare data on these species with data on sperm storage in *Homo sapiens*, given that human cultures worldwide have predominantly monogamous or polygynous mating systems. A ram stores 126 billion sperm in the terminal segments of both epididymides, 300× more gametes than a human male. A male rhesus monkey has a storage capacity of 13 billion sperm, slightly less than 31× the human storage capacity of 0.42 billion. At sexual rest, the terminal segments of the epididymides of buck rabbits contain 4× more sperm than those of a man.

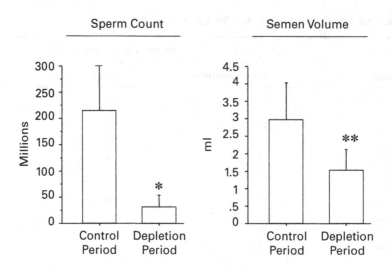

Figure 6.7 Effects of repeated ejaculations (by masturbation) upon semen volume and sperm counts in men. During the depletion period, when ejaculatory frequencies increased to two or three times daily, sperm counts and semen volumes decreased markedly. *$P < 0.05$; **$P < 0.01$. Data (means + SEM) are for six subjects. (From Dixson, 2012.)

What happens to these epididymal stores of sperm in response to frequent ejaculations? Experimental investigations of this question in human males, chimpanzees and rams have produced some useful insights. Freund (1963) measured sperm counts in six men who donated semen samples twice weekly (the 'control period') and then two or three times daily for 10 days (the 'depletion period'). Sperm counts in these men declined during the depletion period to an average of 16.1 per cent of the control period levels. Combined data for the six subjects are shown in Figure 6.7. Total sperm counts in their ejaculates ranged from 41.03 to 534.9 million during the control period, and plummeted to 1.94–65.04 million during the depletion phase of the experiment. These profound decreases indicate that the human reproductive system is not well adapted to sustaining sperm numbers during the high levels of sexual activity that occur in polygynandrous primates.

Marson *et al.* (1989) collected semen samples (by masturbation) at hourly intervals from six adult male chimpanzees. Total sperm counts in the initial collections averaged 1278 ± 872 million, decreasing to 587 ± 329 million in the sixth sample collected 5 hours later. Thus, even after multiple ejaculations, sperm counts in chimpanzees greatly exceed those of men. In the wild, chimpanzee males may copulate an average of 0.72 times per hour, during those periods when females have large sexual skin swellings and are maximally attractive (Tutin, 1979). In such circumstances even the impressive epididymal sperm reserves of such males might become depleted, thus disadvantaging them in sperm competition contests. Some males attempt to sequester a female partner away from the group by forming a consortship with her. A dominant male may succeed in mate-guarding a female during the height of sexual skin swelling. DNA typing studies of paternity reveal that this last tactic is highly successful, but also show that many offspring are the result of multiple-partner matings by females and involve post-copulatory sexual selection (Wroblewski *et al.*, 2009).

High frequencies of copulation and multiple-partner matings are also typical of ovine species (e.g. bighorn sheep, *Ovis canadensis*: Hogg, 1984; domestic sheep, *O. aries*: Lindsay and Fletcher, 1972). Rams are affected by their frequent copulatory behaviour; in flocks of domestic sheep, they may lose 15–42 per cent of testicular weight over the course of 7–8 weeks of sexual activity (Knight *et al.*, 1987). They have enormous testes, weighing approximately 500 g and producing 9.5 billion sperm each day (Amann, 1981). However, experiments by Synott *et al.* (1981) showed that 14 rams were only producing 3–557 million sperm per ejaculate after servicing a flock of ewes for 6 days. During the same period, copulatory frequencies declined from an average of 18.4 to 11.5 per day, although some males continued to mate at high frequencies. In 8 of the 14 males studied, sperm counts had fallen below the critical number (approximately 50 million sperm) required to ensure fertility (Synott *et al.*, 1981). Fieldwork on a feral population of domestic sheep, on Soay Island in Scotland, has shown that dominant rams sire fewer lambs as the rutting season progresses. This occurs despite their continued mating success and high frequencies of copulation. Preston *et al.* (2001) note that 'this mismatch between copulation rate and siring success is difficult to explain in terms other than of sperm depletion'.

As Amann (1981) has pointed out, 'Total sperm per ejaculate is influenced by age, season, testicular size, ejaculation interval, and degree of sexual preparation or foreplay prior to ejaculation.' In practice there are very few of the 6000+ species of extant mammals for which such stringent counts of sperm numbers in the ejaculate have been made. In many cases, for example, sperm counts have involved semen samples collected by electro-ejaculation from males whose prior sexual activity was unknown. Amann (1981) questioned the accuracy of counts made on samples collected by masturbation, but these are surely preferable to those involving electro-ejaculation which often underestimate sperm numbers that are released during copulation. The application of an artificial vagina to collect semen samples is also useful as it at least seeks to replicate the act of copulation. However, such techniques are difficult, or impossible, to apply to many species.

Another of Amann's (1981) criteria for accurately assessing the total numbers of sperm per ejaculate, the 'ejaculation interval', is also poorly documented for most mammals, with the notable exception of laboratory rodents and some other domesticated species. Hourly frequencies of ejaculation have been recorded for males of a number of non-human primate species, however. Data for free-ranging and captive groups are shown in Table 6.4, which also includes information for a substantial number of the American men interviewed by Kinsey *et al.* (1948).

Hourly frequencies of ejaculation in primates that have multimale–multifemale mating systems (and hence a high likelihood of post-copulatory sexual selection) average 0.879 per hour. This includes the chimpanzee and bonobo, as well as various macaques and baboons. By contrast, the average ejaculatory frequency for primates

Table 6.4 Hourly frequencies of ejaculation in primates that have multimale–multifemale (MM), polygynous (PG) or monogamous (MG) mating systems

Species	Ejaculations per hour		Mating system
	Range	Mean	
Lemur catta	1–1.75	1.35	MM
Callithrix jacchus	0.095–0.202	0.155	MG
Aotus lemurinus	–	0.07	MG
Papio ursinus	–	0.75	MM
P. cynocephalus	0.41–1.46	0.83	MM
Mandrillus sphinx	0–3	0.85	MM
Macaca mulatta	0–0.69	0.38	MM
M. fascicularis	1–1.33	0.69	MM
M. radiata	0.44–2.44	0.97	MM
M. arctoides	0–11	1.91	MM
M. sylvanus	0–4.14	2.28	MM
M. nigra	–	0.63	MM
M. thibetana	0–0.9	0.45	MM
Erythrocebus patas	0.19–0.74	0.43	MM*
Theropithecus gelada	–	0.18	PG
Hylobates syndactylus	–	0.005	MG
Pan paniscus	0.19–0.42	0.27	MM
P. troglodytes	0.03–1.14	0.52	MM
Gorilla gorilla	0.32–0.38	0.35	PG
Homo sapiens	0–0.119	0.025	PG/MG

E. patas is primarily a polygynous species, but in this case data were collected during a period when influxes of additional males during the mating season had created a multimale–multifemale group. (From Dixson, 1995b.)

that are monogamous or polygynous is 0.131 per hour. Such is the case, for example, in gibbons, gorillas and human beings. Scores for species in these two groups differ statistically (Mann–Whitney U test: $P < 0.001$; Dixson, 1995b).

During ejaculation, sperm stored in the terminal segment of the epididymis enter the vas deferens, whence they are transported very rapidly, by peristaltic contractions of its muscular walls, to the urethra. Sexual selection has influenced the thickness of the musculature of the vas deferens, as will be discussed in the next chapter. However, the question naturally arises as to how sperm are moved from the terminal segment of the epididymis into the proximal vas deferens at ejaculation. Might sexual selection have influenced this process, given the huge numbers of gametes that must be transported in those species where sperm competition occurs? Figure 6.8 shows the human testis, efferent ducts and epididymis. Serial sections of the epididymis indicate its thickness, from the initial segment through to its terminal portion near its confluence with the vas deferens. The lumen of the epididymis is considerably wider at its terminal end, and a layer of sub-epithelial smooth muscles is present, indicated by the black shading in Figure 6.8. Presumably it is the contractions of these smooth muscles which force sperm from the epididymis into the vas deferens during copulation. No

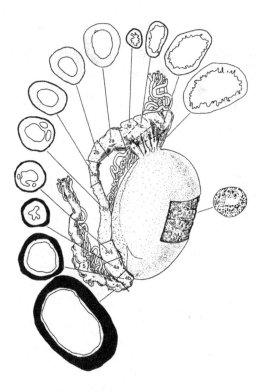

Figure 6.8 The human testis and epididymis. Note the increased thickness of the layer of smooth muscles (shaded black) in the wall of the cauda epididymis, and the greater size of its lumen near its junction with the vas deferens. (From Holstein, 1969.)

quantitative comparisons of the thicknesses of these muscles in mammals that vary in relative testes sizes and mating systems have yet been reported. However, I note that smooth muscles are very well developed in the terminal epididymis of the rat (Reid and Cleland, 1957), whilst in the chimpanzee (Smithwick and Young, 1997) they appear to be thicker than is the case for the human male.

Sexual Selection and Sperm Morphology

Throughout the animal kingdom, spermatozoa exhibit huge morphological diversity (Pitnik *et al.*, 2010), and mammals are no exception to this rule. Some examples of the variations of size and shape exhibited by mammalian sperm are shown in Figures 6.9 and 6.10. The vermiform spermatozoan of a monotreme, the echidna (*Tachyglossus aculeatus*), is included in Figure 6.9. Monotreme spermatozoa more closely resemble those of birds and reptiles than those of other mammals. By contrast, the sperm of marsupials and placental mammals are much more clearly delineated into three regions: the head, the midpiece and the flagellum or principal piece.

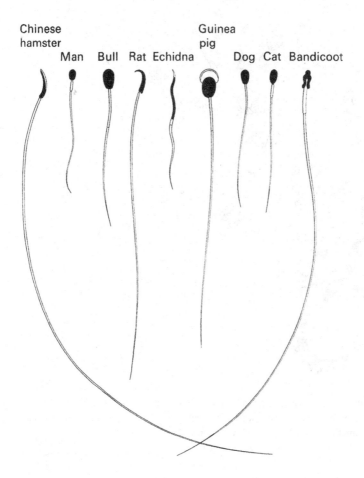

Figure 6.9 Examples of the morphological diversity displayed by mammalian spermatozoa. (After Austin, 1976.)

Sperm heads vary greatly in shape among mammals; in the musk shrew (*Suncus murinus*), for example, the sperm head is dominated by an enormous, fan-shaped acrosome (Figure 6.10A). The rat, like many other murid rodents, has a hook-shaped acrosome, whereas in the plains mouse (*Pseudomys australis*) the sperm head is more complex, as it bears three prominent apical hooks (Figure 6.10B). Interspecific variability in the shape of the sperm head is pronounced in this genus of Australian rodents (Bedford and Hoskins, 1990). Figure 6.10D shows a pair of spermatozoa of the Virginia opossum, joined together by their heads and swimming in unison. 'Binary sperm' of this kind occur in most of the South American marsupials, as discussed below.

The sperm midpiece is roughly cylindrical in shape in most mammals; it contains mitochondria arranged in a spiral around the axoneme. Sperm midpiece volumes vary considerably; the possible significance of such differences for mitochondrial loading and sperm motility are discussed later in this chapter. The sperm mitochondria of

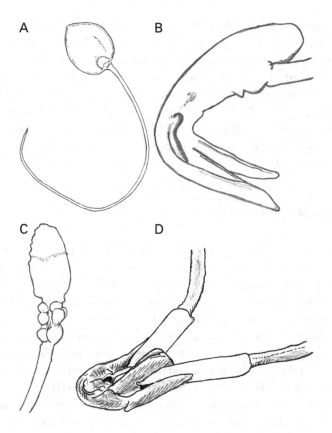

Figure 6.10 A: The spermatozoan of the musk shrew (*Suncus murinus*), which has a greatly expanded, fan-shaped acrosome. **B:** Sperm head of the plains mouse (*Pseudomys australis*) to show the large dorsal and (paired) ventral hooks. **C:** Common dolphin (*Delphinus delphis*). In cetaceans the mitochondria of the sperm midpiece are spherical and arranged in tiers.
D: Virginia opossum (*Didelphis virginiana*). Sperm pairing such as this occurs in the majority of American marsupials. (Author's drawings from photographs in Bedford and Hoskins, 1990 (**A, D**); Safaris *et al.*, 1981 (**B**) and Plön and Bernard, 2006 (**C**).)

cetaceans are most unusual, however, as they are spherical, and arranged in tiers or columns (e.g. in the common dolphin: Figure 6.10C). This arrangement is probably unique among mammals (Plön and Bernard, 2006), but its functional significance is not understood.

In order to gain access to ova, spermatozoa must negotiate a variety of anatomical and physiological challenges as they pass through the female reproductive tract. Moreover, given that the sperm of rival males sometimes compete for access to a given set of ova, it is likely that selection might occur for traits that secure a greater advantage in sperm competition, as well as via cryptic female choice. In addition to specializations of the sperm head and midpiece, such as those described above, sexual selection might also influence the evolution of sperm length. The lengths of mammalian sperm certainly exhibit some surprising differences. Longest of all are the sperm of the honey possum (*Tarsipes rostratus*), a tiny Australian marsupial that could sit comfortably in the palm of one's hand. Yet it has the longest sperm of any mammal (342.6 μm). This dwarfs the sperm of much larger taxa, such as the humpback whale, which has spermatozoa that are just 52.5 μm long (Bedford and Hoskins, 1990; Cummins and Woodall, 1985). The following sections consider the role that sexual selection may have played in the evolution of various morphological traits, including sperm length, sperm midpiece volume and acrosomal morphology, as well as the evolution of binary sperm and sperm bundles in some taxa.

The Evolution of Sperm Length

In 1991, Gomendio and Roldan reported that in rodent and primate species where multiple-partner matings by females are most frequent (and hence sperm competition risk is greatest), males tend to have longer sperm. They also found that there is a positive correlation between sperm length and swimming velocity, for the small sample of mammals where adequate information existed. Their findings were consistent with the conclusion that if longer sperm swim more rapidly, then they might gain an advantage in sperm competition. However, comparative studies of a wide range of mammals failed to reveal the expected correlation between relative testes sizes and sperm lengths (Anderson *et al.*, 2005; Gage and Freckleton, 2003).

Over the years, it has transpired that relationships between sperm length and sperm numbers are more complex than was initially realized (e.g. Gomendio and Roldan, 2008; Mossman *et al.*, 2008; Roldan, 2019). This topic was broached earlier in this chapter in relation to species differences in the length of the SEC and rates of sperm production in mammals. Sperm competition selects for shorter SEC lengths and hence for faster rates of spermatogenesis. However, Ramm and Stockley (2010) suggested that a trade-off occurs between sperm production and sperm length in mammals; spermatogenesis tends to be slower in mammals that produce longer sperm. They found that there is a positive correlation between SEC lengths and sperm lengths in mammals (Figure 6.5). Given that sperm competition is a 'raffle' that favours the provision of larger numbers of sperm in the ejaculate (Parker, 2016; Pizzari and Parker, 2010), the greater volume of the female tract in large mammals necessarily creates a 'dilution effect' which reduces the density of sperm present prior to fertilization. Lüpold and Fitzpatrick (2015) showed that such dilution effects contribute to a greater investment in smaller gametes with increasing body size in mammals. Larger sperm, by contrast, are more likely to occur under sperm competition in smaller species with less voluminous female tracts. This may go some way towards explaining the extreme differences in sperm size referred to earlier between the diminutive honey possum and the humpback whale.

As well as suggesting that a trade-off occurs between sperm length and rates of spermatogenesis, Ramm and and Stockley (2010) noted that these factors might also affect the evolution of testicular architecture. Lüpold *et al.* (2009) had reported that there is a marked positive correlation between sperm length and seminiferous tubule diameter in New World blackbirds (Family Icteridae). They concluded that 'in vertebrates in which spermatogenesis occurs radially within the seminiferous tubules, longer sperm require wider tubules'. In a preliminary study of this question, I compared seminiferous tubule diameters and sperm lengths for 82 mammalian genera representing the monotremes (1 order: 2 genera), marsupials (3 orders: 11 genera) and placental mammals (11 orders: 69 genera). In accord with the findings of Lüpold *et al.*, this showed that sperm length correlates strongly with tubule diameter ($r_s = 0.44373$; $n = 82$; $P < 0.001$; two-tailed test: author's unpublished results).

Do longer sperm swim faster? Holt *et al.* (2010) conducted *in vitro* experiments to measure possible effects of sperm length upon sperm motility using glass columns and a 'swim-up' technique. For all three mammals tested (brown hares, pigs and cattle), flagellar lengths were somewhat greater in the most successful sperm during these swim-up trials (Figure 6.11). Holt *et al.* noted, however, that linear swimming speeds depend upon the beat frequencies of their flagella, as well as upon flagellar length. This naturally leads us to a discussion of sperm energetics, and the role played by the mitochondria of the sperm midpiece in sperm motility.

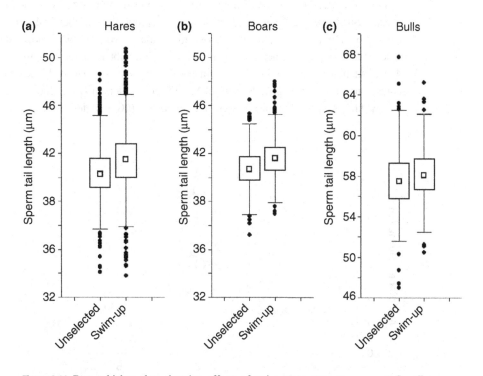

Figure 6.11 Box–whisker plots showing effects of swim-up treatments on sperm flagellar length in (a) hares, (b) pigs and (c) cattle. Small squares = median values; boxes = 25th and 87th percentiles, and whiskers = the non-outlier range. Filled circles = outliers. (After Holt *et al.*, 2010.)

The Sperm Midpiece and Sperm Energetics

The regular beating action of the sperm flagellum falls under the joint control of its component parts, the midpiece and the principal piece, but these operate via different regulatory systems (Suarez *et al.*, 2007). The sperm midpiece contains the mitochondria, which form a helical array, tightly wound around the central strut (axoneme) of the flagellum. Mitochondrial energy production by the midpiece involves oxidative phosphorylation to produce adenosine triphosphate (ATP), whereas in the sperm principal piece energy for motility is generated by glycolysis (Cummins, 2010). The extent to which these two processes govern sperm motility varies considerably among mammals (Bedford and Hoskins, 1990), and it remains to be established how far such variations might reflect phylogenetic factors or the effects of post-copulatory sexual selection. It is known, however, that ATP plays a crucial role in sperm motility, and that 'sperm of species that consume ATP at a faster rate are able to achieve higher swimming velocities' (Touremente *et al.*, 2019).

The possible role that the size of the midpiece might play in sperm competition has been assessed by examining correlations between its volume and measurements of relative testes size. In the first of these studies (Anderson and Dixson, 2002), we reported a significant correlation between midpiece volume and relative testes size for 21 primate species. Subsequently, Gage and Freckleton (2003) reported that they had found no such correlation in mammals. Figure 6.12 shows the results of work that we conducted using an independent data set generated by measuring sperm obtained (at post mortem) from 494 adult males representing 71 genera and 123 species of placental mammals in the collections of the Zoological Society of San Diego (Anderson *et al.*, 2005). The lengths and widths of sperm midpieces were measured for 100 gametes from each male, and

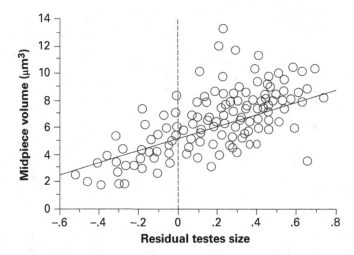

Figure 6.12 Positive correlation between sperm midpiece volumes and residuals of testes size for 123 species of mammals. (From Dixson, 2009, after Anderson *et al.*, 2005.)

midpiece volumes were calculated using the formula for the volume of a cyclinder. Measurements of sperm midpiece volumes correlated strongly with residuals of testes size for this sample of mammals ($P < 0.001$; Figure 6.12).

The implication of these findings is that mammals with larger testes (and thus with a greater likelihood of engaging in sperm competition) tend to have sperm midpieces of greater volume because mitochondrial loading and energy production are enhanced under these conditions. However, it must be acknowledged that correlations do not necessarily reflect the existence of causal relationships. Considerable scatter is apparent among the data for species plotted in Figure 6.12; thus, other factors probably influence relationships between relative testes sizes and sperm midpiece volumes.

Measures of overall midpiece volume include its outer coating and the central axoneme, as well as the mitochondria. It is thus not a perfect measure of mitochondrial loading by any means, but it is likely to be more accurate than relying on linear measurements. Midpiece length has been reported to correlate positively with swimming velocity in mouse sperm (Firman and Simmons, 2010), but not in red deer stags, where sperm with shorter midpieces have greater swimming speeds (Malo *et al.*, 2006). In passerine birds, Immler and Birkhead (2007) found no consistent relationship between sperm midpiece lengths and sperm competition, whereas Rowe *et al.* (2015) reported that in passerines 'elevated levels of sperm competition were associated with more rapid phenotypic divergence in sperm midpiece, flagellum, and total sperm length'. One study in which the volume of the sperm midpiece, rather than its length, was calculated involved *in vitro* experiments of fertilization in a fish species, the stickleback (Bakker *et al.*, 2014). Results showed that sperm with a longer flagellum were faster to achieve fertilizations, but had a shorter activity span than sperm with larger midpiece volumes. The latter remained capable of achieving fertilizations for a longer period of time, therefore.

Comparative studies of mitochondrial activity in the sperm of chimpanzees and men have produced some useful insights concerning the role of the midpiece in sperm energetics (Anderson *et al.*, 2007). Living sperm from five chimpanzees and four men were treated with JC-1, a fluorescent dye that stains metabolically active mitochondria red/orange. Intensity of staining provides a measure of mitochondrial membrane potential. Results showed that fluorescence intensities were markedly higher in the sperm of chimpanzees (Figure 6.13). These differences persisted when sperm had undergone (*in vitro*) capacitation, a process which normally takes place in the female reproductive tract and which prepares sperm physiologically to fertilize ova. Whereas JC-1 staining tended to decrease after capacitation in human sperm, this was not the case in the chimpanzee (Figure 6.13). Capacitated sperm are capable of exhibiting vigorous *hyperactivated motility*, which normally occurs as sperm ascend the oviduct prior to fertilization (Yanagimachi, 1994). These JC-1 studies strengthen the conclusion that differences in sperm midpiece volumes may indeed relate to differences in mitochondrial loading and sperm bioenergetics. There is also evidence from research comparing human and macaque sperm that genetic and ultrastructural differences between their midpieces are consistent with observed differences in sperm motility and sperm competition between the two species (Zhou *et al.*, 2015).

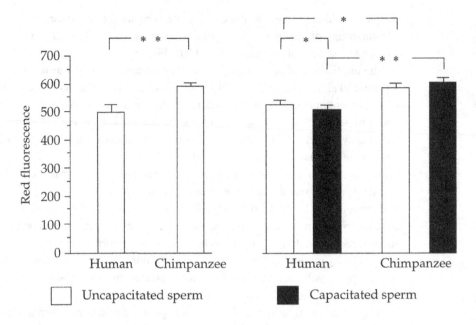

Figure 6.13 Left: Red fluorescence values for JC-1 stained sperm samples from men and chimpanzees, as measured using flow cytometry. **Right:** Effects of *in vitro* induction of capacitation upon JC-1 staining (red fluorescence) of human and chimpanzee sperm. *$P < 0.05$; **$P < 0.01$. (From Dixson, 2009; after Anderson *et al.*, 2007.)

Altruistic Sperm? Sperm Bundles, Binary Sperm and Sperm Hooks

If close degrees of relatedness predispose individuals to altruism, why not search for examples in sex cells, specifically sperm?

Trivers, 1985

Robert Trivers cited several fascinating examples of cooperative behaviour among closely related spermatozoa in various invertebrates, and Pitnik *et al.* (2010) have described many more in their wide-ranging review of sperm morphological diversity. For example, some molluscs produce a giant type of 'helper sperm' (a spermatozeugma), which plays no part in fertilization; instead, it transports hundreds of tiny fertilizing sperm, and releases them as it moves through the female's reproductive tract. Some male butterflies and moths produce two types of gametes: fertilizing (eupyrene) sperm and anucleate (apyrene) sperm. In certain lepidopterans the apyrene sperm are absorbed by the female, and they may delay her from re-mating, or be necessary for eupyrene sperm fertility (Pitnik *et al.*, 2010).

Examples of cooperation among spermatozoa within a single ejaculate are unusual among mammals, but cases of gametes forming 'bundles' or pairs (binary sperm) have been described in monotremes and American marsupials, respectively. A controversial

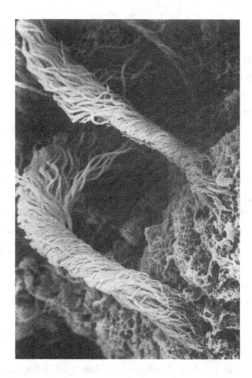

Figure 6.14 Echidna sperm bundles. A scanning electron micrograph of sperm bundles in the terminal segment of the epididymis. The sperm are wrapped around one another in a helical manner. (From Djakiew and Jones, 1983.)

third example concerns the formation of 'trains' of sperm, linked together by a curved apical hook on the sperm head, as occurs in some murid rodents.

During their passage through the epididymis, the spermatozoa of monotremes form into bundles (Figure 6.14), a process which has been studied in most detail in the short-beaked echidna (Djakiew and Jones, 1983). More recently, Johnston *et al.* (2007) collected semen from a tame echidna which had been conditioned to develop a penile erection and to ejaculate without recourse to using invasive procedures, such as electro-ejaculation. Semen collected from this male contained large numbers of highly motile sperm bundles consisting of up to 100 spermatozoa. Johnston *et al.* noted that 'the rostral tips of the sperm heads were joined by an electron-dense amorphous cementing material and were stacked tightly adjacent to each other'. Sperm motility was coordinated and larger bundles moved more rapidly than those containing fewer gametes.

It is likely that post-copulatory sexual selection has led to the evolution of sperm bundles in monotremes. Both the echidna and platypus have very large testes in relation to their body weights (Rose *et al.*, 1997), and the echidna is known to maintain large extra-gonadal stores of spermatozoa (Djakiew and Jones, 1981). We have also seen in earlier chapters that phallic morphology is complex in the echidna, that copulations are prolonged, and receptive females are often pursued by multiple males prior to a mating event. Johnston *et al.* (2007) suggest that sperm bundles might provide males with some advantage in sperm competition, as their superior motility may allow them to secure priority of access to ova. They also speculate that sperm might be stored in the female tract, as occurs in many avian species. This is a fascinating idea which emphasizes the requirement for more detailed histological investigations of the female echidna's reproductive tract in order to search for possible storage mechanisms.

In most American marsupials spermatozoa become joined together in pairs during their passage through the epididymis (Bedford and Hoskins, 1990). Such is the case, for example, in the Virginia opossum (*Didelphis virginiana*), in which the paired sperm heads are joined together in the acrosomal region (Figure 6.10D). The ultra-structural linkages between sperm heads exhibit some interesting taxonomic differences in opossums (Temple-Smith and Grant, 1986) but, as far as is known, all members of the Orders Didelphimorphia and Paucituberculata produce binary sperm. Only *Dromiciops gliroides*, the sole surviving member of the Order Microbiotheria, produces single sperm, as do all of the Australian marsupials to which *Dromiciops* is closely related.

It has been suggested that sperm pairing serves to protect the acrosome of each partner (Bedford *et al.*, 1984; Phillips, 1970), until the gametes separate in the oviduct, prior to fertilization. Bedford and Hoskins (1990) noted that '*Didelphis* spermatozoa, which are ejaculated in very low number, are remarkably efficient in terms of their ability to reach and survive in the oviduct during the fertilization period.' Indeed, the most likely explanation for the evolution of sperm pairing is that it increases the efficiency with which gametes move through viscous environments, such as those they encounter in the female reproductive tract (Moore and Taggart, 1995). Clearly, this ability might prove advantageous in relation to sperm competition and, for *D. virginiana* at least, there is evidence that litters are frequently sired by two or more males (Beasely *et al.*, 2010). Correct alignment of the sperm heads and their acrosomes during pairing in the epididymis is essential if the gametes are to move rapidly in a coordinated fashion (e.g. in *Monodelphis domestica*: Taggart *et al.*, 1993). Perhaps, therefore, the variations in the ultrastructure of paired sperm recorded by Temple-Smith and Grant (1986) are the results of sexual selection, the most effective ultrastructural solutions that ensure coordinated motility differing slightly between taxa.

The third example of possible cooperative behaviour between spermatozoa produced by the same male concerns the functions of the apical hooks that occur on the sperm of many murid rodents. Moore *et al.* (2002) reported that the sperm of woodmice (*Apodemus sylvaticus*) form into 'trains' consisting of some hundreds or thousands of gametes, linked together by the large hooks on the sperm heads. Train formation was associated with increased motility, and also with the premature occurrence of acrosome reactions in many of the sperm. These observations concerned sperm *in vitro*; to my knowledge, it is not known if trains of sperm form *in vivo*, within the reproductive tract of the female woodmouse.

Subsequent to the above report, Immler *et al.* (2007) compared the shapes of apical hooks on the sperm of 37 species of murid rodents. This study showed that the degree of curvature of the apical hooks of these species is positively correlated with their relative testes sizes, and hence with the likelihood of sperm competition (Figure 6.15). The authors concluded that apical hooks are adaptations for sperm competition and that sperm cooperation is likely to be widespread in rodents. Similar results for a smaller sample of murid rodents have also been reported by Sandera *et al.* (2013).

However, two further studies have raised doubts concerning the functions and evolution of apical hooks. Firstly, Firman *et al.* (2011) measured sperm morphologies in lines of house mice that reproduced either under conditions of enforced monogamy or sperm competition (via multiple-partner matings). After 16 generations of selection, morphometric analyses showed that there were no differences between these two lines in the degree of curvature of their sperm hooks. Firman and Simmons (2009) had previously compared sperm hook morphologies of seven island populations of house mice that were known to differ in sperm competition risk (Firman and Simmons, 2008). Sperm hook morphology did not vary according to the degree of sperm competition risk in these populations. Secondly, Touremente *et al.* (2016) re-examined the functions of apical hooks in forming sperm 'trains'. In a comparative study involving 25 species (20 of which have sperm with apical hooks), they found

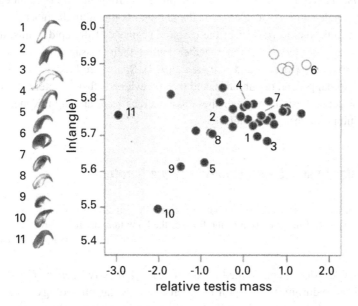

Figure 6.15 Significant positive relationship between the curvature of the apical hooks of sperm and relative testis mass in murid rodents. The pictures of sperm heads represent the range of hook design across species: (**1**) *Rattus tuneyi*, (**2**) *Mastomys coucha*, (**3**) *Leopoldamys sabanus*, (**4**) *Niviventer cremoriventer*, (**5**) *Bandicota bengalensis*, (**6**) *Apodemus argenteus*, (**7**) *Maxomys surifer*, (**8**) *Acomys cahirinus*, (**9**) *Paruromys dominator*, (**10**) *Bunomys fratrorum*, (**11**) *Notomys alexis*. Open circles mark species belonging to the genus *Apodemus*. (From Immler *et al.*, 2007.)

that, in most cases, more than 92 per cent of spermatozoa did not aggregate to form trains. *A. sylvaticus* proved to be an exception in this respect, as approximately 50 per cent of its sperm formed aggregations.

Of course, negative evidence cannot be final, so that alternative explanations for the functions and evolution of sperm hooks in rodents also deserve careful consideration. Perhaps these hooks enable sperm to attach more efficiently to the epithelium lining the isthmus of the oviduct (Smith and Yanagimachi, 1990; Suarez, 1987). Montoto *et al.* (2011) discuss the possibility that 'the presence of a hook may modify the head in such a way that would help the sperm swim faster'. Or hooks might be used to penetrate the zona pellucida of the ovum during fertilization (Flaherty *et al.*, 1983). At the time of writing, a comprehensive explanation for the evolution of these interesting structures remains elusive.

In addition to the examples described above, unusual associations between sperm have been noted in several species of placental mammals, the functional significance of which remain unknown. Sperm of some species exhibit 'stacking', and become associated in rouleaux during their passage through the epididymis. This is the case in the guinea pig (Martan and Shepherd, 1973), flying squirrel (Martan and Hruban, 1970), naked-tail armadillo (Heath *et al.*, 1987) and slow loris (Phillips and Bedford, 1987). In this last example, only one loris was examined, a preserved specimen of *Nycticebus coucang* in which sperm were present in rouleaux in the caput epididymis but only single gametes were stored in the terminal segment. In the other three species, sperm in rouleaux are present in the terminal segment of the epididymis, and in the guinea pig they remain joined together during their passage through the female reproductive tract (Martan and Shepherd, 1973). Sperm are linked together via their peri-acrosomal plasma membranes, and there is evidence that a protein (WH-30) may serve for cell adhesion. Whether these associations have any significance for sperm competition remains to be determined.

Testicular Descent and Evolution of the Scrotum

Descent of the testis into an accommodating scrotal sac remains as one of the more puzzling aspects of the evolution of the form of the body in many mammals.

Bedford, 1978a

In 1926, Carl Moore contributed a paper to *The Quarterly Review of Biology* which has had an enduring effect upon research on testicular physiology, as well as the formulation of theories concerning the origins of the mammalian scrotum. Moore demonstrated that, following transfer of the testes to the abdominal cavity (e.g. in rams and guinea pigs), spermatogenesis was severely compromised. He ascribed this to the deleterious effect of higher body temperatures in the abdomen. In other experiments, he had shown that wrapping insulating material around the scrotum of the ram, and thus raising scrotal temperatures, resulted in degeneration of the seminiferous tubules.

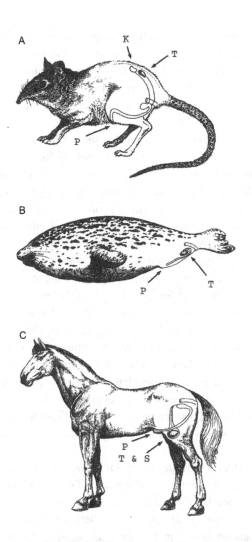

Figure 6.16 Positioning of the testes in ascrotal and scrotal mammals. (**a**) Rufous elephant shrew (*Elephantulus rufescens*): the testes are not descended (testicond). (**b**) Harbour seal (*Phoca vitullina*): the testes are descended but they are ascrotal. (**c**) Horse (*Equus caballus*): the testes are descended and a scrotum is present. T, testis; K, kidney; P, penis; T&S, testes in scrotum. (From Werdelin and Nilsonne, 1999.)

Descent of the testes is a process that begins during foetal development. The testes initially occupy a position close to the kidneys; indeed, they remain in this testicond state throughout life in a number of mammals, including most members of the Afrotheria (e.g. in elephant shrews: Figure 6.16a). Spermatogenesis proceeds normally under these conditions, however, despite retention of the testes deep within the body cavity. In other mammals the degree of descent that occurs during development varies and does not necessarily result in their deposition in a scrotum. Thus, they may descend to the posterior end of the abdominal cavity (e.g.

in cetaceans) or close to its ventral wall (as in hedgehogs and seals: Figure 6.16b). In those species where a scrotum is present, it may be non-pendulous, as in members of the Suidae and Equidae (Figure 6.16c) or pendulous, as in sheep and primates (Carrick and Setchell, 1977). A pendulous scrotum also occurs in many marsupials, but it is situated anterior to the penis; the reverse of the arrangement that pertains in placental mammals.

Several theories have been advanced to account for the evolutionary origin and functions of the mammalian scrotum, and one in particular will be discussed here. This posits that storage of gametes in the terminal segment (cauda) of the epididymis has played a key role in the evolution of the scrotum. Michael Bedford (1978a) advanced this hypothesis and provided cogent evidence in support of it. He suggested that testicular descent into a scrotum has occurred primarily in order to facilitate movement of the terminal segment of the epididymis to a cooler location. From this perspective, 'testicular descent is seen as a merely mechanistic event which enables the cauda epididymis to project from the body'. Thus, within the scrotum, the terminal segment of the epididymis forms a loop situated at the lowest point of the testis and closest to the exterior where lower temperatures prevail (for examples, see Figures 6.6B,C). In the rat, the terminal segment is 3–4°C cooler than the testis (Brooks, 1973). Moreover, in some species, loss of hair on the lower part of the scrotum may help to cool the underlying terminal segment; Bedford demonstrated that such hair loss is not accidental, as it is controlled by androgens. In species that are testicond, or which show varying degrees of testicular descent but lack a scrotum, the epididymis is often in advance of the testis itself, and its terminal region is positioned closer to the body wall (e.g. see Figure 6.6E, which shows the testis and elongated epididymis of an elephant shrew).

Bedford (1978a) also noted that if the testes of scrotal mammals are relocated to the abdominal cavity then sperm stored in the terminal segment of the epididymis die after a few days. If the epididymis alone is reflected to the inguinal canal, leaving the testis in the scrotum, then sperm in the initial and intermediate segments continue to undergo maturation, but gametes stored in the terminal segment do not survive. These experiments, which involved rabbits and rats, showed that effects of abdominal temperatures on the epididymis concern only its storage functions, and not its maturational functions (Bedford, 1978b). Why these adaptations should have arisen during therian evolution has not been fully explained. Regarding the presence of a scrotum in some taxa, but not in others, Bedford (1978a) discussed the possibility that differences in copulatory frequencies might be involved, with males of many scrotal mammals being required 'to ejaculate fertile semen repeatedly within a limited period'. He did not address the issue of sperm competition but, at the time Bedford's papers on the evolution of the scrotum were written, these matters were rarely discussed by mammalian gamete biologists.

Turning now to the subject of phylogenetic analyses that have attempted to map the evolution of the scrotum, Werdelin and Nilsonne (1999) concluded that the presence of a scrotum is the primitive state among mammals, and that the scrotum originated 'in concert with the evolution of endothermy'. Their view was that evolution has proceeded from possession of a scrotum to its loss in various groups, 'but never the reverse'. Kleisener *et al.* (2010), by contrast, concluded that testicondy is plesiomorphic for mammals in general, and that the scrotum arose at least twice: once in the Marsupialia and once in the Boreoeutheria. Subsequently it was lost in many groups.

More recently, some clarity has been brought to these debates, as a result of research by Sharma *et al.* (2018), who studied the phylogenetic distribution of two genes that are involved in the control of testicular descent. These genes (*RXFP2* and *INSL3*) play important roles in the development of the gubernaculum, the ligament which guides the testis during its descent. Comparative studies of 71 species of placental mammals showed that inactivation of *RXFP2* and *INSL3* has occurred independently in four testicond lineages of the Afrotheria: the tenrecs, golden moles, elephant shrews and sirenians (i.e. the manatees and dugong), but not in other groups of placental mammals (Figure 6.17). Sharma *et al.* concluded that testicular descent represents the ancestral state in the Placentalia as a whole, and its loss occurred later, in the different afrotherian lineages. Note, however, that in Figure 6.17 the aardvark is

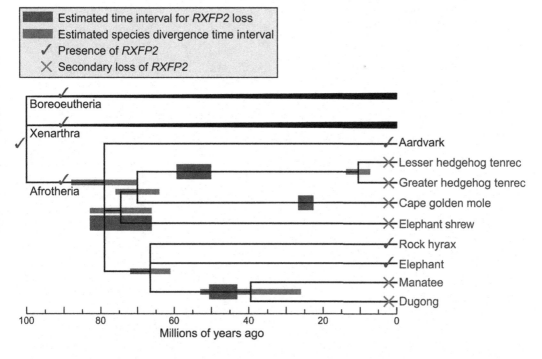

Figure 6.17 Evolution of the *RXFP2* gene in the Afrotheria, and estimated time intervals during which *RXFP2* came under neutral evolution (indicated by the black boxes). The gene was lost independently at different time points. Grey boxes represent estimates for species divergence times. With the exception of the aardvark, the species shown are all testicond. (From Sharma *et al.*, 2018.)

shown as having an intact *RXFP2* gene. This is not unexpected, as the aardvark is the only afrotherian which exhibits (partial) testicular descent. More surprising is the fact that the elephant and hyrax still have intact *RXFP2* and *INSL3* genes. Indeed, the exact genomic basis of testicondy in these two orders of the Afrotheria remains to be determined.

7 The Accessory Reproductive Glands and Ducts

The male accessory glands contain a rather bewildering array of chemical constituents,
and we still remain rather ignorant of the physiologic function of many of the components

Setchell *et al.*, 1994

In addition to spermatozoa, the products of a number of androgen-dependent accessory reproductive glands are transferred to the female during copulation. These include secretions of the vesicular glands and the prostate (which includes the coagulating glands in some taxa), the Cowper's, or bulbourethral, glands and ampullary glands. The accessory reproductive glands differ in their taxonomic distribution, sizes and secretory functions. These differences are discussed here, in relation to possible evolutionary effects of sexual selection at copulatory and post-copulatory levels. Although we are currently far from understanding the physiological significance of most of their secretions, some functions of the accessory glands are becoming clearer. This is particularly true of the processes that control seminal coagulation, and the production of 'copulatory plugs'. Seminal coagulation and plug formation play important roles in sperm transport and survival. Much of this chapter focuses on these topics.

Phylogenetic Distribution of the Accessory Reproductive Glands

Figure 7.1 shows the phylogenetic distribution of the major accessory reproductive glands in the 19 orders of the Placentalia, and the 7 orders of the Subclass Marsupialia taken as a whole. This represents a revision of the schema originally presented by Price and Williams-Ashman (1961). A revision was necessary in order to include current data, and to take account of major changes in the classification of placental mammals that have occurred during the intervening years.

The bulbourethral (Cowper's) glands are phylogenetically ancient structures, being present in monotremes, marsupials and in most orders of the Placentalia. They are especially prominent in marsupials, where between one and three pairs are present in various taxa, whilst a single pair only is present in monotremes and in most placental mammals. Rudimentary structures that may be homologous with the prostate gland occur in the platypus and echidna (Griffiths, 1978; Temple-Smith, 1973), whereas all the marsupials and placental mammals possess well-developed prostate glands. The vesicular glands are found only in placental mammals, although they are absent in some groups (e.g. in cetaceans and many carnivores: Price and Williams-Ashman, 1961) and vary greatly in size among members of the other orders. The ampulla, and its associated glandular tissues, is also restricted to certain orders of the Placentalia, but data on some taxa are still lacking. Two marsupial species have 'convoluted secretory segments' at the distal end of the vas deferens (Tyndale-Biscoe and Renfree, 1987), but these are not currently thought to represent homologues of the ampulla.

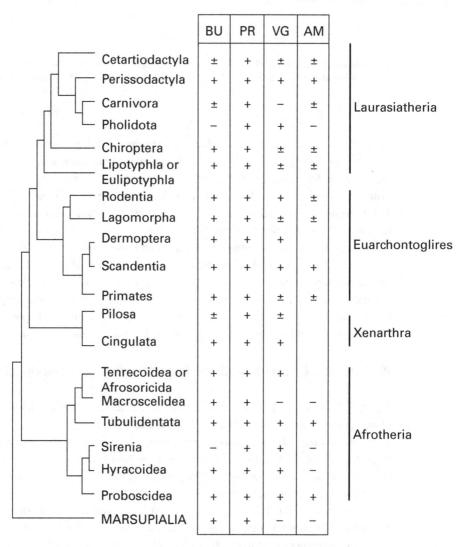

	BU	PR	VG	AM
Cetartiodactyla	±	+	±	±
Perissodactyla	+	+	+	+
Carnivora	±	+	−	±
Pholidota	−	+	+	−
Chiroptera	+	+	±	±
Lipotyphla or Eulipotyphla	+	+	±	±
Rodentia	+	+	+	±
Lagomorpha	+	+	±	±
Dermoptera	+	+	+	
Scandentia	+	+	+	+
Primates	+	+	±	±
Pilosa	±	+	±	
Cingulata	+	+	+	
Tenrecoidea or Afrosoricida	+	+	+	
Macroscelidea	+	+	−	−
Tubulidentata	+	+	+	+
Sirenia	−	+	+	−
Hyracoidea	+	+	+	−
Proboscidea	+	+	+	+
MARSUPIALIA	+	+	−	−

Laurasiatheria, Euarchontoglires, Xenarthra, Afrotheria

Figure 7.1 Phylogenetic distribution of the major accessory reproductive glands in placental mammals and marsupials. BU, Bulbourethral glands; PR, prostate; VG, vesicular glands; AM, ampullary glands. + indicates that a gland is present; − that it is absent or vestigial, and ± that a gland occurs in some members of the order but is absent, or vestigial, in others. (Updated and modified from Price and Williams-Ashman, 1961; the phylogeny is from Archibald, 2011.)

Examples of the anatomical arrangements of the accessory glands of various mammals are shown in Figure 7.2. These examples illustrate the morphological variability of the various glands, and their anatomical positions relative to the vasa deferentia and to the urethra (whence semen is transported during ejaculation). Hamilton (1990) has stressed that, in addition to the intra-pelvic organs, such as the prostate and vesicular glands, it is appropriate to include the excurrent ducts (such as the epididymis and vas deferens) in discussions of the accessory reproductive system. The passage of spermatozoa through the epididymis was considered in the last chapter, up to the point of gamete storage in its terminal segment. During sexual activity, rapid transport of sperm from the terminal segment of the epididymis to the urethra is undertaken by the vas deferens. This is the most muscular tubular duct in the body, and the role played by sexual selection during the evolution of its musculature is discussed below.

Rapid Sperm Transport: The Vas Deferens and Sperm Competition

There are three layers of smooth muscles in the wall of the vas deferens: outer and inner layers of longitudinal muscles are separated by a central layer of circular muscles (Figure 7.3). The lumen of the vas deferens is narrow and lined with ciliated, secretory epithelium. A complicating factor is the occurrence of regional differences in the muscle coat and the epithelial lining of the vas deferens throughout its length. These differences have been fully documented in relatively few mammalian species (e.g. rat: Hamilton and Cooper, 1978; rhesus and stump-tail macaques: Ramos, 1979). Major differences in epithelial structure occur between the proximal and distal regions of the vas deferens. Longitudinal folding of the epithelium is much more complex towards the urethral end of the vas deferens; stereocilia are shorter and more irregular, and epithelial cells contain many more cytoplasmic granules which are lacking at the epididymal end of the duct. It is also the case that the circular muscle layer becomes progressively thicker, whilst the inner longitudinal layer of muscles decreases in thickness, towards the urethral end of the vas deferens (Batra, 1974).

A spindle-shaped thickening of the terminal region of the vas deferens, the ampulla, is present in most orders of the placental mammals. Very large ampullae occur in some species; for example, they are 25 cm long in the horse, 13 cm in camels, 8 cm in elephants and 7 cm in red deer (Setchell et al., 1994). Unfortunately, the exact functions of the ampulla remain obscure. The richly folded secretory epithelium and expanded volume of the ampulla indicates that it is an important glandular structure and, in some species (e.g. Alston's brown mouse, Figure 7.2B), enlarged ampullary glands protrude onto the wall of the urethra. Few studies have examined the chemical nature of ampullary secretions as it is difficult to obtain samples that are uncontaminated by fluid from the vas deferens. In the zebra, jackass and other equids the ampulla

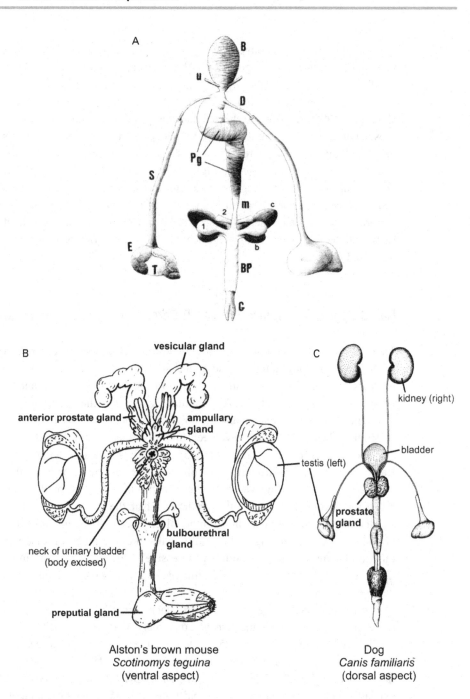

Alston's brown mouse
Scotinomys teguina
(ventral aspect)

Dog
Canis familiaris
(dorsal aspect)

Figure 7.2 Male reproductive tracts of **A:** a marsupial, the yapok (*Chironectes minimus*), and two placental mammals, **B:** Alston's brown mouse (*Scotinomys teguina*) and **C:** the domestic dog (*Canis familiaris*), to show the various accessory reproductive glands. Abbreviations: T, testis; E, epididymis; S, spermatic cord; D, ductus deferens; u, ureter; B, urinary bladder; Pg, three segments of the prostate gland; m, membranous urethra; c, ischiocavernosus muscle; b, bulbospongiosus muscle; 1, lateral bulbourethral gland; 2, medial bulbourethral gland; BP, penile shaft; G, glans. (**A** is from Nogueira *et al.*, 2004; **B** and **C** are from Miller, 2010, after Carleton *et al.*, 1975 and Raynaud, 1969.)

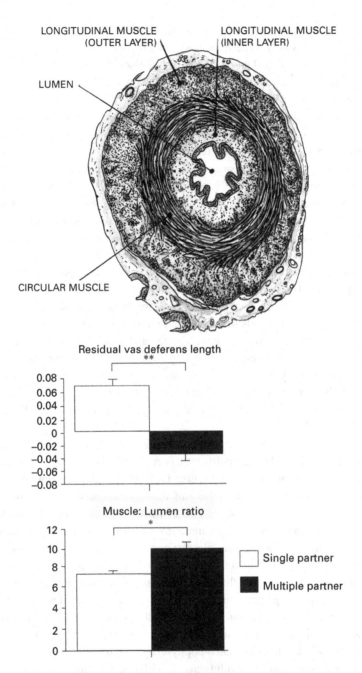

Figure 7.3 Upper: Transverse section through the human vas deferens, to show the thicknesses of its two longitudinal muscle layers and the intermediate layer of circular muscles. (From Dixson, 2009; author's drawing, after Bloom and Fawcett, 1962.) **Lower:** The vas deferens is shorter (in relation to body size) and more muscular (the ratio of muscle wall thickness: diameter of lumen) in mammals where females mate with multiple partners, and sperm competition risk is greatest (black bars) than in species with single-partner mating systems (open bars). $*P < 0.05$; $** P < 0.01$. (From Dixson, 2009.)

secretes large amounts of ergothioneine (Leone, 1954). The reasons for this have long remained a mystery. One hypothesis, arising from research on the domestic horse, posits that the antioxidant properties of ergothioneine may afford sperm some protection against reactive oxidative species (ROS) that are present in the uterine endometrium of the mare (Coutinho da Silva *et al.*, 2008).

Returning to the question of variability in the musculature of the vas deferens, measurements of its length and the thicknesses of its three layers of smooth muscles have revealed that these traits are correlated with sperm competition risk in mammals. Anderson *et al.* (2004a) conducted a morphometric study of the vasa deferentia of 103 species representing 69 genera of placental mammals and one marsupial (*Phascolarctos*: the koala). Most of the species measured were artiodactyls, perissodactyls (four equids) and primates, as well as a single carnivore (the jaguar) and a rodent (the capybara). Results showed that the vas deferens is on average 33 per cent shorter, and its muscular walls are 45 per cent thicker, in those genera and species where females mate with multiple partners, and where sperm competition pressures are greatest. The outer and inner longitudinal muscle layers of the vas deferens are thickened under these conditions, whereas the thickness of the circular muscle layer is reduced. Thus, mammals that have multiple-partner mating systems, and larger testes in relation to body weight, have shorter and more muscular vasa deferentia than mammals where single-partner mating systems and smaller relative testes sizes are the norm. In polygynandrous mammals, the ratio of vas deferens muscle wall thickness to lumen diameter averages 9.9 ± 0.7, as compared to 6.8 ± 0.6 in genera that have monogamous or polygynous mating systems (Figure 7.3B). The ratio in human males is 6.31.

It is not known precisely how the three muscle layers in the wall of the vas deferens operate during sperm transport. In the oesophagus, peristalsis involves sequential contractions of the outer layer of longitudinal muscles. These act in blocks, to concentrate the activity of the inner circular muscle layer, as it in turn contracts to force a bolus of food down to the stomach. The thickening of the longitudinal muscles in the mammalian vas deferens might also increase the efficiency of the circular muscles in some way, and thus make it possible to reduce their bulk. Although the functions of the inner longitudinal muscle layer are not fully understood, it is possible that they might assist in transporting sperm in the reverse direction, so that gametes that are not voided during ejaculation are returned to the cauda epididymis. Prins and Zaneveld (1980) demonstrated this in their radiographic studies of fluid transport in the vas deferens of the rabbit. They injected small volumes of ethiodiol (iodinated poppyseed oil) into the vas deferens of buck rabbits at its junction with the epididymis. Copulation resulted in rapid emptying of the contents of the vasa deferentia. However, 10 minutes after ejaculation had occurred, transport of ethiodiol back into the epididymis had begun. Over the next 24 hours, all of the ethiodiol had returned to the terminal segment of the epididymis. Electrophysiological experiments (Kihara *et al.*, 1995) have also demonstrated that rapid two-way transport of a dye may be induced between the terminal segment of the epididymis and the vas deferens.

Recovery of non-ejaculated sperm from the vas deferens might be especially beneficial to those species in which males ejaculate frequently, and where re-storage of gametes in the terminal segment of the epididymis is adaptive in relation to sperm competition. For example, in species where males make a series of intromissions (e.g. copulatory pattern no. 10, which occurs in some monkeys, and pattern no. 14, in some rodents), the mount series is sometimes disrupted or abandoned prior to ejaculation. It is possible that sperm are moved along the vas deferens in cohorts during each intromission so that numbers are maximized prior to ejaculation (see Figure 4.4). If indeed transfer of spermatozoa from the epididymis to the vas deferens does occur in this way, then the ability to recoup sperm after an abortive mount series would prevent wastage of gametes.

Are sperm stored only in the terminal segment of the epididymis, or might they sometimes be stored in the vas deferens? There is one clear case of a specialized storage organ that occurs in the vas deferens, although others may remain as yet undiscovered. In the common shrew (*Sorex araneus*), a swelling of the vas deferens, situated proximal to the ampulla, acts as a secondary sperm storage organ. Suzuki and Racey (1984) point out that this secondary storage organ is situated higher up in the body than the terminal segment of the epididymis, which lies beneath the skin, and is subject to a cooler environment. The situation in the shrew is intermediate between that which pertains in testicond and scrotal mammals, as is shown in Figure 7.4. This compares the sites of sperm storage in a testicond mammal (a hyrax) with the common shrew, and a typical scrotal species (a rabbit).

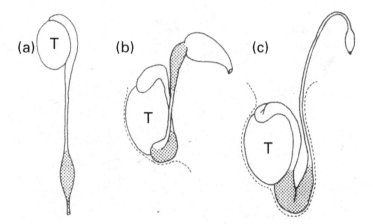

Figure 7.4 Sperm storage sites (stippled areas) in relation to the position of the testes in (**a**) hyrax: a testicond mammal; (**b**) common shrew, in which a secondary store occurs in the distal vas deferens, and (**c**) rabbit: a scrotal mammal. T, testis. (From Suzuki and Racey, 1984.)

The Vesicular and Prostate Glands: Effects of Sexual Selection

Historically the vesicular glands were called 'seminal vesicles' in the mistaken belief that they act as storage organs for spermatozoa. They function as secretory organs, however, and in many placental mammals the vesicular glands make a major contribution to the fluid portion of the ejaculate. In the human male, for example, they provide 60 per cent of the fluid, and 30 per cent is produced by the prostate gland (Harper, 1994).

Each vesicular gland consists of a single coiled tube, which may be branched, and which is sometimes folded upon itself to form a lobulated mass. An outer fibrous coat and a thick layer of longitudinal and circular muscles form the wall of the tube, which is lined with a secretory epithelium. An example of a large and complex type of vesicular gland is provided in Figure 7.5, which shows a dissection of the reproductive organs of a male drill (*Mandrillus leucophaeus*). The drill and the mandrill, like the macaques and most of the baboons and mangabeys, have multiple-partner mating systems, and males of all these species have very large vesicular glands. The same is

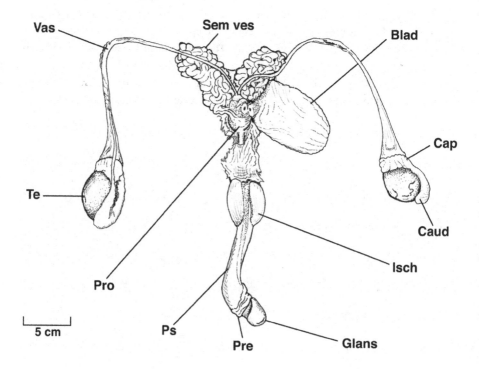

Figure 7.5 Dissection (dorsal view) of the reproductive tract of an adult male drill (*Mandrillus leucophaeus*). The neck of the bladder has been transected, and the bladder reflected to one side. Blad, bladder; Cap, caput epididymis; Caud, cauda epididymis; Glans, glans penis; Isch, ischiocavernosus muscle; Pre, prepuce; Pro, prostate; Ps, shaft of penis; Sem ves, vesicular glands; Te, testis; Vas, vas deferens. (From Dixson, 2015b.)

true of the chimpanzee and bonobo, whereas in gorillas, which are polygynous, they are small. This pattern of size differences relative to mating systems extends across the Order Primates as a whole, as is made clear in Figure 7.6. This shows the sizes of the seminal vesicles (rated on a four-point scale) for 27 genera of primates. Those genera

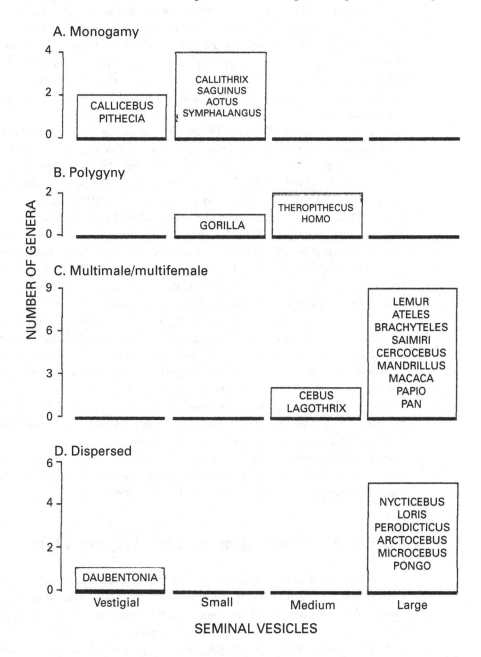

Figure 7.6 Vesicular gland size and mating systems in 27 genera of the Primates. (From Dixson, 2015b, after Dixson, 1998b.)

that have polygynandrous (i.e. multimale–multifemale or dispersed) mating systems have larger vesicular glands than the monogamous and polygynous taxa. They also have larger testes in relation to body weight, and exhibit higher frequencies of ejaculations (Dixson, 1998b).

The vesicular glands produce secretions that are rich in fructose, proteins and other constituents. Coagulation of semen, and the formation of copulatory plugs in some taxa, is due in part to proteins secreted by these glands, as is discussed below. Given that the vesicular glands are physiologically 'costly' structures, it is reasonable to suppose that natural selection may have favoured reductions in their size under conditions where copulations are infrequent and and the need for coagulum formation is reduced. This is likely to be the case for some monogamous primate taxa, such as *Callicebus*, *Aotus* and *Callithrix* in Figure 7.6. The case of the aye-aye (*Daubentonia madagascariensis*) must be different, however, as this non-gregarious Malagasy lemur, which has a dispersed mating system (Sterling, 1993), engages in prolonged copulations and exhibits genital traits indicative of sperm competition (Dixson, 2012). Yet the vesicular glands of the aye-aye are atrophic. Hill (1953) noted that the glans penis of Daubentonia resembles that of members of the Family Canidae. It is possible, therefore, that a copulatory lock also occurs in the aye-aye. Canids also lack seminal vesicles, as is true of some rodents in which prolonged locks occur during copulation (Dewsbury and Hodges, 1987; Hartung and Dewsbury, 1978). Under these conditions, where emission is also prolonged, the penis, rather than the presence of a copulatory plug, may serve to prevent backflow of semen.

At the time when the data shown in Figure 7.6 were obtained, relatively little information was available concerning the sizes and functions of mammalian vesicular and prostate glands in relation to post-copulatory sexual selection. However, research on rodents (Ramm *et al.*, 2005) and a variety of other mammals (Anderson and Dixson, 2009) confirms that prostate weights, as well as the weights of the vesicular glands, correlate positively with measurements of relative testes size. Mammals which have the largest testes in relation to body weight (and hence high levels of sperm competition) also have the largest vesicular and prostate glands (Figure 7.7). It is relevant to mention that, in the human male, the vesicular and prostate glands are quite small in relation to body size. This finding is consistent with a history of monogamy and/or polygyny during human evolution (Dixson, 2009).

Coagulation of Semen and the Formation of Copulatory Plugs

In many placental mammals copulation results in an interaction between proteins produced by the vesicular glands and an enzyme (vesiculase) secreted by the prostate to cause the coagulation of semen. Removal of the cranial lobe of the prostate prevents this seminal coagulation (e.g. in the rhesus monkey: Greer *et al.*, 1968). In rodents such as the rat and guinea pig, clotting enzymes (which include a transglutaminase) are produced by specialized lobes of the prostate: the coagulating glands (Notides and Williams-Ashman, 1967; Williams-Ashman *et al.*, 1977). Mixing fluid from the rat

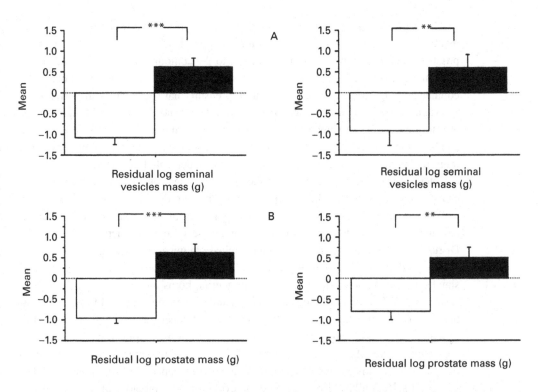

Figure 7.7 Weights of **A:** vesicular glands and **B:** prostate glands in mammals (89 species, representing 60 genera and 8 orders of placental mammals and marsupials). Data are means ± SEM residuals of prostate and seminal vesicles weights. Mammals having large relative testes sizes (i.e. data points fall above the regression line in double logarithmic plots of testes weight versus body weight) are indicated by black bars. Mammals having small relative testes sizes are indicated by open bars. Analyses are at the genus level (left) and species level after comparative analysis by independent contrasts (right). $**P < 0.01$; $***P < 0.001$. (From Anderson and Dixson, 2009.)

coagulating gland with rhesus monkey vesicular glandular secretions also results in coagulum formation (Van Wagenen, 1936).

In marsupials, where only the prostate and Cowper's (bulbourethral) glands are present, very little information concerning the physiology of seminal coagulation has been published. Tyndale-Biscoe and Renfree (1987) state that macropods are the only marsupials to produce a true copulatory plug. Coagulation apparently is under the sole control of the prostate gland (Rodger and White, 1975; Roger and Hughes, 1973). However, Johnston *et al.* (1997) noted that coagulation and plug formation occurred when semen was collected (by artificial vagina) from koalas, and the Cowper's glands are involved in this process (Johnston, personal communication). The role of the Cowper's glands in bringing about seminal coagulation in other marsupials is uncertain, but the large size of these glands, and the fact that three pairs are present in some marsupials (such as the koala), is intriguing.

The degree to which semen coagulates varies considerably among the placental mammals. In muroid rodents, for example, rapid hardening of semen occurs to produce a copulatory plug that moulds itself to the contours of the vagina and cervix (Baumgardner *et al.*, 1982; Hartung and Dewsbury, 1978). This 'close fit' between the copulatory plug and the cervix is required to ensure that sperm are transported from the vagina into the uterus (Blandau, 1945; Matthews and Adler, 1977), and perhaps also to prevent loss of semen from the vagina (Mann and Lutwak-Mann, 1951). One ancillary function of the multiple intromission copulatory pattern employed by some muroid rodents is to break up, or loosen, plugs deposited by previous males. In Chapter 5 it was noted that, in the rat, the penile muscles control reflexive movements of the glans penis that gradually break up copulatory plugs (see Figure 5.23).

Ablation of the vesicular and coagulating glands in rats renders males infertile, although their copulatory performance is otherwise normal (Cukierski *et al.*, 1991). Disruption of the clotting enzyme transglutaminase in mice, by deleting a gene required for its production, abolishes the ability of males to produce copulatory plugs and significantly impacts sperm transport to the uterine horns and oviducts of the female (Dean, 2013). Depletion of the accessory glandular secretions required for plug formation can occur in intact males, when copulatory frequencies are high enough. For example, the coagulating glands of male rats are almost empty after 4–6 hours of copulatory activity (Hawkins and Geuze, 1977), hence the importance of larger prostates and vesicular glands in rodents that engage in sperm competition (Ramm *et al.*, 2005).

Sexual selection has also influenced the evolution of copulatory plugs in primates. Male ring-tailed lemurs, for example, produce plugs that range in volume from 1578 to 5013 mm^3. They also vary in shape, elongated or smaller rounded plugs being most common (Parga *et al.*, 2006). Males dislodge or remove copulatory plugs deposited by their rivals (Parga, 2003). Ring-tailed lemurs have a multimale–multifemale mating system and a short mating season, during which individual females are receptive for less than 24 hours. Males copulate frequently (Koyama, 1988) and DNA typing studies have shown that extra-group males, as well as residents, may sire offspring (Parga *et al.*, 2016). Dunham and Rudolph (2009) posit that in those mammals where mate competition is intense, yet body size is not sexually dimorphic, copulatory plugs may represent an alternative or 'passive mate-guarding strategy' by males. Results of their comparative analysis of 62 primate species are consistent with the conclusion that copulatory plugs occur more frequently in primates that lack sexual dimorphism, in which females have short periods of sexual receptivity and males have penile spines. Some caution is advisable, however, when considering these results. Despite the use of statistical procedures to control for phylogeny, the substantial number of prosimians (one-third of the data set) included in the study is problematic. Most prosimians are less sexually dimorphic than the anthropoids. Males of most prosimian species also have large penile spines, and females exhibit limited periods of oestrus (whereas monkeys and apes do not).

The degree of seminal coagulation that occurs in primates varies in ways that are consistent with differences in their mating systems (Figure 7.8). None of the primates for which adequate information exists exhibits a complete absence of seminal

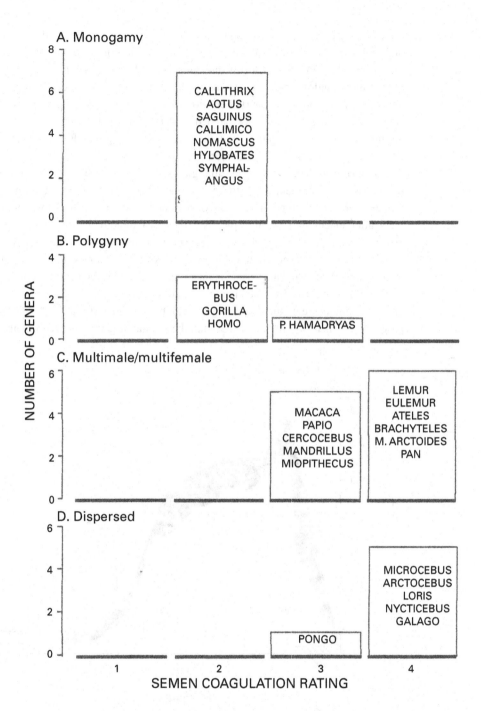

Figure 7.8 Semen coagulation ratings for 27 primate genera. Coagulation of semen occurs rapidly after ejaculation in most cases, but is more pronounced (coagulation ratings 3 and 4) in genera that have multimale–multifemale and dispersed mating systems, as compared to those having monogamous or polygynous mating systems ($P < 0.001$). (From Dixson, 2015b, after Dixson and Anderson, 2002.)

coagulation. However, in monogamous species such as gibbons and owl monkeys, and polygynous species such as gorillas, males produce only slightly gelatinous ejaculates. The same is true for the human species. By contrast, in those primates that have polygynandrous mating systems, males produce a pronounced coagulum or, in some cases, a more solid or rubbery copulatory plug. For example, mouse lemurs, ring-tailed lemurs, lorises, black-handed spider monkeys, muriquis and chimpanzees all produce copulatory plugs, and they all have polygynandrous mating systems (Dixson, 2012; Dixson and Anderson, 2002).

Secretions produced by the vesicular glands of some primates are alkaline, whereas the vaginal environment tends to be more acidic. Vaginal pH in the human female ranges from 3.5 to 4.0 before coitus (Masters and Johnson, 1966). However, immediately after ejaculation, vaginal pH rises to approximately 7.0 due to the buffering action of seminal fluid. This assists sperm survival and motility in the vagina, an effect which can last for several hours (Figure 7.9). Among placental mammals, the pH of semen varies between 7 and 8, and is thus capable of buffering acidic conditions in the vagina (this subject is discussed in more detail in Chapter 8). Some mammals that lack vesicular glands (e.g. the Iberian lynx and bottlenose dolphin in Table 8.4) also produce semen with a pH of 7–8, so that the prostate gland is likely to be the source

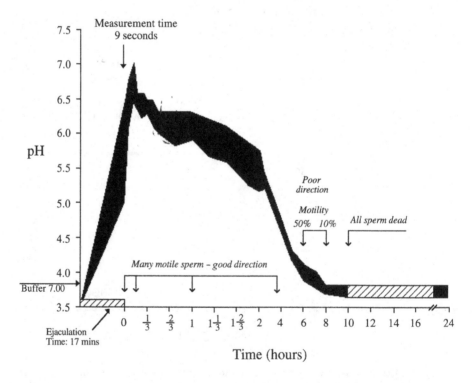

Figure 7.9 Buffering action of human seminal fluid upon vaginal pH and its relationship with sperm motility after intercourse. (From Dixson, 2012, redrawn from Masters and Johnson, 1966.)

of semen alkalinity in such cases. Indeed, in cetaceans, the prostate is the only accessory reproductive gland that is present in males.

A coagulum may promote gamete survival by retaining sperm in an alkaline environment, rather than exposing them directly to the hostile conditions of the vagina. Under conditions of intense sperm competition, further specializations might have occurred to cause hardening of semen, and plug formation. In the black-handed spider monkey, for example, the copulatory plug promotes the passage of highly motile, linearly moving sperm through the cervix. The plug buffers vaginal pH and also raises the temperature of the vagina (Hernández-López *et al.*, 2008). Sperm survival in the vagina and prompt trans-cervical sperm transport are important in the context of multiple-partner matings by females and resultant sperm competition between rival males. At the present time, such findings provide the most likely explanation for the evolution of greater seminal coagulation and copulatory plug formation in polygynandrous mammals.

An alternative but not mutually exclusive hypothesis is that mammalian copulatory plugs might obstruct semen deposition and/or sperm transport by a second male. In experiments using guinea pigs, the first male to mate and to deposit a copulatory plug blocked the ability of a second male to sire any of the resulting offspring (Martan and Shepherd, 1976). In the guinea pig 'the plug may be formed even within the uterus' (Walton, 1960), which might offer some greater advantage as a barrier to the sperm of rival males. An extreme example of copulatory plug formation concerns the banner-tailed kangaroo rat (*Dipodomys spectabilis*), a polygynandous rodent which occurs in the western USA and Mexico. The copulatory plug of this species, described by McCreight *et al.* (2011), fills the entire vagina and its fornices and extends, via a 'filamentous extension', through the cervical canal, to occupy both uterine horns (Figure 7.10A).

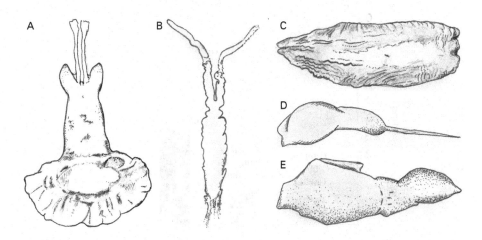

Figure 7.10 Examples of rodent copulatory plugs. **A:** Banner-tailed kangaroo rat, *Dipodomys spectabilis*. **B:** Guinea pig, *Cavia porcellus*. **C:** Paca, *Cuniculus paca*. **D:** Black-wristed deer mouse, *Peromyscus melanocarpus*. **E:** Large vesper mouse, *Calomys callosus*. (A–C, Author's drawings from photographs in McCreight *et al.*, 2011, Walton, 1960 and Eberhard, 1996. **D** and **E** were redrawn from Barmgardner *et al.*, 1982.)

However, this does not guarantee that an individual male's gametes will gain sole access to the female's reproductive tract, or prevent sperm competition, because DNA typing of plugs has revealed the presence of genetic material from as many as three males (McCreight *et al.*, 2011).

McCreight *et al.* suggest that expansion of the copulatory plug of the kangaroo rat, as it solidifies, may force sperm through the cervix and into the uterus. Matthews and Adler (1977) had previously examined this question during a series of experiments on plug formation and sperm transport in the rat. They recorded that the copulatory plugs deposited by male rats were approximately 10 mm long and 3 mm wide. The tight fit of the copulatory plug within the vagina, and the pressure exerted on the cervix, determined the efficiency with which sperm were transferred to the uterine horns, a process which took 6–10 minutes. Males that succeeded in depositing tight-fitting plugs transferred an average of 34 million sperm, by comparison with 8 million sperm when plugs were less well-positioned. Further, the tight placement of plugs also

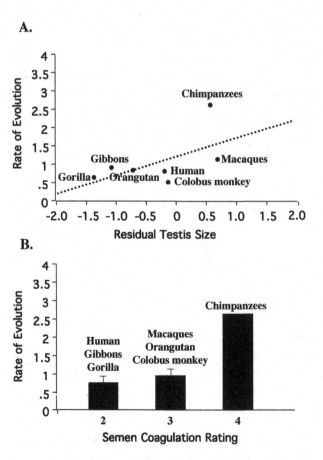

Figure 7.11 Correlations between the rate of evolution of the semenogelin 2 gene and **A:** relative testes sizes, **B:** semen coagulation ratings, in monkeys, apes and humans. (From Dixson, 2009; redrawn from Dorus *et al.*, 2004.)

depended upon the female partner, as well as the male remaining immobile during ejaculation, so that cryptic female choice may also have influenced mating success. Matthews and Adler also studied the ability of intromissions by rival males to dislodge plugs and interfere with sperm transport. These effects were most pronounced when such matings occurred within a few minutes of plug deposition, while sperm transport was still in progress. Clearly, these observations have important implications regarding sperm competition.

Molecular research has revealed that there is a relationship between sexual selection for the coagulation of semen and the rate of evolution of genes that encode semenogelin 2, the vesicular protein which undergoes coagulation by prostatic enzymes (Dorus *et al.*, 2004; Jensen-Seaman and Li, 2003). Dorus *et al.* compared the rates of evolution of the semenogelin 2 gene in 12 primate species, including the great apes and human beings. They found that rates of evolution were accelerated in those species in which sperm competition was most advanced, as reflected by larger residuals of testes size, higher semen coagulation ratings and more frequent multi-partner matings by females. Thus, the rate of semenogelin 2 gene evolution in *Homo sapiens* is consistent with that of other monogamous or polygynous primates, but notably less than that of macaques or chimpanzees, which have polygynandrous mating systems (Figure 7.11).

Table 7.1 Examples of some of the seminal vesicle secretory (SVS) proteins that have been identified in the seminal fluid of muroid rodents

Species	SVS Protein No. 1	2	3	4	5	6
Rattus norvegicus	*	*	*	*	*	X
Mus musculus domesticus	*	*	X	*	*	*
Mus musculus castaneus	*	*	*	*	X	X
Mus macedonicus	X	*	X	*	X	X
Mus spicilegus	X	*	X	X	X	*
Coelomys pahari	*	*	*	X	X	*
Apodemus sylvaticus	*	*	X	*	*	X
Pseudomys australis	X	*	*	*	X	X
Acomys cilcicus	X	*	X	X	X	*
Meriones unguiculatus	X	*	*	X	X	X
Microtus agrestis	X	*	*	*	*	X
Clethrionomys glareolus	*	*	X	X	X	*
Phodopus sungorus	X	*	X	X	X	*
Phodopus roborovskii	X	*	X	X	X	*
Peromyscus californicus	X	X	*	X	*	*
Peromyscus leucopus	*	*	*	X	X	*
Peromyscus maniculatus	*	*	*	X	X	*
Peromyscus polionotus	*	*	*	X	X	*

* This SVS protein is definitely present; X, this SVS protein is absent or present at very low levels. (Data are from Ramm *et al.*, 2009.)

Ramm *et al.* (2008) have confirmed that post-copulatory sexual selection affects the evolution of genes encoding seminal coagulation proteins. Their studies included the seminal vesicle secretory 2 gene of rodents. In muroid rodents, seminal vesicle secretory (SVS) proteins make up the bulk of the secretions contributed to the semen by the vesicular glands. Seven of these proteins have been studied in mice and in other muroids (Ramm *et al.*, 2009, 2015). The SVS2 protein is important for copulatory plug formation, and proteins SVS 5 and SVS 6 are thought to fulfil other functions (yet to be elucidated) relevant to sperm competition. Table 7.1 shows the results of proteomic studies to determine the distribution of SVS proteins in 18 species of muroid rodents. The functions of most of these proteins are not known; nor are they the only polypeptides that are secreted by the vesicular glands. Setchell *et al.*'s (1994) observation that 'the accessory reproductive glands contain a rather bewildering array of chemical constituents' still rings true today.

As well as affecting seminal coagulation, sperm transport and survival, the secretions of the accessory reproductive glands have the potential to interact with, and to influence, the female's physiology in multiple ways. These topics are addressed in the next two chapters, both of which focus upon copulatory behaviour and post-copulatory sexual selection primarily from the perspective of female mammals.

8 Cooperation, Conflict and Cryptic Female Choice

> Sperm progression to the Fallopian tubes is not an efficient process when viewed quantitatively. Not only do most spermatozoa fail to reach and enter the tubes, but the hazards of sperm loss associated with internal fertilization in mammals may not be appreciably less than those found under conditions of external (aquatic) fertilization in many lower species.
>
> Hunter, 1995

Ronald Hunter (1995) summarized the many hazards that mammalian spermatozoa encounter during their passage through the female reproductive tract (Figure 8.1). Most of the sperm perish, being engulfed by an army of leucocytes, or entrapped by mucus, so that they advance no further than the cervix, uterus or uterotubal junction. Some of them fail to undergo physiological changes, triggered by the female's physiology, that are essential if they are to fertilize ova (e.g. capacitation, hyperactivation of sperm motility and the acrosome reaction). Hence, only a small fraction of male gametes that enter the female tract will reach her oviducts and, of these, only one will unite with each ovum to bring about fertilization (Table 8.1).

Hunter attributed the release of such large numbers of spermatozoa to the requirement that enough of them might survive and gain access to the isthmus of the oviduct prior to ovulation. He also dealt with the consequences of competitive matings by males in relation to the timing of ovulation. The possible effects of post-copulatory sexual selection require additional consideration, however. Thus, rival males might gain a reproductive advantage by ejaculating larger numbers of sperm and also gametes that are better adapted to survive the rigours of the female's tract (sperm competition: Parker, 1970). This may be the reason why a polygynandrous species, such as the chimpanzee, ejaculates in excess of 1200 million sperm (Marson et al., 1989), compared to 280 million in its monogamous human relative. It is also possible that many of the hazards to gamete survival and transport listed in Figure 8.1 might positively, or negatively, bias the fate of spermatozoa that originate from different males, via cryptic female choice.

Comparative Anatomy of the Female Reproductive System

Given that the female's reproductive system is the arena in which copulatory and post-copulatory sexual selection takes place, it is necessary to take into account the

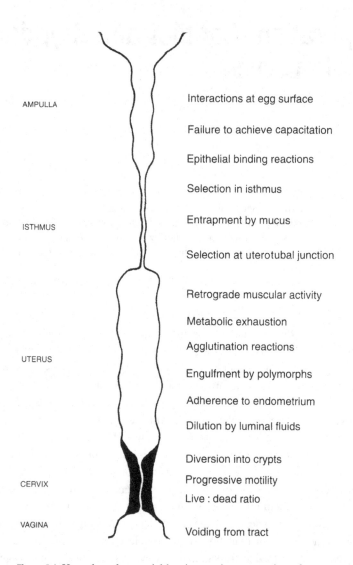

AMPULLA

Interactions at egg surface

Failure to achieve capacitation

Epithelial binding reactions

Selection in isthmus

ISTHMUS

Entrapment by mucus

Selection at uterotubal junction

Retrograde muscular activity

Metabolic exhaustion

Agglutination reactions

UTERUS

Engulfment by polymorphs

Adherence to endometrium

Dilution by luminal fluids

Diversion into crypts

CERVIX

Progressive motility

Live : dead ratio

VAGINA

Voiding from tract

Figure 8.1 Hazards and potential barriers to the progression of spermatozoa through the female reproductive tract, from the vagina to the ampullary–isthmic junction of the the oviduct. (After Hunter, 1995.)

differences in reproductive anatomy that characterize female monotremes, marsupials and placental mammals. In the monotremes, as represented by the platypus in Figure 8.2, there are two ovaries, oviducts and uteri; both sides of the system communicate with the urogenital sinus which, in turn, opens to the exterior via the cloaca. Only the left ovary of the platypus is functional, a trait which it shares with many avian species, whereas in the echidna both ovaries are active. Monotremes produce large, yolk-laden ova, 4.0 mm in diameter in the case of the echidna. Fertilization takes place in the oviduct, after which the ovum becomes enclosed

Table 8.1 Many are called but few are chosen. Numbers of spermatozoa ejaculated, sites of deposition and numbers of sperm in the ampulla of the oviduct in mammals

Species	No. of spermatozoa per ejaculate	Site of sperm deposition	Sperm nos. in ampulla
Human	280 million	Vagina	200
Mouse	50 million	Uterus	<100
Rat	58 million	Uterus	500
Rabbit	280 million	Vagina	250–500
Ferret	–	Uterus	18–1600
Guinea pig	80 million	Vagina/uterus	25–50
Domestic cattle	3000 million	Vagina	A few
Sheep	1000 million	Vagina	600–700
Pig	8000 million	Uterus	1000

Data are from Harper (1982, 1994).

in an eggshell. The egg then enters the uterus where it remains for 21–23 days (Griffiths, 1998).

Where female marsupials and placental mammals are concerned, developmental differences in the positioning of the ureters, in relation to the genital ducts, result in major differences in genital anatomy between the two groups (Tyndale-Biscoe, 2005). Female marsupials have two lateral vaginae, as well as a central canal which remains closed in most species, except when the female gives birth. The reason for these peculiar anatomical arrangements is that, during foetal life, the developing ureters migrate inside and above the genital ducts, so that they pass in between the developing genital ducts, preventing their fusion. Two lateral vaginae thus develop in female marsupials. In placental mammals, by contrast, the developing ureters migrate outside, and below, the genital ducts, so that the latter are free to fuse in the midline, forming the uterus and a single median vagina (Figures 8.2 and 8.3).

Anatomical differences between the female genitalia of monotremes, marsupials and placental mammals may, in turn, be linked directly with certain features of masculine genital morphology and copulatory behaviour. The following discussion is largely speculative, but it is consistent with the observed facts of reproductive anatomy.

The male platypus has an elongated phallus with a bilobed glans; the left lobe of which is markedly larger than the right (Figure 5.15). Only the left ovary is functional in the platypus and Temple-Smith and Grant (2001) suggest that the enlarged left lobe of the glans may make direct contact with the opening of the left uterus during copulation. As far as is known, there is no distinct 'cervix' in monotremes. A rosette of foliate papillae emerges from the tip of the glans during the erection, and this may assist the male platypus to deposit sperm directly into the left uterus. The volume of the ejaculate is very small in male monotremes, given that males lack a functional prostate gland, and the accessory reproductive glands are represented by a single pair of Cowper's (bulbourethral) glands which open into the penile canal.

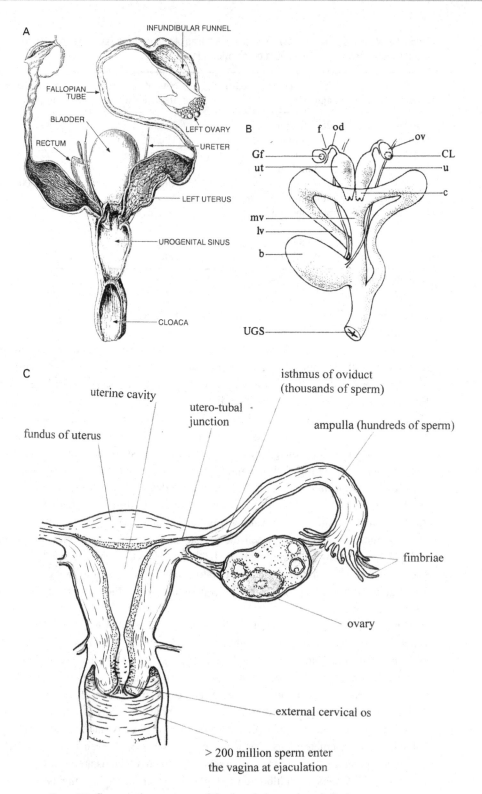

Figure 8.2 Comparative anatomy of the female internal genitalia in monotremes, marsupials and placental mammals. **A:** Platypus (after Griffiths, 1998). **B:** Tammar wallaby

Intrauterine insemination of the ejaculate may be highly advantageous under such conditions. The male echidna also has a complex glans penis, each half of which bears a pair of rosette-like structures. During erection, one pair of rosettes remains fully enlarged and rotates in order to become aligned with the openings of both uteri, as was discussed in Chapter 5 (see Figure 5.15).

Turning to the marsupials, the presence of two lateral vaginae is matched by the occurrence of a bifid glans penis in males of many taxa. Might this represent a case of coevolution between the female and male genitalia? The presence of two lateral vaginae is a plesiomorphic trait for the marsupials as a whole, governed by the developmental factors described above. However, where the penis is concerned, it is possible that the simple (non-bifid) condition is plesiomorphic, as suggested by Hershkovitz (1992). Thus, the distal end of the penis is initially non-bifid in young males of various South American genera, but gradually bifurcates as they mature. The possibility that each branch of the bifid penis might enter the ipsilateral vagina during copulation cannot be discounted, therefore, as the information required to settle this question is lacking.

The presence of a central birth canal in female marsupials (Figure 8.2B) also requires consideration here. The birth canal only becomes patent during parturition and closes up thereafter, except in some of the macropods and in the honey possum (Tyndale-Biscoe and Renfree, 1987). In these cases, the birth canal remains patent and the term 'pseudo vagina' is sometimes applied to this structure. However, there is little evidence as to whether it is involved in copulation. Females may sometimes bleed from the urogenital sinus after mating (koala: Johnston *et al.*, 2000a; macropods: Tyndale-Biscoe and Renfree, 1987), which might be due to damage to the lining of the pseudo vagina.

In the tammar wallaby (*Macropus eugenii*), the lateral vaginae act as conduits for spermatozoa and females often mate with several males during a postpartum oestrus. Up to 100 ml of coagulated semen is stored within the vaginal complex (Tyndale-Biscoe and Rodger, 1978). The lateral vaginae exhibit peristaltic movements that probably serve to mix and transport semen to their distal ends, where each vagina expands to form a vaginal cul-de-sac, separated from its neighbour by a median septum. The cervices of both uteri open into the vaginal culs-de-sac. Tyndale-Biscoe and Rodger (1978) demonstrated experimentally that 2–5 hours after mating much greater numbers of sperm have entered the cervical canal of the non-parturient uterus. They also determined that 'the differential distribution of spermatozoa in post partum animals was due to failure of transport in the recently pregnant side of the tract, rather than attraction of spermatozoa to the ovulation side'. Sperm transport by the lateral vaginae and uptake by the cervix thus falls, at least in part, under female control. Whether cryptic female choice occurs, favouring the gametes of any particular

Figure 8.2 (cont.) (after Tyndale Biscoe and Renfree, 1987). b, bladder; c, cervix; CL, corpus luteum; f, fimbrium; Gf, Graafian follicle; lv, lateral vagina; mv, median vagina; ov, ovary; od, oviduct; u, ureter; UGS, urogenital sinus; ut, uterus. **C:** Human (after Dixson, 2009).

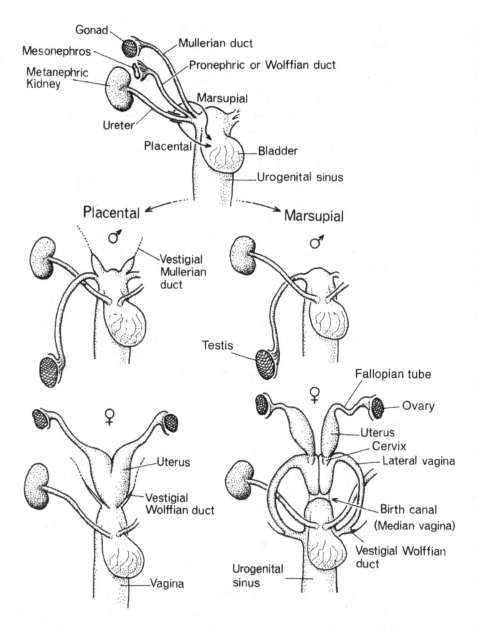

Figure 8.3 Differences in embryonic development, involving positioning of the ureters and genital ducts, determine major differences in genital morphology between marsupials and placental mammals. Further explanation is provided in the text. (After Tyndale-Biscoe, 2005.)

male, remains unknown. It should also be recalled here that, in marsupials, fertilization of ova occurs at the top of the oviduct (Tyndale-Biscoe, 2005), rather than at the isthmic–ampullary junction, as is the case for most of the eutherian mammals that have been studied thus far.

The unusual vaginal anatomy of marsupials almost certainly limits the possibilities for direct contact between the distal end of the penis and the uterine cervices during copulation. I know of no case in which intrauterine insemination has been identified in a marsupial species. Occurrences of copulatory plugs are also unusual, except in some of the macropods. Among the placental mammals, by contrast, intrauterine insemination occurs in a variety of taxa, as do copulatory plugs that assist sperm transport from the vagina to the uterus. It appears likely that the presence of a single vagina and cervix in placental mammals has facilitated the evolution of specializations of distal penile morphology that facilitate contact with the cervix (e.g. urethral processes, projecting bacula and other traits discussed in Chapter 5), especially so in those taxa where females mate with multiple partners. Induced ovulation, due to penile stimulation, is also known to occur in a number of placental mammals but is rare among marsupials. One known exception concerns the koala (*Phascolarctos cinereus*), although in this case it is possible that chemical cues in the semen combine with mechanical stimuli to trigger ovulation (Johnston *et al.*, 1997, 2004).

The Female Genitalia: Copulatory and Post-copulatory Sexual Selection

The following sections focus on the possible effects of cryptic female choice in determining the fate of sperm (resulting from multiple-partner matings) as they pass through the female's reproductive system. Most of this discussion concerns placental mammals, as much less is known about this subject where monotremes and marsupials are concerned. In truth, research on cryptic female choice in various groups of invertebrates (especially arthropods) has progressed much further than work on mammals (e.g. Aisenberg and Eberhard, 2009; Briceño and Eberhard, 2009; Eberhard, 1996, 2011; Eberhard and Huber, 2010; Peretti and Aisenberg, 2015). The same caveat applies to studies of sexually antagonistic coevolution (e.g. Arnqivst and Rowe, 2005). Hence, where it may be helpful to readers, the limited information available for placental mammals will be compared to some results of more advanced work on invertebrates.

Cryptic female choice and sperm competition are not mutually exclusive phenomena. When a female mates with multiple partners, the potential is created for competition to occur between the sperm of rival males for access to her ova. However, sperm do not have direct access to her ova; they must travel (or be transported) through her reproductive tract in order to reach the oviducts, where fertilization occurs. The potential for cryptic female choice thus also arises throughout this process, beginning in the vagina and cervix, and culminating in the oviduct, with the fertilization of ova. This discussion begins by considering those events that occur during and immediately after mating.

Copulatory Courtship: Reflexive Responses to Penile Stimuli

Eberhard (1985) proposed that, during copulation, the penis may act as an 'internal courtship device' and that runaway sexual selection by cryptic female choice favours those males that possess the most effective morphological or stimulatory phallic traits. Females benefit from such cryptic choices because their male offspring will inherit these advantageous traits. Runaway sexual selection and divergent evolution of penile morphology thus occurs under these conditions. Eberhard noted that 'Different species are thought to diverge because of the improbability that female choice will focus on exactly the same sets of male characteristics in different populations.' Examples of complex, species-specific penile morphologies in mammals were discussed in Chapter 5.

Female discrimination may involve responses to the tactile stimulation received, the degree of mechanical 'fit' between the genitalia of both sexes, or some combination of these factors. Eberhard also noted that once discrimination becomes established, 'selection would favour any male that was better able to meet the female's criteria (by squeezing her harder, touching her over a wider area, rubbing her more often, and so on). The ability to "convince" the female would become in itself an important determinant of male fitness'.

Copulatory courtship and cryptic choice in mammals may therefore include responses shown by females to tactile stimulation, both at the genital level (vagina, clitoris, cervix) and elsewhere via other types of stimulation provided by males during or after mounting. Table 8.2 lists some examples of reflexive genital responses that occur during mating in female mammals.

Much less attention has been paid to the study of such sexual reflexes in females than is the case where male mammals are concerned. The human female provides an exception to this rule, doubtless because of the clinical relevance of such observations. Bancroft (2009) and Levin (2020) have provided excellent overviews of this aspect of human sexuality. Only a few examples are cited here.

In women, the vagino-cavernosus reflex involves contractions of the bulbocavernosus (BC) and ischiocavernosus (IC) muscles in response to distension of the vagina. Shafik (1993) proposes that, during intromission, the pressure exerted by such contractions may

Table 8.2 Examples of reflexive responses shown by female mammals to penile and associated tactile stimuli provided by males during copulation. The functions of these reflexes are discussed in the text

Species	Reflex	Source
Human	Vagino-cavernosus reflex	Shafik, 1993
Rabbit	Vagino-cavernosus reflex	Cruz *et al.*, 2010
Human	Vagino-levator reflex	Shafik, 1995
Human	Clitoro-pelvic reflex	Gillan and Brindley, 1979
Human	Orgasm	Masters and Johnson, 1966
Stump-tail macaque	Orgasm	Slob *et al.*, 1986
Marmoset	Copulatory response	Dixson, 1986
Rat	Lordosis	Pfaff, 1980
Dog	Bulbocavernosus reflex	Hart, 1978
Cat	Post-copulatory after reaction	Hart, 1978
Cat	Vaginal sphincter contractions	Lagunes-Córdoba *et al.*, 2009
Pine marten	Post-copulatory after reaction	Grant and Hawley, 1991
Koala	Post-copulatory 'convulsions'	Smith, 1980

enhance erection of both the clitoris and the penis, and may also assist in 'milking' any semen that remains in the urethra when the penis is withdrawn. The vagino-levator reflex causes elevation of the uterus ('tenting') and increases in vaginal volume ('ballooning') to better accommodate the penis (Shafik, 1995). Female orgasm, the homologue of ejaculation in the male, involves contractions of the outer third of the vagina and also the uterus (Masters and Johnson, 1966). It is uncertain whether orgasmic responses play a role in sperm transport, however, as is discussed later in this chapter.

Further examples of sexual reflexes that are elicited by copulatory stimulation in female mammals mostly involve research on domesticated species, with some information also on the non-human primates (Table 8.2). Orgasmic responses occur in macaques and chimpanzees, for example (Dixson, 2012) and in the case of the stump-tail macaque (*Macaca arctoides*) uterine contractions have been recorded during orgasm (Slob *et al.*, 1986). In the marmoset (*Callithrix jacchus*) the tactile stimulation that results from intromission causes the female to struggle, turn her head, open her mouth and terminate copulation once ejaculation has occurred (Dixson, 1986). These responses are blocked by intravaginal application of a local anaesthetic (lidocaine), but not by its application to the external genitalia, including the clitoris. Intromission duration also increases markedly, and copulation is terminated by the male partner, rather than by the female (Figure 8.4).

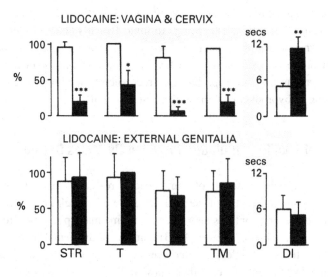

Figure 8.4 Effects of local anaesthesia of the genitalia upon behavioural responses shown during copulation by female common marmosets (*Callithrix jacchus*). Data are mean (± SEM) percentages of control tests (open bars) or lidocaine-treated tests (solid bars) during which females showed struggling movements (STR), head-turning (T), opening the mouth (O) or termination of the mount after ejaculation (TM). Intromission durations (DI) are in seconds. Application of lidocaine intravaginally in eight females (upper histograms) had profound effects upon these behavioural responses, whereas anaesthesia of the external genitalia, in the same subjects (lower histograms), was without effect. *P = 0.03; **P = 0.01; ***P = 0.004. (After Dixson, 1986.)

Domestic cats and many other felines exhibit an 'after reaction' to copulation which consists of vigorous rubbing and rolling behaviour (Diakow, 1971; Mellen, 1993). After reactions have also been observed in some other carnivores, including mustelids (e.g. the pine marten, *Martes martes*: Grant and Hawley, 1991, and the American mink, *Mustela vison*: Enders, 1952). Female African civets (*Civettictis civetta*) exhibit 'wildly excited post-copulatory rolling' (Ewer and Wemmer, 1974). In one of the marsupials (the koala: *Phascolarctos cinereus*), the female also exhibits post-copulatory 'convulsions' during which her head is thrown back and 'her loins contract sharply about once a second' (Smith, 1980). Cats, mustelids and koalas are all induced ovulators; the question of possible linkages between after reactions and the neuroendocrine regulation of induced ovulation are discussed in the next chapter.

It is not known whether the copulatory and post-copulatory reactions described above might be akin to the orgasmic contractions of the vagina and uterus which occur in women during orgasm (Masters and Johnson, 1966). Some years ago an important function was attributed to female orgasm in relation to human sperm competition by Baker and Bellis (1993), but there is, as yet, no convincing evidence that female orgasm plays any role in post-copulatory sexual selection in human beings, or in other primates (Dixson, 2009, 2012; Lloyd, 2005). It is interesting that positron emission tomography (PET) scan studies have shown that manual stimulation of the clitoris (resulting in orgasm) or the penis (resulting in ejaculation) activates exactly the same areas of the brain (in the dorsolateral and ventrolateral pontine tegmentum) in women and men (Huynh *et al.*, 2013). This brings to mind Beach's (1976) observation that neural mechanisms mediating sexual responses typical of one sex may also be capable of expression in the opposite sex, given favourable conditions for their elicitation. Thus Donald Symons (1979) was probably correct when he interpreted human female orgasm as being a 'byproduct of female bisexual potential'.

Other Types of Tactile Stimulation Provided By Males During Copulation

During copulation, male mammals of some species restrain females by using their jaws to grip the skin on the nape of the neck. The use of a 'neck grip' during mating occurs in many carnivores, but it is also present in some marsupials, bats, rodents and primates (Figure 8.5; Table 8.3). Ewer (1973) pointed out that female carnivores, such as cats, cheetahs, lions and polecats, often use the neck grip when transporting their young offspring. When held in the mother's jaws in this way, the youngsters exhibit a reflexive response that results in them being immobilized. The use of a neck grip in sexual contexts by males is thus an example of exploiting a 'sensory trap' by activating an immobilization response. Eberhard (1996) noted that 'evolution of male traits involved in triggering cryptic female choice processes seem particularly likely to involve the use of sensory traps'.

In many hoofed mammals (i.e. perissodactyls and artiodactyls), 'the male's scent, vocalizations, and/or tactile contacts may release a kind of immobilization reflex in the female' (Walther, 1984). In the black rhino, for example, the male rests his chin on the

Table 8.3 Examples of mammals in which males 'neck-grip' females during copulation

Common name	Latin name	Source
Marsupials		
Striped possum	*Dactylopsila trivirgata*	McKenna, 2005
Koala	*Phascolarctos cinereus*	Smith, 1980
Paucident planigale	*Planigale gilesi*	Whitford *et al.*, 1982
Dibbler	*Parantechinus apicalis*	Wolfe *et al.*, 2000
Tasmanian devil	*Sarcophilus harrisii*	Eisenberg *et al.*, 1975
Carnivores		
Least weasel	*Mustela nivalis*	East and Lockie, 1965
Wolverine	*Gulo gulo*	AFD
Sea otter	*Enhydra lutris*	AFD
Jungle cat	*Felis chaus*	Mellen, 1993
Snow leopard	*Panthera uncia*	Lanier and Dewsbury, 1976
Bats		
Little brown bat	*Myotis lucifugus*	Barclay and Thomas, 1979
Broad-nosed bat	*Scoteinus balstoni*	Ryan, 1966
Big brown bat	*Eptesicus fuscus*	Mendonça *et al.*, 1996
Short-tailed fruit bat	*Carollia perspicillata*	Knörnschild *et al.*, 2014
Livingstone's fruit bat	*Pteropus livingstonii*	Courts, 1996
Shrews (Eulipotyphla)		
Common shrew	*Sorex araneus*	Crowcroft, 1957
Short-tailed shrew	*Blarina brevicauda*	Rood, 1958
Rodents		
Cape mole-rat	*Georhychus capensis*	Bennett and Jarvis, 1988
Desert kangaroo rat	*Dipodomys deserti*	Butterworth, 1961
Primates		
Garnett's galago	*Otolemur garnettii*	Dixson, 2012
Spectral tarsier	*Tarsius spectrum*	Hidayatik *et al.*, 2018

AFD, author's observations, using videotaped recordings.

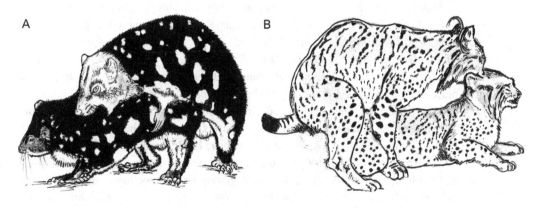

Figure 8.5 Neck grips by males occur during copulation in diverse taxa. **A:** Tiger quoll (*Dasyurus maculatus*). **B:** Iberian lynx (*Lynx pardinus*). (Author's drawings, from photographs.)

female's back, at the base of her tail, prior to making a mount attempt. Moreover, males may mount as many as 20 times over the course of several hours before copulation takes place (Goddard, 1966). Similar pre-copulatory 'chinning' behaviour has also been recorded for white rhinos (Owen-Smith, 1975). Chinning and mounting without copulation form a behavioural sequence that tests the female's receptivity: placing pressure on her lower back, and seeking to activate the immobilization reflex. The bull moose (*Alces alces*), for example, walks steadily behind the female, chinning her, and may then mount if she slows her pace and shows other indications of being receptive. The bull mounts anywhere from 1 to 14 times, however, before performing a rapid copulation, lasting for 5 seconds (Ballenberghe and Miquelle, 1993). Males of many African ungulates also exhibit chinning behaviour and/or multiple mounts prior to intromission; examples discussed by Estes (1991) and Walther (1984) include waterbuck, oryx, addax, sitatunga, eland and the African buffalo.

In the domestic pig (*Sus scrofa*), a complex amalgam of stimuli (chemical, vocal and tactile cues) provided by the boar serve to elicit the sow's immobilization reflex (Signoret, 1970). However, in about 50 per cent of sows, exerting pressure on the lower back of the sow is sufficient to elicit the immobilization response. Warthogs (*Phacochoerus africanus*) also exhibit chinning behaviour; the boar massages the female's body with his snout disc and rests his chin on her back before he mounts (Frädrick, 1974).

In many invertebrates, males stroke, lick, tap, or rub the female's body, limbs or head during the act of mating. Eberhard (1991, 1994) found that such behaviour commonly occurred during or immediately after copulation. His large-scale surveys produced correlational evidence for the existence of cryptic female choice in many insects and spiders. No surveys of comparable magnitude have been conducted on mammals. Where *pre-copulatory courtship* is concerned, Darwin (1871) noted that 'With mammals the male appears to win the female more through the law of battle than through the display of his charms.' The same reservation may apply to the (non-genital) aspects of copulatory courtship in mammals. However, some possible examples of tactile courtship during copulation are described below.

Males of a number of carnivorous marsupials (Dasyuromorphia) rub the chin and throat from side to side, against the female's neck during copulation (e.g. in *Sminthopsis murina*: Fox and Whitford, 1982; *Ningaui* spp.: Fanning, 1982; *Planigale gilesi*: Shimmin et al., 2002). Shimmin et al. also observed male *P. gilesi* scratching the female's rump with their hind feet during mating. Turning to the placental mammals, the male striped skunk (*Mephitis mephitis*) raises one hind foot and scratches at the female's vulva during mounting, prior to attaining intromission. This causes the female to raise her hindquarters and deflect her tail, which in turn facilitates the male's attempts to intromit (Ewer, 1973; Wight, 1931). Males of some other carnivore species lick or nip the female's ears during mating (e.g. in the fossa and the lion; author's observation); male grizzly bears sometimes attempt to chew the female's ears (Mundy and Flook, 1964). In the New Zealand fur seal (*Arctocephalus forsteri*) the male rubs his neck against the shoulders and neck of the female (Stirling, 1971).

Among the primates, Schulze and Meier (1995) reported that male slender lorises (*Loris tardigradus*) display lateral head movements, rubbing the chin and throat against the female's back during copulation (see Figure 3.8E). In many monkeys and apes, visual communication, rather than tactile cues, may be more relevant to this discussion. Thus, facial displays and eye-contact proceptivity play an important role during pre-copulatory communication, and may continue to be displayed during the act of mating. Female monkeys of a number of species turn to look back at the male and engage him in eye contact during copulation. Such mutual eye contact is particularly marked in the orang-utan, bonobo and gorilla during copulations that take place in a ventro-ventral position (Dixson, 2012).

In muroid rodents, such as rats, hamsters and gerbils, the male palpates the female's flanks rapidly with his forepaws and thrusts against her perineum during mounting. These tactile stimuli induce the sexually receptive female to display lordosis. This in turn facilitates the attainment of intromission, during which penile stimulation of the vagina and cervix further amplifies the lordotic response (as, for example in the rat: Figure 8.6). Many examples may be cited of mammals in which males clasp the female firmly around the waist during mating. Such behaviour might simply serve to restrain the female and assist the male in maintaining the mounting position. It is possible, however, that by clasping a receptive female the male activates reflexes that cause her to remain immobile. In the kinkajou (*Potos flavus*), for example, 'the male clasps the female with his hands turned so as to bring the enlarged and pointed radial sesamoid bone into contact with her body, and rubs her flanks' (Ewer, 1973).

Copulatory Courtship: The Mechanical 'Fit' Between Genitalia

Conflicts can occur between the sexes, both during and after the act of mating (Arnqvist and Rowe, 2005). Nonetheless, females and males share some common goals. Partners of both sexes need to mate successfully, and to produce offspring that will perpetuate their genes. Cases where the divergent interests of males and females may lead to copulatory (and post-copulatory) conflicts will be discussed in a moment. First, however, let us acknowledge that coevolution of genital traits can occur in a positive way; not *everything* is the result of a sexual arms race. Among placental mammals, for example, there is a positive relationship between the length of the penis and the length of the female reproductive tract, measured from its external opening (introitus) to the point where ejaculation occurs. In most cases the latter measurement equates to the length of the vagina. There are exceptions, however, as in the spotted hyena, where intromission takes place via the clitoris, or the pig, where the spiral-shaped distal part of the penis is inserted into the cervical canal. Figure 8.7 compares penile length and overall length of the relevant portion(s) of the female tract in 20 species of cetartiodacyls, perissodactyls, carnivores and primates. There is a strong positive correlation between the two measurements ($r_s = 0.90895$; $P < 0.001$; two-tailed test).

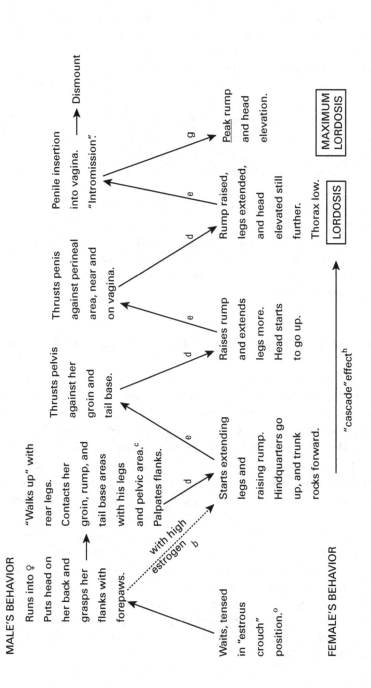

Figure 8.6 Lordosis behaviour in the female rat involves a sequence of reflexes, with corresponding responses made by the male (from Pfaff, 1980).

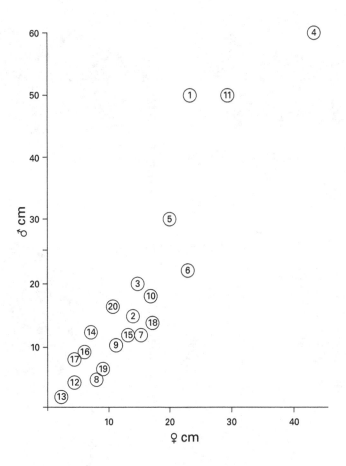

Figure 8.7 Length (cm) of the erect penis and length of those portion(s) of the female reproductive tract that receive the penis during copulation. **1**, Cattle; **2**, defassa waterbuck; **3**, sheep; **4**, pig; **5**, horse; **6**, harbour porpoise; **7**, bottlenose dolphin; **8**, short-beaked common dolphin; **9**, harbour seal; **10**, spotted hyena; **11**, Indian elephant; **12**, ring-tailed lemur; **13**, common marmoset; **14**, black-crested mangabey; **15**, mandrill; **16**, rhesus macaque; **17**, stump-tail macaque; **18**, chimpanzee; **19**, western lowland gorilla; **20**, human. Further details are provided in Appendix 3.

A special case of coevolution of the male and female genitalia concerns those Old World monkeys and chimpanzees in which females develop large sexual skin swellings during the follicular and peri-ovulatory phases of the menstrual cycle. Examination of these swellings in a number of species (Figure 8.8) leads one to infer that the posterior projection of the lower (pubic) region of the female's sexual skin increases the operating depth of the vagina. This being so, then such swellings may effectively increase the distance that males must negotiate to place their ejaculates at the external cervical os. Measurements of the genitalia of chimpanzees support this conclusion. The operating depth of the vagina increases by 50 per cent when the sexual skin is swollen. Males vary in their ability to position their copulatory plugs close to the cervix under these conditions (Dixson and Mundy, 1994), as is shown in

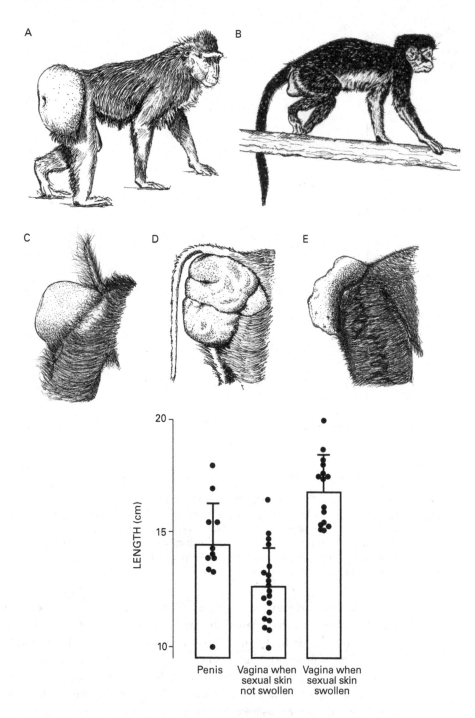

Figure 8.8 Upper: Lateral views of sexual skin swellings in five species of Old World anthropoids. **A:** *Macaca nigra*. **B:** *Miopithecus talapoin*. **C:** *Mandrillus sphinx*. **D:** *Papio hamadryas*. **E:** *Pan troglodytes*. (From Dixson, 2015b.) **Lower**: Measurements of penile erection and vaginal length (when the female sexual skin is not swollen and when it is at maximal swelling) in chimpanzees (*P. troglodytes*). Data are shown for individual animals, with the overall means and standard deviations indicated by the histograms and bars. (From Dixson, 2012; after Dixson and Mundy, 1994.)

the lower part of Figure 8.8. Thus, although female swellings evolved primarily to act as sexually attractive visual signals of female fertility (Dixson, 1983b; Nunn, 1999), cryptic female choice may also have occurred, selecting for elongation of the penis.

The huge diversity of mammalian penile morphology was reviewed in Chapter 5. There it was concluded that it is the distal region of the penis that has undergone the greatest evolutionary changes as a result of copulatory and post-copulatory sexual selection. The obvious question that arises is whether corresponding morphological changes have occurred in the female genitalia, and especially in the vagina or cervix. The answer is that vaginal morphology often remains little affected in many species where males have complex penile morphologies. This is the case, for example, in the great majority of carnivores, bats, rodents and primates for which vaginal morphology has been described in sufficient detail. In these cases it is likely that copulatory courtship involves female discrimination on the basis of tactile stimuli provided by the male. The female's nervous system is thus the arbiter of such stimuli, rather than mechanical discrimination involving the shape of the vagina. Evidence that supports this conclusion concerns the importance of vaginal and other types of reflexive responses during mating in female mammals (e.g. see Tables 8.2 and 8.3).

Eberhard (1985) noted that the occurrence of 'diverse male genitalic morphologies but uniform female morphologies is a common pattern' in many groups of invertebrates as well as 'in rodents, and probably other mammals'. I have encountered only a few exceptions to this rule among mammals. For example, in the dugong (*Dugong dugon*), Hill (1945) reported that:

The most striking feature in the vaginal interior is the arrangements in the vault. Extending from the summit of the vault, ventrally for almost half the length of the ventral wall, is a raised shield-shaped keratinized area, broad near the vault and narrowing to a point caudally. It is abruptly marked off from the rest of the vaginal mucosa.

In the black-handed spider monkey (*Ateles geoffroyi*), Wislocki (1936) noted that: 'Corresponding to the cornified barbs described on the penis, adult females possess similar but smaller barbs in the vagina.' Fooden (1971) also reported the presence of cornified spines lining the wall of the vagina in the Assam macaque (*Macaca assamensis*), suggesting that these structures might interact, during copulation, with the penile spines of the male. Another example of possible coevolution of the genitalia involving vaginal specializations concerns the squirrel *Tamiasciurus douglasii* (Smith, 1968). Females of this species have a coiled vagina and the male's elongated penis contains a much reduced baculum. The exact mechanics of copulation in this squirrel remain unknown. Coiling of the vagina also occurs in the northern short-tailed shrew (*Blarina brevicauda*). This species displays a copulatory lock, during which the 'S'-shaped glans penis and its filiform tip are thought to become lodged within the coiled vagina (Pearson, 1944).

The vaginal morphology of whales, dolphins and porpoises also calls for comment here, as muscular transverse folds, sometimes called 'pseudo cervices' project from the vaginal walls, in some cases forming spiral arrays (Figure 8.9). Possession of these muscular folds is a plesiomorphic trait, shared by both the baleen and toothed whales.

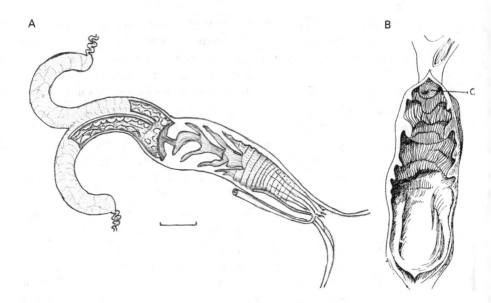

Figure 8.9 Dissections of the lower part of the reproductive tract of female cetaceans, to show the transverse vaginal folds. **A**: long-finned pilot whale (*Globicephala melas*). Scale = 1 cm. (After Harrison, 1949.) **B**: A porpoise (*Phocoena* sp.). C, cervix. (After Slijper, 1962.)

However, there are marked phylogenetic differences in the sizes and numbers of these unusual structures among the various taxa. Similar, transversely oriented folds also occur in the vagina of the hippopotamus, the closest surviving phylogenetic relative of the extant cetaceans. Yet, as far as I have been able to determine, transverse vaginal folds are lacking in other aquatic, or amphibious mammals, such as the sirenians, pinnipeds, otters, beavers and coypu.

The possible functions of the vaginal folds in cetaceans have been much debated. Meek (1918) was one of the earliest workers to suggest that they might serve important copulatory functions. He suggested that during intromission:

the penis will have to pass through a number of the folds at least, and it is probable, therefore, that they have been developed for the purpose of promoting the discharge. It will be noted that the folds are directed downwards and they are highly muscular. It is possible, therefore, that the folds are expanded and contracted, and depressed and raised, and such movements would have the effect of sending the spermatic fluid upwards, towards the uterus.

Slijper (1962) later summarized the information then available as follows:

These peculiar folds, which are not found in any other mammals, may serve for keeping water out of the womb, and also for providing extra space to allow the foetus to be born. They may also play some part during copulation.

Robeck (1994), based upon his studies of reproductive physiology and artificial insemination in captive cetaceans, noted that the entrance of seawater into the vagina during copulation would be likely reduce the viability of spermatozoa. The vaginal folds may therefore play a protective role in this context.

Has the evolution of the vaginal folds of cetaceans been affected by post-copulatory sexual selection? Convincing answers to this question remain elusive (Orbach *et al.*, 2017a, 2020), due in part to the difficulties of quantifying the morphological complexity of the folds and their actions in living animals. Comparative measurements of the morphology of the vaginal folds in a sufficient number of cetacean species may help to resolve this problem (Orbach *et al.*, 2017b). Clearly, this will be a challenging task, especially when attempting to make measurements of the largest whale species.

The ability of the mammalian penis to function as an 'internal courtship device' is likely to involve its mechanical interactions with the cervix, as well as the vagina. Cryptic female choice may thus have resulted in coevolution of complexity of the penis and the cervix. The penis may stimulate the os cervix during pelvic thrusting movements, for example. Chapter 2 established that pelvic thrusting is widespread among mammals, and that it occurs during four of the five most frequent copulatory patterns displayed by males.

In those ungulates where an elongated urethral process is present, it may become mobile during ejaculation, distributing semen around the external cervical os (e.g. in the goat *Capra aegagrus hircus*: Hafez, 1968). During semen collections by artificial vagina, coiling of the distal penis has been observed in cattle (Seidel and Foote, 1969), as well as rotatory movements of the penile tip in dromedaries, *Camelus dromedarius* (Al-Eknah *et al.*, 2001).

Examples of more invasive phallic specializations that serve for intracervical or intrauterine insemination were discussed in Chapters 5 and 7. During intrauterine insemination in the pig (*Sus scrofa*), the male's filiform spiral penis becomes lodged within the sow's cervix during prolonged copulations, whereas in the horse (*Equus caballus*), semen is conveyed via the urethral process of the penis into the cervical canal and uterus (Glover, 2012). In hystricognath rodents, such as the agoutis and cavies, an intromittent sac, situated just below the urinary meatus of the glans penis, is everted during erection (e.g. in Azara's agouti: Figure 5.16); its large spines and spikes are well positioned to stimulate the vagina and cervix during copulation. Intrauterine insemination is known to occur in some of the histricognaths (e.g. in the guinea pig: Walton, 1960).

Elongation of the penile bone (baculum) has been linked to post-copulatory sexual selection in a number of taxa. The distal pole of the baculum projects beyond the tip of the penis in some primates (e.g. greater galago: Figure 5.19), carnivores (e.g. the fossa: Figure 5.12) and rodents (e.g. the springhare: Coe, 1969). Anatomical comparisons between the male and female genitalia of these species indicate that the tip of the baculum may be inserted into the external cervical os during mating. I am unable to confirm this for the fossa, as I can find no published description of the female's internal genitalia. However, the penis is greatly elongated in this species.

There are cases in which the penis does not penetrate the cervical canal during mating, but reflexive movements of the glans and deposition of a copulatory plug result in semen being transported into the uterus. As discussed in the last chapter, expansion of the copulatory plug as it hardens is thought to force semen through the cervical canal. This occurs in the Norway rat (Matthews and Adler, 1977; Sachs, 1983), and perhaps also in the kangaroo rat (McCreight *et al.*, 2011).

Diversity of distal penile morphology among closely related species is sometimes matched by species-specific variations in cervical morphology. One particularly striking example of this phenomenon concerns monkeys belonging to the genus *Macaca*, 20 species of which are distributed throughout Asia and South-East Asia, while a single species, the Barbary macaque (*Macaca sylvanus*), occurs in the Atlas Mountains of North Africa. Macaques live in multimale–multifemale groups. Their mating systems are polygynandrous, and males have relatively large testes, and morphologically complex penes; traits that are consistent with the effects of post-copulatory sexual selection (Dixson, 2012). The morphology of the female genitalia also varies in the different species groups of macaques, as is shown in Figure 8.10. In the *silenus–sylvanus* and *fascicularis* species groups (as exemplified by *M. mulatta* in Figure 8.10), the cervix is of moderate size, and its canal is 'S'-shaped due to the presence of dorsal and ventral colliculi. In the *sinica* species group, the cervix is hypertrophic, the colliculi are massive and the cervical canal is tortuous. The *arctoides* group contains the single species *M. arctoides*, in which the cervix lacks colliculi so that its canal is relatively straight. However, the entrance to the vagina is narrow, due to the presence of a dorsal collicle. The elongated glans of the penis fits through this

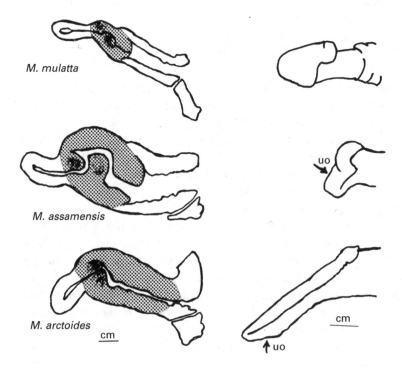

Figure 8.10 Comparative morphology of the female and male genitalia in three macaques. Shaded areas indicate the extent of the uterine cervix; uo, opening of the urethra. (From Dixson, 2012; redrawn and modified from Fooden, 1991.)

narrow opening during intromission and a partial genital lock is maintained during copulation (Fooden, 1967; Lemmon and Oakes, 1967).

Interactions between the cervix and the penis described in the preceding paragraphs may include elements of conflict between the goals of the two sexes, resulting in sexually antagonistic coevolution (Arnqvist and Rowe, 2005; Eberhard, 2004). This might arise, for example, when phallic specializations include traits (such as penile spines) that have the potential to damage the cervix or vagina. For example, Bermant and Westbrook (1966) noted that repeated intromissions by male rats sometimes caused bleeding to occur from the vagina. Hardy and DeBold (1972) recorded the presence of red blood cells in vaginal smears after copulation. In this connection, it is interesting to note that mechanical stimulation of the vagina and cervix in rats has the capacity to block behavioural responsiveness to painful stimulation (such as pinching the female's paw: Komisaruk and Sansone, 2003).

The cervix acts in part as a muscular valve which protects the internal environment of the uterus from outward harm, including possible incursions by bacteria and other pathogens. In many mammals the cervical canal contains a maze of diverticula (e.g. in the cow: Figure 8.11) and these have the capacity to deploy vast numbers of leucocytes that remove pathogens by phagocytosis. In the sheep, the cervix is a long fibrous structure and a series of 4–7 annular folds effectively blocks its central lumen so that it is not possible to insert a catheter during artificial insemination procedures in this species (Fair *et al.*, 2019). Whether it might be possible for a ram to insert the filiform urethral process of the penis into the proximal part of the cervical canal during ejaculation is not known.

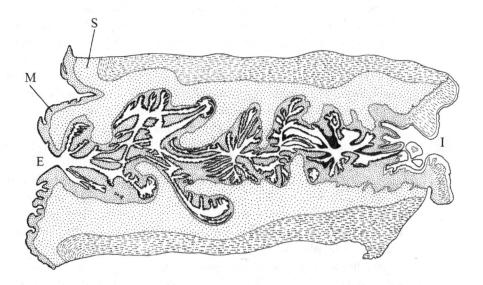

Figure 8.11 A sagittal section through the cervix of the cow, to show its complex internal structure. E, external and I, internal opening of the cervix; M, mucous membrane; S, submucous tissue. (From Harper, 1982.)

Males of those species that are able to deposit their sperm deeper into the cervix, or directly into the uterine cavity, may gain a reproductive advantage over their competitors. However, circumventing the protective barrier imposed by the cervix may impose a cost upon females, for example by causing post-copulatory inflammation of the uterus (e.g. in horses: Katila, 2012) or increasing risks of disease transmission. In this context, it is noteworthy that basal white cell counts are higher in those primate species where females commonly engage in multiple-partner (MP) matings than in species where single-partner (SP) matings are the norm. This may be the result of selection to combat sexually transmitted infections (STIs: Anderson et al., 2004b; Nunn et al., 2000). In the study by Anderson et al., primate genera with MP mating systems ($n = 17$) had average white blood cell counts of 13,200 $\pm$ 322 cells per microlitre, as compared with 8490 $\pm$ 3005 per microlitre in eight genera having SP mating systems ($P < 0.01$). Red cell counts, by contrast, did not differ between these two groups. Subsequent research by Wlasiuk and Nachman (2010) has shown that immunity genes which interact closely with pathogens have undergone more rapid evolution in those primates that have MP mating systems, as is consistent with the STI hypothesis outlined above.

Much more is known about sexually antagonistic coevolution among the invertebrates than is the case for mammals; indeed, it may be useful at this point to consider a few examples. Hypodermic insemination, by which males inject their sperm directly into the female's body cavity, occurs in a number of insects, including bed bugs (Family Cimicidae). The male bed bug employs a sharp, hollow paramere to inject his sperm, which then move through the haemocoel to reach the ovaries. However, in some species females have evolved a specialized paragenital structure, the ectospermalege. Males inject females only at this site, whence their sperm can more readily gain access to the ovaries (Figure 8.12A). From the female perspective, the ectospermalege is adaptive as it lessens the risk of damage inflicted by males that would otherwise inject sperm at random sites (Carayon, 1966). Eberhard (1985) cites a remarkable example, originally described by Mann (1962), of parallel evolution in this regard, involving rhynchobdellid leeches of the Genus *Piscicola*. Leeches are hermaphroditic, and in the rhynchobdellids one individual places a spermatophore on the body of another. The spermatophore penetrates the body wall and releases its sperm into the interior. However, *Piscicola* has developed a specialized paragenital structure (analogous to the ectospermalege of bedbugs) where spermatophores are deposited, rather than at random sites on the body (Figure 8.12B).

Sexually antagonistic coevolution may also involve chemical cues that are present in semen, and which affect the female's physiology or behaviour in ways that are costly to her despite their reproductive benefits to the male. For example, male fruit flies (*Drosophila melanogaster*) are known to transfer more than 120 such seminal proteins to females during copulation (Chapman, 2018). Seminal proteins affect diverse functions, including the female's immune responses, egg production and sperm storage. The peptide Acp70A, produced by the male fruit fly's accessory reproductive glands, stimulates increased egg production by the female, while at the same time reducing her sexual receptivity. Exposure to this 'sex peptide' is physiologically costly to the female, however, as it shortens her lifespan (Chapman, 2018;

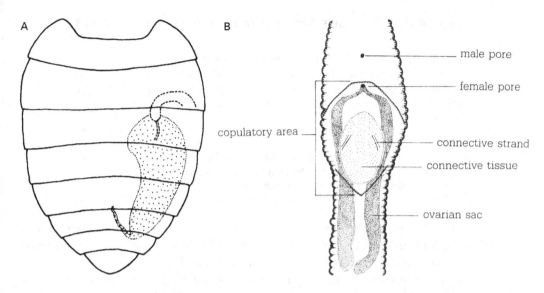

Figure 8.12 Female control of sperm deposition and transport, via paragenital structures in a bedbug and a leech. **A:** In bedbugs of the Genus *Stricticimex*, external and internal structures (the female 'spermalege' organs) route sperm directly to the oviduct. (After Carayon, 1966.) **B:** In the fish leech (*Piscicola geometra*) spermatophores are deposited in a specialized copulatory area, whence sperm migrate via the underlying tissues to the ovarian sacs. (After Mann, 1962.)

Chapman *et al.*, 1995). Morimoto *et al.* (2019) have studied the effects of deleting the sex peptide receptor in females upon their sexual behaviour and reproductive success. Under these conditions, female fruit flies remain sexually receptive; multiple-partner matings are thus more frequent and post-copulatory sexual selection is strengthened. Some males are able to mate repeatedly with individual females and to increase their paternity share.

These studies, and many others that involve invertebrates, should provide ample food for thought for mammalian reproductive physiologists. As discussed in Chapter 7, the accessory reproductive glands of mammals have long been known to secrete a 'bewildering array of chemical constituents' (Setchell *et al.*, 1994). Yet, with a few notable exceptions, the functions of these chemicals remain unknown. No mammalian equivalent of a 'sex peptide' has yet been discovered. The duration of female sexual receptivity is reduced by copulatory stimuli in some species, including guinea pigs (Goldfoot and Goy, 1970), hamsters (Carter, 1973; Huck and Lisk, 1986), rats (Blandau *et al.*, 1941; Hardy and DeBold, 1972), ring-tailed lemurs, greater galagos (Dixson, 2012; Stockley, 2002) and white-tailed deer (White *et al.*, 1995). However, in most cases mechanical stimulation of the vagina and cervix is primarily responsible for producing such effects. While it is true that chemical cues in semen can induce ovulation in some taxa (notably in camelids: Ratto *et al.*, 2019), whether chemical cues might play a role in reducing the duration of sexual receptivity in mammals remains to be established.

Cryptic Female Choice: Sperm Survival, Storage and Transport

Females in animals with internal fertilization have partial or complete control over many processes that can influence a male's chances of fathering their offspring. In an analogy with sporting events, both the characteristics of the playing field on which males are competing and many of the rules by which they must abide are set by the female.

Eberhard (1996)

Surprisingly little is known about what happens to the various components of the ejaculate after deposition in the vagina. It is clear, however, that the ejaculate is not particularly welcome in the female reproductive tract.

Arnqvist and Rowe (2005)

From the moment that spermatozoa enter the female reproductive tract, their survival is determined by the vaginal environment, or (for those species that are intrauterine inseminators) by the environment within the uterus. The evolution of the uterus and cervix in marsupials and placental mammals and the requirement to protect and nurture offspring in the uterus throughout foetal life has led to the development of mechanisms to repel unwanted incursions by bacteria and other pathogens. This is particularly the case in placental mammals, given that their gestation periods are so much longer than those of marsupials, thus placing the offspring at potentially greater risk. In the monotremes, by contrast, the eggshell provides the main protection for the developing offspring, and its sojourn in the female reproductive tract does not require implantation of the zygote or the development of a placenta.

The spermatozoa and accessory glandular secretions that comprise the ejaculate are antigenic, so they constitute a challenge to the female immune system. The arrival of hundreds of millions of spermatozoa, suspended in seminal fluid, in the female tract thus provokes a number of cellular and humoral responses. Phagocytes are released in huge numbers, and these engulf sperm, including immotile or morphologically abnormal gametes. Many spermatozoa are voided from the reproductive tract (Bedford, 1982; Drobnis and Overstreet, 1992; Hogarth, 1982; Overstreet, 1983). These processes represent the first stage in winnowing out less-viable sperm, and thus may constitute mechanisms of cryptic female choice. The seminal plasma contains prostaglandins, proteins, zinc and other trace elements that possess immunosuppressant qualities, as well as polyamines that may counteract the effects of proteolytic enzymes in the female tract (Arnqvist and Rowe, 2005; Hogarth, 1982; Leonhard-Marek, 2000; Mann and Lutwak-Mann, 1981). Sexually antagonistic coevolution may thus have occurred between the immunological and other defence mechanisms deployed by females and countermeasures to increase sperm survival involving the secretions of the male accessory reproductive glands (e.g. the prostate, bulbourethral glands and seminal vesicles). Indeed, the reason for the evolution of such a diverse array of accessory male reproductive glands may relate back to the origins of viviparity in the ancestors of the marsupials and placental mammals, and to the uterine, cervical and immunological specializations that accompanied the transition to viviparous modes of reproduction.

Apart from the female's immune defences, an additional challenge to sperm survival concerns the acidity of the vagina. In the human female, for example, vaginal pH averages 4.5, whereas optimum sperm survival and motility requires neutral or slightly alkaline conditions. As was discussed in Chapter 7, Masters and Johnson (1966) reported that immediately after ejaculation vaginal pH rose to approximately 7.0 in women, due to the buffering effect of seminal fluid. Marked improvements in sperm survival resulted (see Figure 7.9). Not all primates have such low vaginal pH values as human beings, however. This is the case, for example, in *Macaca nemestrina* (pH = 7.6), *Papio anubis* (5.0–5.6), *P. cynocephalus* (5.5) and *Ateles geoffroyi* (6.5). These measurements were all made at around the time of the pre-ovulatory oestrogen peak (Miller *et al.*, 2016). Indeed, human beings are most unusual among mammals in general in having such a low vaginal pH. Elizabeth Miller and her colleagues have examined this phenomenon in detail. They point out that the vaginal biome in human beings is dominated by bacteria belonging to the Genus *Lactobacillus*, unlike other mammals in which lactobacilli rarely account for more than 1 per cent of the overall bacterial population. Miller *et al.* (2016) propose that the large amount of starch included in human diets favours the proliferation of lactobacilli and results in lower pH values than in other mammals (Figure 8.13).

Although the vaginal biome and very low vaginal pH values of women are unusual among mammals, and the ability of human semen to buffer vaginal pH is pronounced, it is likely that semen also serves to raise vaginal pH and assist sperm survival and motility in many other mammals. Twelve of the 22 species represented in Figure 8.13 have average pH values of less than 7, so that mating with males having higher pH values in their semen should be expected to produce some buffering effect. Indeed, measurements of seminal pH in a variety of placental mammals have provided remarkably consistent results, with pH values averaging between 7 and 8 in most cases (Table 8.4).

Sperm motility is important in assisting sperm survival and migration from the vagina into the cervix. However, it is the rhythmic contractions of the female's reproductive tract that are mainly responsible for transporting the male gametes to the oviducts. At the level of the uterus, for example, oestrogen stimulates contractions of the uterine myometrium, which increase in strength during oestrus (e.g. in the ewe: Ramondt *et al.*, 1994). Events that occur during copulation are also important in this context; thus, oestrogens are also present in boar semen (Langendijk *et al.*, 2005). Given that a large volume of semen is deposited directly into the sow's uterus during copulation, oestrogens provided by the male may thus augment uterine contractions that control sperm transport. In addition, sows exhibit large increases in circulating oxytocin in response to mating, beginning 2 minutes after the onset of ejaculation and lasting for up to 40 minutes (Claus and Schams, 1990). Copulatory increases in circulating oxytocin have also been measured in female goats (McNeilly and Folley, 1970) and in women (Carmichael *et al.*, 1987). Thus oxytocin, which causes smooth muscle contractions, might also affect sperm transport. Wildt *et al.* (1998) have shown experimentally that exogenous oxytocin stimulates uterine contractions in women.

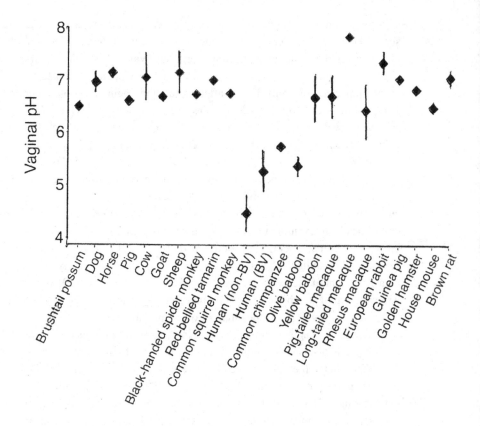

Figure 8.13 Measurements of human vaginal pH compared to data on other mammals. Diamonds indicate overall mean values for each species and standard deviations are shown as vertical bars. Data for a group of women with bacterial vaginosis (BV) are shown separately from a non-BV group. (Modified and redrawn from Miller *et al.*, 2016.)

As Martin (2013) has pointed out: 'when moving unaided, human sperm can swim about 7 inches per hour. At that rate it would take at least 45 minutes to cover the distance from the neck of the womb to the lower end of the oviduct'. In reality, the first cohort of sperm reaches the human oviduct anywhere between 5 and 45 minutes after insemination (Settlage *et al.*, 1973). A similar phase of rapid sperm transport to the oviducts after copulation has also been described in a number of mammals, taking several minutes in rabbits, 2–13 minutes in cows,15 minutes in guinea pigs, mice, rats and sows, and a minimum of 6 minutes in sheep (Harper, 1982, 1994). It has often been stated that sperm conveyed during this initial rapid transport phase are unlikely to fertilize ova, as they arrive in the oviduct and are voided into the peritoneal cavity well before ovulation has occurred. However, it should be kept in mind that in mammals which lack rigidly controlled periods of female receptivity ('oestrus'), rapid sperm transport might favour males of polygynandrous species that succeed in mating closest

Table 8.4 pH of semen in placental mammals

Species	Latin name	pH range (mean)	Source
Chinchilla	*Chinchilla lanigera*	7.0–7.6 (7.3)	Busso *et al.*, 2005
European rabbit	*Oryctolagus cuniculus*	(7.48)	Fallas-López *et al.*, 2011
Domestic pig	*Sus scrofa*	6.7–8.3 (7.5)	McPherson *et al.*, 2014
Chacoan peccary	*Catagonus wagneri*	(7.7)	Goblet *et al.*, 2018
Red deer	*Cervus elaphus*	6.07–8.69	Giżewski, 2004
Domestic goat	*Capra aegagrus hircus*	(7.4)	Türk *et al.*, 2011
Banteng	*Bos javanicus*	(7.04)	Sarsaifi *et al.*, 2013
Malayan tapir	*Tapirus indicus*	7.0–8.0 (7.7)	Tipkantha *et al.*, 2011
Rhinoceros spp.*		7.9–9.0 (8.5)	Roth *et al.*, 2005
Domestic horse	*Equus caballus*	(7.62)	Dowsett and Knott, 1996
Iberian lynx	*Lynx pardinus*	7.5–8.3 (8.0)	Gañán *et al.*, 2009
Coati	*Nasua nasua*	7.0–8.5 (7.8)**	
		8.0–9.0 (8.5)***	Barros et al., 2009
Bottlenose dolphin	*Tursiops truncatus*	(7.0)	Van der Horst *et al.*, 2018
African elephant	*Loxodonta africana*	(7.4)	Howard *et al.*, 1984
Indian elephant	*Elephas maximus*	(7.6)	Imrat *et al.*, 2013

* Roth *et al.* reported a single average pH measurement for *Rhinoceros unicornis*, *Diceros bicornis* and *Ceratotherium simum*.
** pH of samples collected from animals under ketamine anaesthesia;
*** pH of samples collected under tileamine zolazepam anaesthesia.

to ovulation. This might be the case, for example, in some primate species, such as macaques and chimpanzees (Dixson, 2018). This could only apply, however, if sperm transported rapidly to the oviduct could then remain there long enough to undergo capacitation, which is essential for fertilization to occur.

Once the rapid transport phase is over, the majority of sperm are transported more slowly through the female tract, and they interact extensively with its epithelial lining and mucus secretions as they do so. Temporary storage of sperm in crypts, or attachment to epithelial surfaces, occurs at certain points in the cervix, uterus, uterotubal junction and oviduct, depending upon the species considered. The vast majority of sperm will fail to fertilize ova; there are thus many possibilities for cryptic female choice to occur during sperm transport and storage, as is discussed in the sections that follow.

The ability of spermatozoa to enter the cervix is greatly facilitated by changes in the composition of the cervical mucus at around the time of ovulation. Rising levels of oestrogen stimulate the formation of large amounts of a more watery type of mucus, and in some species the cervical canal widens, so that quantities of mucus protrude from the os cervix into the upper vault of the vagina (Katz *et al.*, 1997; Suarez and Pacey, 2006). For example, the water content of human cervical mucus rises to 98 per cent during the peri-ovulatory period and contains a glycoprotein which gives the mucus an elastic quality ('spinnbarkheit') so that it readily forms into long fibrils (Yudin *et al.*, 1989). Motile sperm are better able to penetrate and swim through mucus of this type; human sperm move through cervical mucus at 0.1–3.0 mm per minute when observed *in vitro* (Harper, 1982). Many sperm that migrate from the vagina are guided along mucus strands to enter the cervical crypts, where they are stored and subsequently released over the course of several days (Harper, 1982; Moghissi, 1984). Insler *et al.* (1980) estimated that 100,000–200,000 sperm were present in the cervical crypts of women 2 hours after artificial insemination, most of the gametes having passed through the cervix to enter higher levels of the tract. Gould *et al.* (1984) recovered human sperm from the cervical mucus (not from the crypt contents) for up to 5 days after insemination. Fertilizing capacity was detected for up to 3 days; the upper limits for sperm survival and fertilizing ability are not known, however.

The cervical crypts probably play an important role as temporary storage sites for sperm in many mammals. Tyndale-Biscoe and Rodger (1978), for example, noted that sperm are stored in the cervices of tammar wallabies and released gradually during the first 24 hours after copulation. Figure 8.14 shows the results of a histological study carried out by Hafez and Jaszczak (see Hafez, 1973) to examine sperm migration through the cervix of the rhesus macaque (*Macaca mulatta*) after copulation. Cervical morphology varies considerably among macaque species, all of which mate polygyn-andrously as discussed earlier. In female rhesus macaques the cervical canal is long and serpentine when viewed in sagittal section. By one hour after copulation, sperm-atozoa are distributed in a gradient, with largest numbers in the lowest limb of the 'S'-shaped cervical canal and its associated crypts. Much smaller numbers of sperm occupy the canal and crypts of the distal cervix, closer to its internal os and to the uterine cavity. In addition to the effects of sperm motility, the female's anatomy and physiology probably play a major role in determining gamete distribution. Thus, in their histological study of a closely related macaque species (*M. fascicularis*), Jaszczak and Hafez (1972) noted that 'although spermatozoa appeared to migrate at random, they were often densely crowded in strands of mucus. Some strands of mucus containing spermatozoa disappeared into the crypts of cervical mucosa, while others continued through the internal os to the uterus'.

The possibilities for sperm selection to occur at the level of the cervix are also illustrated by Mullins and Saacke's (1989) study of the bovine cervix. Figure 8.11 shows the internal structure of a cow's cervix, viewed in sagittal section. This two-dimensional representation of the cervix only partially captures its anatomical com-plexity, however. Mullins and Saacke used serial sections of the bovine cervix to create a three-dimensional model of its overall structure. They found that deep longitudinal grooves are present, which lead directly from the external os cervix to the uterus. Mucus deep within these grooves is less dense than that which fills the cervical canal during the follicular phase of the ovarian cycle. Motile sperm that gain access to these deep grooves are probably better able to reach the uterus than those that become entrapped in denser mucus, within the central lumen of the cervix.

Mechanisms of sperm transport and storage have been studied in very few carni-vores; the most detailed research has involved the domestic dog (*Canis familiaris*: England *et al.*, 2006). Unusual features have been described in both sexes of this

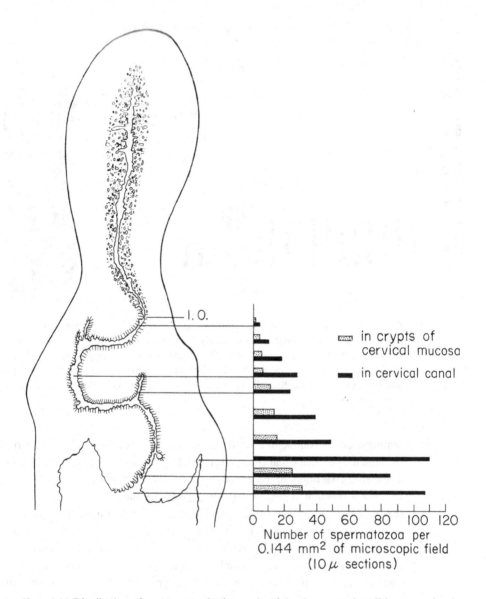

Figure 8.14 Distribution of spermatozoa in the cervix of the rhesus monkey (*Macaca mulatta*) one hour after copulation. Open bars, numbers of sperm in the cervical crypts; closed bars, numbers of sperm in the cervical canal. IO, internal cervical os. (After Hafez, 1973.)

species, some of which are likely to apply to canids in general. Females ovulate immature primary oocytes, which are not ready for fertilization until 2–3 days later; the oocytes of dogs may thus remain viable for 7–8 days after ovulation. Once sperm have entered the female tract they too have an extended lifespan (up to 11 days: Doak *et al.*, 1967). The female's cervix remains open throughout oestrus, and

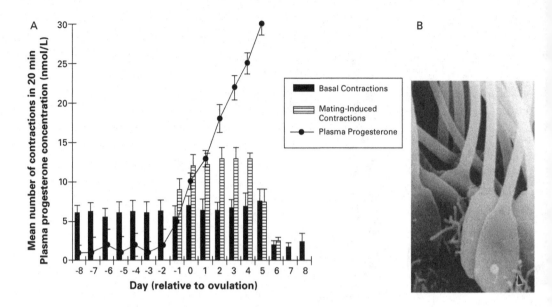

Figure 8.15 A: Numbers of spontaneous and mating-induced uterine contractions in female domestic dogs (*Canis familiaris*) and levels of plasma progesterone in relation to the estimated day of ovulation. Data are means ± SEM for uterine contractions per 20 minutes, and nanomoles per litre of progesterone. **B:** A scanning electron micrograph showing sperm heads attached to uterine epithelial cells 12 hours after copulation in the domestic dog. (After England *et al.*, 2006.)

mating-induced contractions of the vagina and uterus enhance the transport of semen through the cervical canal (Figure 8.15A). Large numbers of spermatozoa then attach to the epithelial lining of the uterus (Figure 8.15B), while others are transported to the uterotubal junction. Thus, in dogs, it is primarily the uterus and uterotubal junction that act as temporary storage sites for spermatozoa, rather than the cervical crypts and isthmus of the oviduct, as is the case in bovids, primates and many other mammals.

Spermatozoa do not pass freely from the uterus into the oviduct; the uterotubal junction acts as a filtering mechanism and temporary storage site for sperm in ways that are not fully understood and which differ among species. The structure of the uterotubal junction has been documented in very few mammals. For a review that deals mainly with domesticated species (e.g. the horse, pig, cow, sheep, rabbit and dog), readers may consult Hook and Hafez (1968). These authors also described its structure in two of the non-human primates (*Macaca nemestrina* and *M. mulatta*) and reviewed the available literature on other mammals (including rodents). A number of accounts are available concerning the human uterotubal junction (e.g. Fadel *et al.*, 1976). Most recently, Penfold *et al.* (2019) have described the anatomy and histology of the uterotubal junction of the cheetah (*Aconomyx jubatus*). This last report is unusual, however, as few data are available on the anatomy and physiology of the uterotubal junction in any of the non-domesticated species. Further comparative research is badly needed in this area.

There is some experimental evidence indicating that the human uterotubal junction might act reflexively as a one-way valve, allowing sperm to enter the isthmus of the oviduct (Shafik, 1996). In cattle, a vascular plexus in the wall of the junction can become filled with blood and compress the lumen, thus acting as a valve (Wrobel *et al.*, 1993). In the uterotubal junction of the sow, an infundibular–cornual ligament contracts rhythmically during the peri-ovulatory period. This may be a mechanism for filtering or transporting sperm (Persson and Rodriguez-Martinez, 1990). Normal motility can be important if sperm are to pass through the uterotubal junction (golden hamster: Smith *et al.*, 1988; rat: Gaddum-Rosse, 1981). Proteins on the sperm head are also important, such as ADAM3 in the mouse (Yamaguchi *et al.*, 2009), and sperm may attach temporarily to the uterotubal epithelium.

Sperm are also stored in the distal uterotubal junction in dogs (England *et al.*, 2006), in pigs (Viring *et al.*, 1980) and also in the alpaca, where the uterotubal junction serves as the major site of sperm storage (Bravo *et al.*, 1996). These authors conducted experiments to determine the time course for the transport of sperm and ova after copulation in the alpaca. The data concerning sperm transport and storage are shown in Figure 8.16. Alpacas are induced ovulators and intrauterine inseminators; ovulation occurs 24 hours after copulation. The majority of spermatozoa are stored in the uterotubal junction, and some have also entered the oviduct by 6 hours after copulation. Maximum numbers of sperm are present in the isthmus of the oviduct by 18 hours and continue to be present at lower numbers for up to 30 hours. Few spermatozoa were recovered from the ampulla of the oviduct (the presumptive site of fertilization) during these experiments. Numbers averaged 108 (maximum 416) in alpacas, as is consistent with data for other placental mammals (Table 8.1). The exact timing of fertilization was not determined, but fertilized ova at the morula (4–8 blastomere) stage were recovered 4 days after copulation, which was the earliest time at which samples were collected.

After spermatozoa have passed through the uterotubal junction, they interact in complex ways with the physical and chemical milieu of the oviduct. As sperm enter the isthmus, their progress is slowed by mucus in its lumen, and they become attached temporarily to epithelial cells. This process has been studied in a few domestic livestock species and in some laboratory mammals, but very little is known concerning sperm–oviductal interactions in the majority of mammals. In cattle, seminal plasma proteins on the surface of the sperm acrosome bind to fucose-containing ligands on cilia lining the isthmus (Figure 8.17). A number of proteins (annexins) also form part of the receptor mechanism (Ignotz *et al.*, 2007). A reservoir of inactive gametes is thus produced and, as the time for ovulation to occur approaches, they gradually undergo important changes (capacitation and flagellar hyperactivation) that prepare them to pass onward to the ampulla of the oviduct, to undergo the acrosome reaction and to fertilize ova (Suarez, 2007, 2008a, 2010).

In some marsupials, spermatozoa are trapped temporarily in specialized mucosal crypts in the isthmus rather than attaching to the oviductal epithelium. This is the case in the Virginia opossum (*Didephis virginiana*: Rodger and Bedford, 1982), and in dasyurids such as the agile *Antechinus* (*A. agilis*: Shimmin *et al.*, 1999) and the

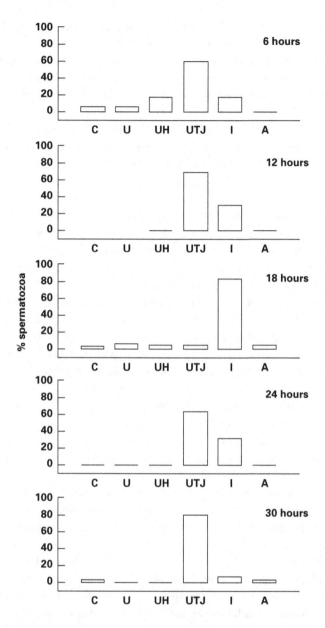

Figure 8.16 Percentage of spermatozoa present in the cervix (C), uterus (U), uterine horns (UH), uterotubal junction (UTJ), isthmus (I) and ampulla (A) of female alpacas at different times after copulation. (After Bravo *et al.*, 1996.)

fat-tailed dunnart (*Sminthopsis crassicaudata*: Bedford and Breed, 1994). Storage crypts also occur in shrews (Order Eulipotyphla) and these exhibit some unusual variations (Figure 8.18). In the Asian house shrew (*Suncus murinus*: Figure 8.18E) sperm are stored for about 12 hours in isthmic crypts, at which point some are released

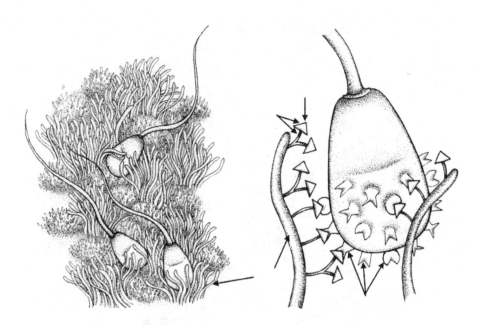

Figure 8.17 Binding interaction between cattle spermatozoa and the oviducal epithelium. **Left:** Low magnification, illustrating that spermatozoa bind primarily to cilia via the acrosomal region of the head. **Right:** High magnification diagram of the binding of bovine seminal plasma proteins (PDC-109, BSP-A3 and BSP-30-kDa) on the plasma membrane overlying the sperm acrosome to fucose-containing ligands on the surface of cilia. (From Suarez, 2007.)

and small numbers of them finally reach the ampulla, where fertilization occurs. In the greater white-toothed shrew (*Crocidura russula*) sperm also exit the isthmic crypts after 12 hours or so; larger numbers migrate to the ampulla where 'most are trapped by a few bubble-like crypts (Figure 8.18D), whilst others pass onwards to the fertilization site at the top of the oviduct' (Bedford *et al.*, 2004). In the North American least shrew (*Cryptotis parva*), which at 7.5 cm long is one of the world's smallest mammals, fertilization also occurs in the upper oviduct. Sperm are not stored in the isthmus; instead, they enter crypts in the ampulla (Figure 8.18C), from which small numbers are released at the time of ovulation. The final example, shown in Figure 8.18B, is the African mouse shrew (*Myosorex varius*), which stores sperm in deep crypts in the isthmus and also throughout the ampulla. The site of ovulation is not indicated in Figure 8.18B, as only a single female has been studied, and in this case sperm were found only in the ampullary crypts (Bedford *et al.*, 2004).

These examples of unusual sperm storage and fertilization sites in shrews provide exceptions to the general rule that, in placental mammals, sperm attach temporarily to the epithelium in the isthmus and fertilization occurs in the ampulla of the oviduct. Among the marsupials fertilization probably occurs at the top of the oviduct, rather than in the ampulla (Tyndale-Biscoe, 2005). As large numbers of spermatozoa pass through the length of the oviduct and enter the peritoneal cavity in many mammals,

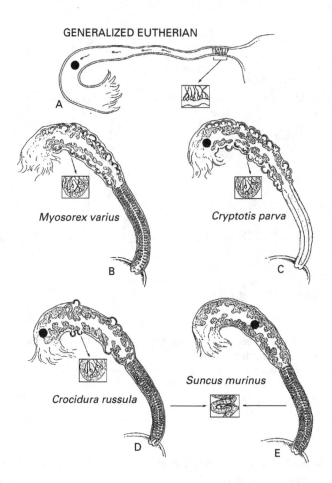

GENERALIZED EUTHERIAN

A

Myosorex varius

B

Cryptotis parva

C

Crocidura russula

D

Suncus murinus

E

Figure 8.18 Distribution of spermatozoa in the oviduct during the pre- and peri-ovulatory (fertilization) period in **A:** a generalized placental (eutherian) mammal, as compared to four genera of shrews (**B–E**), belonging to the Order Eulipotyphla. The inserts show regions where spermatozoa are initially housed, either as free motile cells in crypts (in shrews), or attached to the epithelium (as in most placental species). Subsequently, a few spermatozoa are released around the time of ovulation and migrate to the site of fertilization, indicated by the black circles. (From Bedford *et al.*, 2004.)

the question arises as to whether sperm might enter the follicles in the ovary and fertilize ova *in situ*. Remarkably, this is the case in one group of Afrotherians, the tenrecs (Nicoll and Racey, 1985). Given the extent of mammalian diversity, it is likely that further unusual specializations remain to be discovered.

Much also remains to be learned about how interactions between the oviducts and spermatozoa affect post-copulatory sexual selection. Consider, for example, a female sheep, dolphin, rat or chimpanzee that mates with multiple partners prior to ovulating. Do spermatozoa from all of these males succeed in reaching the oviductal storage site? If so, are gametes of some males more successful than others in undergoing capacitation and hyperactivation? Are the sperm of some males more successful in disengaging from the epithelia of the storage site and ascending the oviduct to encounter the ova? There are currently no definitive answers to these questions.

Experiments using domestic pigs have shown that differential activation or suppression of motility in subpopulations of sperm within the isthmus may play a key role in sperm selection (Satake *et al.*, 2006). The mammalian oviduct has increasingly become recognized as being an important arena for cryptic female choice, as well as for sperm competition (e.g. Holt and Fazeli, 2016). In this regard, it is interesting that the oviducts of mammals differ considerably in their length in relation to body size (Hunter, 1988). Measurements of the (extramural) portion of the oviduct in 48 species, representing 33 genera of mammals (Anderson *et al.*, 2006), have shown that residuals of oviduct length are positively correlated with relative testes sizes (Figure 8.19) and also with sperm midpiece volumes. Perhaps longer oviducts might test the ability of the gametes of rival males to migrate from the isthmus of the oviduct to the site of fertilization in the ampulla.

In addition to its anatomical and physiological specializations, the oviduct may possess genetic mechanisms for filtering and and screening spermatozoa. In mice, for example, it has been shown that spermatozoa trigger a number of changes in the oviductal transcriptome (Fazeli *et al.*, 2004). Elegant experiments involving bilateral laparoscopic insemination of either X or Y chromosome-bearing sperm into the oviducts of pigs have demonstrated that certain genomic responses are sex-specific (Almiñana *et al.*, 2014). These authors suggest that such sex-specific oviductal responses to spermatozoa might represent 'a gender biasing mechanism controlled by the female'. If this is correct, then cryptic female choice for either X- or Y-bearing sperm might explain adaptive skewing of birth sex ratios in mammals, as is hypothesized to occur if healthy/ high-ranking females benefit from producing more sons than daughters (Trivers and Willard, 1973). Skewing of birth sex ratios has been reported for a number of mammals (Clutton-Brock and Iason, 1986). For example, dominant red deer hinds give birth to more sons (Clutton-Brock *et al.*, 1984), and in wild horses mares in good condition are more likely to produce male foals (Cameron *et al.*, 1999). Yet many other studies have produced inconsistent results (e.g. see Brown and Silk, 2002, for an insightful review of the primate data). However, a meta-analysis by Cameron (2004) concluded that publications dealing with maternal condition at the time of conception strongly support the conclusion that mothers in good condition are more likely to give birth to sons.

Figure 8.20 shows Yanagimachi's (1994) concept of relationships between sperm capacitation, hyperactivation of motility and the acrosome reaction. The phenomenon of capacitation was discovered by Chang (1951) and Austin (1951), who independently reported that a period of exposure to the female reproductive tract and its fluids is necessary for spermatozoa to acquire the ability to fertilize ova. The mechanisms that control capacitation have mainly been studied *in vitro*, but doubts have arisen as to whether the results accurately reflect events that occur in living animals. Hunter and Rodriguez-Martinez (2004), for example, suggest that capacitation 'represents an active and specific coordination within succeeding regions of the female tract and one that is synchronized with the time of ovulation'.

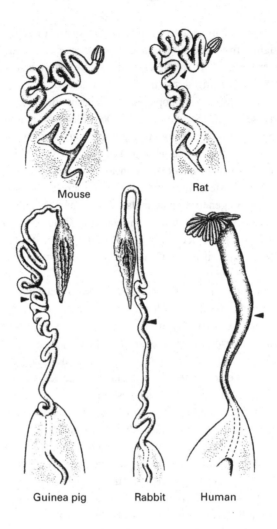

Mouse

Rat

Guinea pig   Rabbit   Human

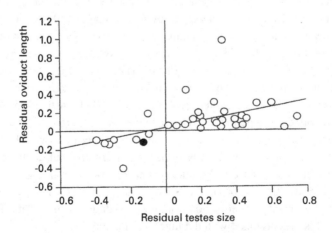

Figure 8.19 Upper: Examples of oviductal morphologies in mammals, to illustrate differences in the length and degree of coiling of the fallopian tubes. The arrows indicate the approximate

Hyperactivation of spermatozoa involves vigorous asymmetrical flagellar movements (Figure 8.20B). This type of motility was initially described in hamster sperm, but was subsequently identified in several other rodent species, as well as in cattle, sheep, dogs, dolphins and primates (Yanagimachi, 1970, 1994). The physiological mechanisms that cause the onset of hyperactivated motility are unknown, but are almost certainly triggered by the female, either by secretions of the oviductal epithelium or via chemical signals released after ovulation from the cumulus cells that surround the ova (Suarez, 2008a).

Hyperactivation may help spermatozoa to break free from their attachments to the epithelium in the isthmus, and to move through the fibroelastic mucus of the oviductal lumen. Sperm thus gradually migrate to the ampulla, partly as a result of their own motility but also as a result of muscular contractions of the oviduct walls (Suarez, 2008b). The ova, meanwhile, are transported by the fimbriae to the entrance of the oviduct, and thence by continued ciliary and muscular action to the ampulla. The numbers of fimbriae and their lengths vary considerably among species. For example, in guinea pigs and rabbits they are elongated, whereas the ostium of the human oviduct is surrounded by much shorter fimbriae (see Figure 8.19). The hormonal control of the ciliation of the fimbriae and mechanisms of 'ovum pickup' have been studied in various domesticated mammals. However, phylogenetic differences in fimbrial morphology and their possible functional significance (e.g. in monotocous versus polytocous taxa) remain to be explored.

The oviduct and the ovum and its vestments all play crucial roles in guiding spermatozoa to the site of fertilization; both thermotaxis and chemotaxis have been implicated in this process (Eisenbach and Giojalas, 2006). A temperature gradient occurs in the oviduct (e.g. in rabbits: David *et al.*, 1972; and pigs: Hunter and Nicol, 1986), the ampulla being 1–2°C warmer than the sperm storage site. This temperature difference becomes most pronounced at around the time of ovulation, due to a decrease in temperature at the storage site (e.g. in the rabbit: Bahat *et al.*, 2005). It is likely that thermotaxis may serve as an initial guide for sperm, whereas chemotactic cues probably come into play once the male gametes reach the vicinity of ova (Bahat *et al.*, 2003).

Results of experiments conducted *in vitro* have shown that spermatozoa exhibit chemotaxis towards mammalian follicular fluid. However, follicular fluid is released only once, at the time of ovulation, whereas chemotaxis of sperm *in vivo* would be expected to involve cues that continue for as long as viable ova remain in the oviduct. Indeed, the ovum and the cumulus cells which surround it emit chemical signals that attract spermatozoa (Eisenbach and Giojalas, 2006).

There appears to be a lack of species specificity in the chemotactic responses shown *in vitro* by mammalian spermatozoa to follicular fluids and a variety of chemicals

Figure 8.19 (cont.) position of the junction between the isthmus and ampulla. (From Dixson, 2009; after Harper, 1982.) **Lower:** Correlation between oviductal length and relative testes size in mammals. Data for *Homo sapiens* (●) are included for comparative purposes. (From Dixson, 2009; redrawn and modified from Anderson *et al.*, 2006.)

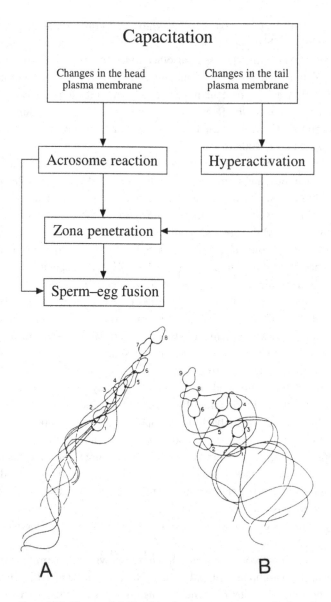

Figure 8.20 Upper: Relationships between sperm capacitation, the acrosome reaction and hyperactivation. (Redrawn from Yanagimachi, 1994.) **Lower:** Diagrams of human sperm (**A**) before and (**B**) after hyperactivation of motility. (From Yanagimachi, 1994; after Morales *et al.*, 1988.)

(Sun *et al.*, 2003). This is very different from the situation that pertains in some aquatic invertebrates where fertilization occurs externally, and where sperm and ova are released into the surrounding water. Cross-species fertilization might easily occur under these conditions, and this may be why species-specific chemotactic mechanisms are well developed (e.g in abalone: Riffell *et al.*, 2004). Sperm chemotaxis also affects individual reproductive success in sea urchins (Hussain *et al.*, 2016), indicating that sexual selection operates at this level. Although internal fertilization in mammals might be expected to reduce the requirement for species-specific chemotactic signals, the Class Mammalia is large and phylogenetically diverse. So few mammals have been studied that the existence of species-specific chemical cues should not be discounted.

Only spermatozoa that have undergone capacitation are capable of exhibiting chemotaxis, and only capacitated sperm are able to fertilize ova. For the very small numbers of spermatozoa that succeed in negotiating the oviduct and contacting ova, one final hurdle remains: to penetrate the layer of cumulus cells and the zona pellucida, and to enter the ovum. Once a sperm attaches to the zona pellucida, the acrosomal contents are released (the acrosome reaction). These contain hydrolytic enzymes that may assist the sperm in penetrating the ovum vestments (Kim *et al.*, 2008). However, it is possible that the mechanical interaction between the sperm and the ovum may be crucial, as Bedford has explained in the following personal communication to the author (see also Bedford, 2008):

I believe that current evidence supports the once-heretical view that sperm penetration of the eutherian zona depends wholly or largely on physical thrust, not to any major extent (and likely not at all) on lysis by acrosomal enzymes, and that this new mode is reflected in the unique design (and oscillating behavior) of the eutherian sperm head.

Hyperactivation of motility may therefore be important in enabling the sperm to thrust its way through the zona pellucida, and to enter the ovum, where the nuclei of the two gametes fuse together (Quill *et al.*, 2003). Only one spermatozoan completes the fertilization process; the ovum blocks further entry of sperm and thus reduces the risk that polyspermy might occur. Although interactions between sperm and ova are often represented as being dominated by the male gamete, the ovum is far from passive during the process of fertilization. Bronson (1998) has even compared fertilization to phagocytosis; the ovum 'incorporates' the sperm, rather than being 'penetrated' by it (Figure 8.21). Therefore, selection of sperm by cryptic female choice might also be possible during the sequence of interactions described above.

Polyovulation and Cryptic Female Choice

The occurrence of polyovulation in females of a small number of species belonging to six orders of mammals was discussed in Chapter 2. Polyovulation has been described in some members of the Order Dasyuromorphia (e.g. the Tasmanian devil: Hughes, 1982), in five species of elephant shrews (Order Macroscelidea) including the round-eared sengi (Schubert *et al.*, 2009), in some rodents (e.g. the plains viscacha: Flamini *et al.*, 2020; Weir, 1971), some tenrecs (Order Afrosorida), two species of bats (Chiroptera) and the pronghorn (Order Cetartiodactyla).

The plains viscacha presents the most extreme example of this unusual phenomenon, as females may release between 50 and 845 ova during a single cycle, yet only

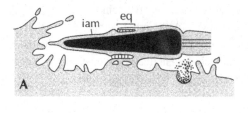

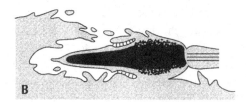

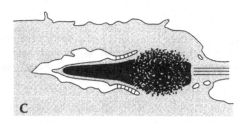

Figure 8.21 Diagram of the adhesion and subsequent incorporation of a mammalian sperm by the oocyte. **A:** Plasma membrane fusion occurs at the equatorial segment (eq) of the acrosome-reacted sperm head and the oolemma. iam, inner acrosomal membrane. **B:** Oolemma microvilli engulf the sperm. Early nuclear decondensation is visible. **C:** The rostral portion of the sperm is engulfed in an oolemma-derived vesicle. (Modified by Bronson, 1998 from Bedford, 1982.)

two offspring are produced (Weir, 1971). Figure 8.22 shows the uterus of of a viscacha containing seven developing embryos, six of which are undergoing resorption. The female thus exerts considerable control over the processes that govern implantation and survival of embryos. Dizygotic twinning is the norm in the plains viscacha (e.g. in 55 of 61 litters examined by Weir, 1971), and also in the pronghorn, big brown bat and those elephant shrews that exhibit polyovulation.

Birney and Baird (1985) attempted to account for the evolution of polyovulation in those taxa where twinning occurs, on the basis that it allows the female to ensure that only one embryo remains in each uterine horn (usually the embryo that is situated closest to the cervix) whilst others are resorbed. This hypothesis is unsatisfactory as it seems unlikely that such high rates of ovulation as those that occur in viscachas could have undergone positive selection solely on this basis. It also fails to account for polyovulation in tenrecs that produce large litters, or in the Tasmanian devil where the

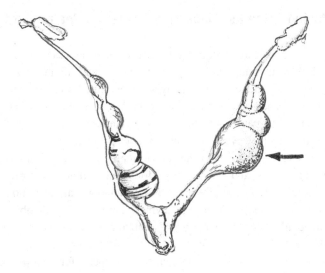

Figure 8.22 The reproductive tract of a pregnant female plains viscacha (*Lagostomus maximus*). The uterine horns contain seven embryos, only one of which is viable (as indicated by the arrow). The others are undergoing resorption. (Author's drawing from a photograph in Weir, 1971.)

average litter size is greater than two and much of foetal development occurs in the mother's pouch (which contains four nipples) rather than in the uterus alone.

Kozlowski and Stearns (1989) examined two further hypotheses that seek to explain the evolution of polyovulation and the over-production of zygotes by some plants and animals. The first hypothesis ('bet-hedging') may apply if the optimal litter size is subject to unpredictable environmental conditions. Females therefore produce excess zygotes so that litter size 'can be flexibly adjusted downward to the optimum number for that attempt'. The second hypothesis (selective abortion) better accounts for culling of embryos at very early stages of development in species where environmental conditions are more predictable. This posits that females produce large numbers of ova and zygotes in order to 'identify those with the highest fitness expectations, then kill or abandon those with lower fitness'.

The selective abortion hypothesis fits closely with the likely operation of cryptic female choice in mammals that exhibit polyovulation. By this mechanism females that mate with multiple partners would be able to dispense with genetically less fit potential offspring at a very early stage of development, whilst favouring the full development of others. Polyovulation may indeed represent an unusual but potentially highly effective type of cryptic female choice. The application of this hypothesis to the five species of elephant shrews in which polyovulation occurs may be criticized on the grounds that they are considered to be monogamous. However, as discussed in earlier chapters, 'social monogamy' does not necessarily equate to 'sexual monogamy' in mammals, and too little is known about sexual interactions and paternity in elephant shrews to conclude that they are monogamous.

Some Concluding Remarks Concerning Long-term Sperm Storage

The examples of sperm storage within the female reproductive tract discussed in this chapter have dealt with retention of spermatozoa at sites in the cervix, uterus, uterotubal junction and oviduct for relatively short periods, lasting in most cases for a few days or a week. The gradual release of sperm from these temporary storage sites ensures that a supply of gametes passes gradually through the oviduct during the female's fertile period. However, in some vertebrates, including many species of reptiles and fish, sperm are stored in the female reproductive tract for much longer periods, lasting for months, and in some cases for years (Birkhead and Møller, 1993; Holt, 2011). Such long-term sperm storage is rare among mammals, however. For example, given their unique status as egg-laying mammals, it is possible that long-term sperm storage might occur in monotremes but, to my knowledge, no evidence for this has yet come to light.

Bats are the only mammals that are known to store sperm for long periods within the female reproductive tract. Thus, in many species of vespertilionids, some rhino-lophids and a few other bat taxa, females store sperm for prolonged periods (Racey, 1979; Wimsatt, 1942, 1944). Many of these bats live at higher latitudes and are seasonal breeders; they mate in the autumn months, but then hibernate over the winter. Females, however, delay ovulation until the following spring (April/May). Fertilization then occurs, using sperm stored during the previous autumn, and the resulting offspring are born during the summer when conditions for their survival are more favourable. Thus, the evolution of sperm storage is linked to female reproductive strategies that separate the events of ovulation from copulation. This gives females maximum control over when fertilization, pregnancy and birth will occur. Some examples of the storage times for spermatozoa in various bat species are shown in Table 8.5, which also presents information about the storage sites involved (in the uterus, uterotubal junction and oviduct).

Table 8.5 Some examples of sperm storage times and storage sites in the reproductive tracts of female bats

Storage time (days)		Storage site	
Pipistrellus ceylonicus	16	*Scotophilus heathi*	UT
Tylonycteris pachypus	21	*Pipistrellus abramus*	UT
Myotis sodalis	68	*Chalinolobus gouldii*	UTJ
Myotis lucifugus	138	*Myotis daubentoni*	UTJ
P. pipistrellus	151	*Miniopterus schreibersi*	UTJ
Eptesicus fuscus	156	*Rhinolophus ferrimequinum*	OV
P. abramus	175	*Myotis natteri*	OV
Nyctalus noctula	198	*Tylonycteris robusta*	OV

UT, Uterus; UTJ, uterotubal junction; OV, oviduct. (Data are from Mori *et al.*, 1982; Racey, 1979; and sources cited therein.)

The vespertilionid bats have large testes in relation to their body weights, and many of them also have multiple-partner mating systems, traits that are indicative of sexual selection by sperm competition (Wilkinson and McCracken, 2003). Males as well as females store spermatozoa; in the common noctule bat (*Nyctalus noctula*), for example, males continue to store sperm in the cauda epididymis during the winter, long after their testes have regressed (Racey, 1974). Indeed, males of a number of species have also been observed copulating with females during the winter months (Racey, 1979). Thus, the sperm stores of female bats may contain gametes originating from a number of males. Given that the survival as well as the release of sperm from storage sites is governed by the female's anatomy and physiology, there is considerable potential for cryptic female choice, as well as sperm competition, to occur.

It used to be thought that prolonged storage of sperm (for up to 30 days) might also occur in hares (Martinet and Raynaud, 1972, 1975). Female hares exhibit superfoetation: the ability of the pregnant female to initiate another pregnancy before the first one is complete. However, experiments by Roellig *et al.* (2010) have shown that although superfoetation certainly does occur in captive and free-ranging European hares, fertilization is not due to long-term storage of sperm. Instead, the pregnant female becomes sexually receptive and mates again and a second litter is sired as a result. The fertilized ova remain in the oviduct until the first litter is born.

9 The Evolution of Mating-induced and Spontaneous Ovulation

> In agreement with other authors we feel that animals cannot be separated into those that ovulate spontaneously and those ovulate reflexly, as there is clearly a continuum
>
> Weir and Rowlands, 1973

In most marsupials and placental mammals such as the primates, perissodactyls and elephants, as well as many rodents and artiodactyls, females ovulate 'spontaneously', meaning that ovulation proceeds in the absence of copulation. However, in certain species, such as rabbits, cats, and ferrets, stimulation provided by the male partner during mating is required to trigger the pre-ovulatory LH surge and thus to induce ovulation. Often, tactile stimulation during mating triggers ovulation, but in certain cases chemical cues, present in the semen, stimulate the LH surge. Examples of this latter type occur in members of the Family Camelidae, which includes the llamas and alpacas, as well as the dromedary and the bactrian camel.

The evolutionary origins of induced and spontaneous ovulation in mammals have been much debated. Some have proposed that induced ovulation may have been the ancestral condition among mammals (e.g. Conaway, 1971; Jöchle, 1975; Ramirez and Soufi, 1994; Zarrow and Clark, 1968). Others have argued that spontaneous ovulation is more likely to represent the basal pattern (Bakker and Baum, 2000; Ewer, 1973; Kauffman and Rissman, 2006). Indeed, the imposition of a rigid dichotomy between spontaneous and induced ovulation is considered to be misleading, as in some mammals both types of ovulation reportedly occur in the same species. These topics are reviewed here, beginning with a discussion of current knowledge concerning the phylogenetic distribution of spontaneous and mating-induced patterns of ovulation throughout the 27 orders of extant mammals.

The Phylogenetic Distribution of Mating-induced Ovulation

Those mammals that are known to exhibit induced ovulation are listed in Table 9.1. The control of ovulation in the monotremes is unknown, which is unfortunate given their unique phylogenetic position as the only surviving egg-laying mammals. It has been suggested that induced ovulation might occur in the short-beaked echidna (Morrow and Nicol, 2009), but definitive evidence is lacking. The great majority of marsupials are spontaneously ovulating species. In 1987, Tyndale-Biscoe and Renfree

Table 9.1 Mammalian species that are known to exhibit mating-induced ovulation. Data sources are from Kauffman and Rissman (2006), unless otherwise stated

Order	Species: common and Latin names
Placental mammals	
Cetartiodactyla	Bactrian camel (*Camelus bactrianus*); dromedary (*Camelus dromadarius*); llama (*Lama glama*); alpaca (*Lama pacos*)
Perissodactyla	Sumatran rhinoceros (*Dicerorhinus sumatrensis*) (Roth *et al.*, 2001)
Carnivora	Domestic cat (*Felis catus*); lion (*Panthera leo*) (Schramm *et al.*, 1994); island fox (*Urocyon littoralis*) (Asa *et al.*, 2007); mink (*Mustela vison*); ferret (*Mustela furo*); black bear (*Ursus americanus*) (Boone *et al.*, 1998); raccoon (*Procyon lotor*); striped skunk (*Mephitis mephitis*); Canadian otter (*Lontra canadensis*)
Eulipotyphla	Short-tailed shrew (*Blarina brevicauda*); least shrew (*Cryptotis parva*); white-toothed shrew (*Crocidura russula*); Asian house shrew (*Suncus murinus*); European hedgehog (*Erinaceus europaeus*)
Rodentia	Collared lemming (*Dicrostonyx groenlandicus*); bank vole (*Clethrionomys glareolus*); European pine vole (*Pitymys subterraneus*); tree mouse (*Phenacomys longicaudus*); California vole (*Microtus californicus**); 13-lined ground squirrel (*Citellus tridecemlineatus*); five-striped Indian ground squirrel (*Funambulus pennanti*); woodchuck (*Marmota monax*)
Lagomorpha	European rabbit (*Oryctolagus cuniculus*); common hare (*Lepus europaeus*)
Marsupials	
Diprotodontia	Koala (*Phascolarctos cinereus*) (Johnston *et al.*, 2000a, 2000b); brush-tailed bettong (*Bettongia penicillata*) (Hinds and Smith, 1992)
Didelphimorphia	Grey short-tailed opossum (*Monodelphis domestica*) (Fadem and Rayve, 1985)

* Kauffman and Rissman (2006) list eight species of the genus *Microtus* that are induced ovulators.

noted that '*Phascolarctos cinereus* may, on further study, turn out to be an exception'. Indeed, subsequent research has shown that the koala is an induced ovulator, as is also the case for the brush-tailed bettong (*Bettongia penicillata*) and the South American grey opossum, *Monodelphis domestica* (see Table 9.1). The Australasian brush-tail possum (*Trichosurus vulpecula*) may represent an additional case but, although the frequency of ovulation is known to increase when captive females are housed with males, whether the act of mating induces ovulation has not been established (Crawford *et al.*, 1998).

Mating-induced ovulation has been identified in some members of at least seven orders of the placental mammals (Figure 9.1). It occurs in many carnivores, including members of Family Felidae, as well as the bears, racoons, weasels, skunks and some otters. Species belonging to Family Canidae, such as dogs and wolves, are spontaneous ovulators, but one case of induced ovulation has been described in the island fox (Asa *et al.*, 2007) and others may exist among the smaller, less gregarious taxa. Rabbits and hares (Order Lagomorpha) are induced ovulators, as may also be the case in their smaller relatives, the pikas. The rodents, which are the closest phylogenetic relatives of the lagomorphs, also include many species of induced ovulators (Table 9.1) and, given the huge size of Order Rodentia, further examples are sure to

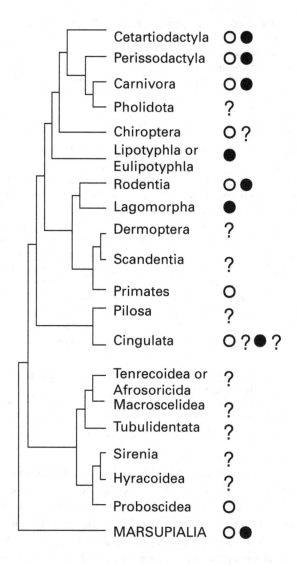

Figure 9.1 Phylogenetic distribution of mating-induced and spontaneous patterns of ovulation in the 19 orders of placental mammals, and in the Subclass Marsupialia considered as a whole. Open circles = occurrences of spontaneous ovulation; closed circles = occurrences of induced ovulation. Note that in some cases only a few species are known to exhibit induced ovulation, e.g. in Order Cetartiodactyla only the camelids are induced ovulators, and in Subclass Marsupialia only three species are currently known to exhibit induced ovulation. Further information is provided in Table 9.1 and in the text.

exist. Induced ovulation has also been identified in a small number of species belonging to the Eulipotyphla (shrews, hedgehogs, moles and solenodons). It may turn out to be widespread throughout the order, but currently only limited information is available concerning the hedgehogs, moles and solenodons.

With few exceptions, spontaneous ovulation is the rule throughout the Cetartiodactyla. The same applies to the perissodactyls, primates and proboscideans. One exception among the perissodactyls concerns the Sumatran rhinoceros (*Dicerorhinus sumatrensis*). This magnificent and endangered rhinoceros (less than 400 of them survive) has rarely reproduced in captivity. However, research on captive rhinos at the Cincinnati Zoo (Roth *et al.*, 2001) established that a surge in LH began 1–2 hours after copulation. The subsequent occurrence of ovulation was confirmed using ultrasonography.

There are still many groups of placental mammals for which information about ovulation is either limited or totally lacking (Figure 9.1). This is the situation for the pangolins, colougos, tree shrews, sloths and anteaters, tenrecs and golden moles, as well as the elephant shrews, aardvark, hyraxes and manatees. Zhang *et al.* (2020), on the basis of their behavioural observations of Sunda pangolins (*Manis javanica*), 'suspect that repeated mating may induce estrus and ovulation in the female'. Likewise, Eisenberg (1975) suspected that female tenrecs 'may be induced ovulators'. Bats (Chiroptera) are presumed to be mainly spontaneous ovulators, but as there are more than 1100 species of them, it would be rash to deny that some of the many unstudied taxa might exhibit mating-induced patterns of ovulation. Likewise, information concerning the 21 species of armadillos is fragmentary; the nine-banded armadillo (*Dasypus novemcinctus*) is probably a spontaneous ovulator (Loughry and McDonough, 2013), whereas the pichi (*Zaedyus pichiy*) may be a mating-induced ovulator (Superina, 2007).

Substantial gaps in knowledge concerning ovulation in many of the lineages discussed above limit the usefulness of phylogenetic approaches when attempting to explain the origins of mating-induced or spontaneous ovulation in mammals. Hopefully, further research will, in time, rectify this situation. It should also be acknowledged that some earlier proponents of induced ovulation as the basic pattern among mammals (e.g. Conaway, 1971; Zarrow and Clark, 1968) were influenced by occurrences of induced ovulation in 'primitive' mammals belonging to what was then the Order Insectivora. Yet, as discussed in Chapter 2, the Order Insectivora has undergone a radical revision, with the tenrecs, golden moles and elephant shrews being reassigned to the Superorder Afrotheria, the treeshrews to the Order Scandentia and the 'flying lemurs' to the Dermoptera. Only the shrews, hedgehogs, moles and solenodons remain in what is now Order Eulipotyphla and, with the exception of some shrews and one species of hedgehog, little is known about occurrences of induced ovulation in the majority of taxa.

Broader phylogenetic comparisons that include other vertebrate groups may help to shed some light on the question of whether spontaneous or mating-induced patterns of ovulation represent the ancestral condition for Class Mammalia. Induced ovulation is absent or occurs only very rarely in most vertebrate groups other than mammals (Bakker and Baum, 2000; Kauffman and Rissman, 2006). Thus, although females ovulate spontaneously in many fish species, the presence of males may stimulate spawning behaviour. Other examples of male-mediated effects upon female reproductive physiology in fish, amphibians, reptiles and birds have been reviewed by Crews and Silver (1985) and Wingfield *et al.* (1994). Some exceptional cases of induced ovulation have been identified in reptiles. Thus, in the red-sided garter snake 'spring mating had a significant effect on ovarian recrudescence' (Mendonça and Crews, 1989). Mating-induced ovulation has also been identified in two chelonians (the loggerhead turtle: Manire *et al.*, 2008; and the ploughshare tortoise: Kuchling, 2015). Given the solitary lives of turtles and tortoises, and the ability of females to store sperm for long periods, the capacity to exhibit either spontaneous or induced ovulation may be a more common strategy among chelonians than is currently realized. In birds, there are cases where the presence of a male partner and the stimulation provided by his (non-contact) displays causes the female to come into breeding condition and to ovulate. In the ring dove (*Streptopelia risoria*), for example, visual and auditory access to intact male partners resulted in ovulation in 13 of 20 females tested, as compared with 3 of 20 females tested with castrated males (Erickson and Lehrman, 1964). Intact males displayed to females, by bow-cooing, nest-cooing and wing-flapping, whereas castrates failed to display. Later work by Cheng *et al.* (1998) showed that an exchange of nest-cooing displays between the sexes is crucial to causing female ring doves to ovulate.

Whether mating-induced ovulation might occur in ratites, geese and ducks, in which males have a phallus, is not known. However, when one considers the evidence pertaining to vertebrates as a whole, it appears that spontaneous ovulation rather than mating-induced ovulation is the norm in fish, amphibians, reptiles and birds. It seems likely, therefore, that the early precursors of the mammals, the therapsids of the Permian Period, would also have been spontaneous ovulators.

It should also be noted here that the onset of female sexual receptivity (oestrus) may be advanced by the presence of males in some mammals. A variety of stimuli may be involved in producing such effects. In domestic sheep, the 'ram effect' involves olfactory and other cues (Martin *et al.*, 1980; Signoret *et al.*, 1984), while in red deer, the roaring vocalizations of stags during the rut coordinate the timing of oestrus in groups of hinds (McComb, 1987). Pheromonal and behavioural stimuli provided by boars stimulate sows to enter oestrus (Signoret *et al.*, 1984). As Bakker and Baum (2000) have pointed out, these kinds of male-induced effects on oestrus onset could have paved the way for the evolution of mating-induced ovulation. If this scenario is correct, however, it is also logical to suggest that male-induced onset of oestrus might also have been associated, at least initially, with spontaneous (steroid-induced) patterns of ovulation, just as in the examples cited above. Mating-induced ovulation might have been an additional development. In the female prairie vole (*Microtus ochrogaster*), for example, chemical cues in the male's urine result in increased secretion of ovarian oestrogen and the onset of female receptivity. However, in this species ovulation is also induced by the male, and occurs 12 hours after mating (Carter and Getz, 1985; Carter *et al.*, 1989).

Ovulation Considered from a Social and Ecological Perspective

Many mammals that exhibit mating-induced ovulation have non-gregarious patterns of social organization. This does not mean that they are totally solitary creatures.

Individuals occupy separate home ranges that overlap to varying degrees with those of conspecifics, so that direct encounters may occur, but scent-marking and vocal signals also play an important role in maintaining social communication. Members of 20 of the 25 genera cited by Kauffman and Rissman (2006) as being induced ovulators are non-gregarious species. Most (23 genera) are also seasonal breeders. It is possible, therefore, that selection might favour the evolution of induced ovulation when the sexes are widely dispersed throughout the environment and encounters are infrequent. However, some caution is necessary when considering this hypothesis, as many mammals that are non-gregarious are spontaneous ovulators, and they appear to have no difficulty in locating partners during the female's (often short) periods of seasonal sexual receptivity. This applies, for example, to many rodents, as well as to nocturnal prosimian primates such as galagos, lorises and mouse lemurs.

Studies of the African mole-rats (Family Bathyergidae) provide a good example of relationships between ecology, social behaviour and the mechanisms that govern ovulation. Mole-rats are burrowing rodents, and most are non-gregarious. Burrowing in search of a potential mate is energetically costly. Periods of high rainfall soften the soil and make burrowing easier, as well as increasing the food available to mole-rats. Non-gregarious mole-rat species that live in areas where rainfall varies throughout the year tend to be seasonal breeders and to exhibit mating-induced ovulation (Faulkes *et al.*, 2010). More social or eusocial mole-rat species are usually spontaneous ovulators and do not have defined breeding seasons (Figure 9.2). Faulkes *et al.* (2010) concluded that induced ovulation is likely to represent the plesiomorphic condition for the African mole-rats, and that spontaneous ovulation has developed as a secondary specialization in species such as the eusocial naked mole-rat (*Heterocephalus glaber*).

Insights From the Fossil Record of Mammalian Evolution

In Chapter 2, it was noted that a rapid diversification of the various orders of placental mammals occurred during the Paleocene and Eocene Epochs, subsequent to the mass extinction event that marked the close of the Cretaceous Period. Some 66 Mya, a huge meteor collided with the Earth, causing major environmental changes that eventually resulted in the extinction of the non-avian dinosaurs. Prior to this, the mammals were represented by a variety of taxa that were probably no larger than extant rats or shrews (Archibald, 2011; Kemp, 2005). An example of an exceptionally complete fossil of one of these small Cretaceous mammals (*Eomaia scansoria*) was discussed in Chapter 2 (see Figure 2.26).

It is possible that the small-bodied Cretaceous eutherians would have occupied ecological niches similar to those filled by today's rodents and by members of the Eulipotyphla, such as the shrews and moles. Many of them may have had non-gregarious types of social organization, therefore, whilst some formed social groups. It is not known whether spontaneous or induced patterns of ovulation predominated among these eutherian mammals. It is unlikely that Cretaceous metatherians would

Control of ovulation in female giant mole-rats

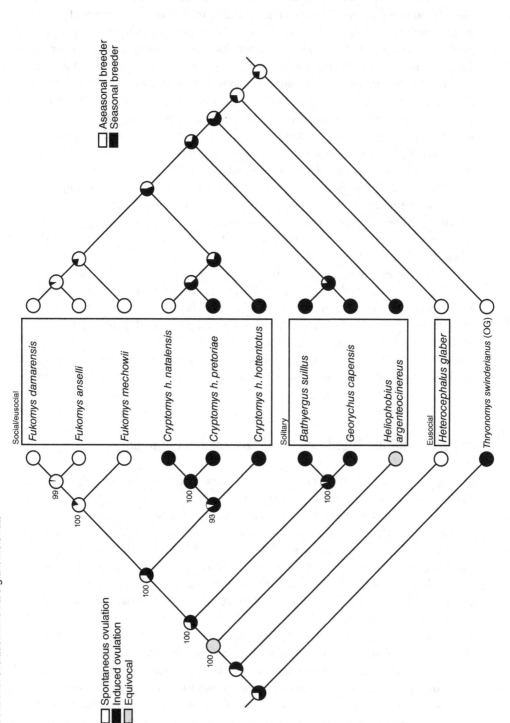

Figure 9.2 Mirrored phylogenetic trees for members of six genera of the African mole-rats, indicating the degree of likelihood of ovulation being either spontaneous or induced (left-hand side of the diagram) and breeding being either seasonal or non-seasonal (right-hand side of the diagram). The African cane rat (*Thryonomys swinderianus*) is included as the nearest out-group (OG) species. The equivocal status of *Heliophobius* is mainly due to lack of data for this species. (From Faulkes *et al.*, 2010.)

have included induced ovulators, given that mating-induced ovulation has been identified in only a handful of the 350+ extant species of extant marsupials. Yet, whatever the case, fossils belonging to none of the 19 orders of the placental mammals alive today have yet been identified in the fossil record of Cretaceous mammals (145–66 Mya). Diversification of placental mammals only took place after the mass extinction, during the Paleocene and Eocene between 66 and 34 Mya, when fossils representing 18 of the extant orders first appear (Archibald, 2011). These changes were, in geological terms, comparatively rapid. It is fruitless to debate whether extant placentals are all the descendants of either spontaneously ovulating or induced ovulating ancestors, given that it is not known which group, or groups, of Cretaceous eutherians gave rise to the Subclass Placentalia. We can say that induced ovulation is likely to represent an ancestral trait for many members of the Carnivora, Rodentia and Lagomorpha, as well as for shrews (Family Soricidae) of the Order Eulipotyphla. Spontaneous ovulation, on the other hand, is likely to represent an ancestral trait in the Cetartiodactyla, Perissodactyla, Primates and Proboscidea. For the remaining orders, there is currently insufficient information upon which to base a judgement.

Pavlicev and Wagner (2016) and Pavlicev *et al.* (2019) take a different view. They conclude that phylogenetic evidence indicates that mating-induced ovulation is plesiomorphic in eutherians, and that 'neuroendocrine mechanisms underlying female orgasm evolved from and are homologous to the mechanisms mediating copulation-induced ovulation'. Spontaneous ovulation is thus posited to derive from this ancestral condition. However, 'in spontaneous ovulators the role of clitoral stimulation for ovulation became vestigial, but maintained traces of the ancestral neuroendocrine reflex even in humans'. Pavlicev and Wagner (2016) assume that 'the clitoris is the main source of the orgasmic induced endocrine surge in all mammals' and suggest that changes in the position of the clitoris during evolution have reduced its sensitivity to copulatory stimulation. Such is proposed to be the case in primates, for example, as the glans clitoris is situated outside the vaginal opening.

There are substantial problems with Palvicev and Wagner's 'ovulatory homologue model of female orgasm'. The phylogenetic evidence they present for induced ovulation being a plesiomorphic trait is far from convincing. There is no evidence that female orgasm plays any role in triggering ovulation in mammals. Nor can one assume that the clitoris is the main sensate focus for induction of ovulation, given that stimulation of the vagina and cervix during mating is clearly involved in some taxa. In his commentary on Pavlicev and Wagner's (2016) paper, Komisaruk (2016) concluded that the model they propose 'depends upon unfounded assumptions, does not address contradictory evidence, and contains significant factual errors'.

The Neuroendocrine Control of Ovulation

The neuroendocrine mechanisms that bring about ovulation share some fundamental similarities in mammals that exhibit either spontaneous or mating-induced ovulation.

In both cases, a surge of LH causes the fully developed ovarian follicles to rupture and to release their ova. The LH surge results from events that occur in the brain and the pituitary gland. The neurons which constitute the hypothalamic 'pulse generator' produce increasing amounts of a decapeptide (luteinizing hormone releasing hormone: LHRH, or GnRH) and this in turn stimulates specialized cells (gonadotrophs) in the anterior lobe of the pituitary gland to secrete a surge of LH. A group of peptides called kisspeptins play an important role in coordinating inputs to the GnRH neurons, including those that arise in the external environment as well as endogenous, hormonal and metabolic signals (Inoue *et al.*, 2011; Roseweir and Millar, 2009).

The crucial difference between the two types of ovulation thus resides in the nature of the stimuli that impinge upon the kisspeptin neurons and GnRH pulse generator. In the case of mating-induced ovulation, somatosensory stimuli provided by males trigger the cascade of events described above, whereas in spontaneous ovulators, endocrine processes involving positive feedback by oestradiol (either alone or in combination with progesterone in some taxa) result in ovulation, irrespective of whether mating occurs. By contrast, positive feedback by ovarian hormones upon LH secretion is lacking, or much reduced, in induced ovulators (Bakker and Baum, 2000).

Given that the neuroendocrine substrates that control spontaneous and induced ovulation share many features, it is not surprising that a continuum might exist between them, and that both types of ovulation can sometimes occur in the same species. For example, among the South American hystricomorph rodents, the chinchilla (*Chinchilla lanigera*) and the casiragua (*Proechimys guairae*) may either ovulate spontaneously or in response to mating (Weir, 1974). Some mammals that are normally induced ovulators may occasionally exhibit a spontaneous ovulation, as is the case in some carnivores. Schramm *et al.* (1994), for example, conducted experiments on five captive female lions. When paired with a vasectomized male all the females ovulated, but when kept in isolation just one of the five females ovulated spontaneously. Domestic cats have long been known to ovulate as a result of copulation (e.g. Johnson and Gay, 1981; Wildt *et al.*, 1980), yet instances of spontaneous ovulation have also been recorded, especially in group-housed animals (Gudermuth *et al.*, 1997; Lawler *et al.*, 1993). Note, however, that in both these studies female cats were housed in groups and in some cases in proximity to males, so that social stimulation among females or distance cues from males might have been sufficient to trigger ovulation.

Although the Norway rat (*Rattus norvegicus*) is a spontaneous ovulator, copulation may, if correctly timed, increase the number of ova released by females. Rodgers (1971) reported this to be the case if matings occurred between 17.50 and 18.30 hours on the afternoon of pro-oestrus. However, subsequent experiments failed to demonstrate the expected post-copulatory increase in LH during this time window (Rodgers and Schwartz, 1973). Older multiparous female rats, nearing the end of their reproductive lives, may fail to ovulate. Davis *et al.* (1977) found that if male rats completed a single mount series with ejaculation, then no embryos were recoverable from the uteri of such older females. However, after three copulatory series an average of 9.37 embryos was counted and this increased to 12.45 after five mount series with ejaculation. These results might have been due to increases in numbers of ova released after copulation, but they could also have been caused by greater survival of embryos. This is because copulation induces surges of prolactin in some rodents (including the rat) and, as discussed in earlier chapters, this facilitates support of the corpus luteum and secretion of progesterone during early pregnancy. Post-copulatory increases in progesterone were measured during Davis *et al.*'s (1977) study.

There is no doubt, however, that female rats are capable of exhibiting mating-induced ovulation in response to experimental manipulations of a most important facet of their external environment, namely the photoperiodic cues that entrain the ovarian cycle. A circadian clock controls the timing of the pro-oestrus LH surge in rats and some other rodents (Turek and Van Cauter, 1994). However, when females are housed under a constant light regime, the cyclical occurrence of ovulation is blocked and, under these conditions, ovulation occurs in response to mating (Brown-Grant *et al.*, 1973; Dempsey and Searles, 1943). The ability to exhibit mating-induced ovulation may thus lie dormant in a spontaneously ovulating species and be activated in response to the changed external conditions.

Somatosensory Feedback and Mating-induced Ovulation

The sensory stimuli required to trigger the pre-ovulatory LH surge vary among species that exhibit induced ovulation. Nor are such cues necessarily confined to penile stimulation of the vagina and cervix. The rabbit provides a good example of a species in which multiple somatosensory cues combine to trigger the pre-ovulatory LH surge (Allen and Adler, 1985; Ramirez and Soufi, 1994). Partial sensory deficits, such as result from local anaesthesia of the vagina (Fee and Parkes, 1930) or removal of primary sensory inputs (visual, auditory, or olfactory: Brooks, 1937) do not, in isolation, prevent ovulation. Ramirez and Soufi (1994) point out that 'in the rabbit and other mammals the male activates areas that are innervated by many nerves including the perineal, pudendal and several somatic nerves originating in the skin of the dorsum, the flanks, and the legs'. Tactile stimulation of the female's back, flanks and perineum by the male rabbit during mounting causes her to elevate her rump and raise her tail; these reflexive responses are essential for the occurrence of intromission. Intromission lasts only a second or two; a single deep pelvic thrust results in ejaculation and the male dismounts. LH begins to rise rapidly in less than 3 minutes after ejaculation, with ovulation occurring about 10 hours later. The effects of copulation on LH secretion when rabbits are pair-tested in captivity are shown in the upper part of Figure 9.3. It should be noted that two of the eight females tested in this study failed to show an LH surge. This is unlikely to reflect what occurs under more natural conditions. When rabbits are housed in social groups, for example, they experience much higher levels of social and sexual activity (Myers and Poole, 1962), all of which might contribute to the induction of ovulation.

Repeated copulations in some induced ovulators produce a cumulative effect; the best-documented example of this type concerns the domestic cat. Mating is also brief

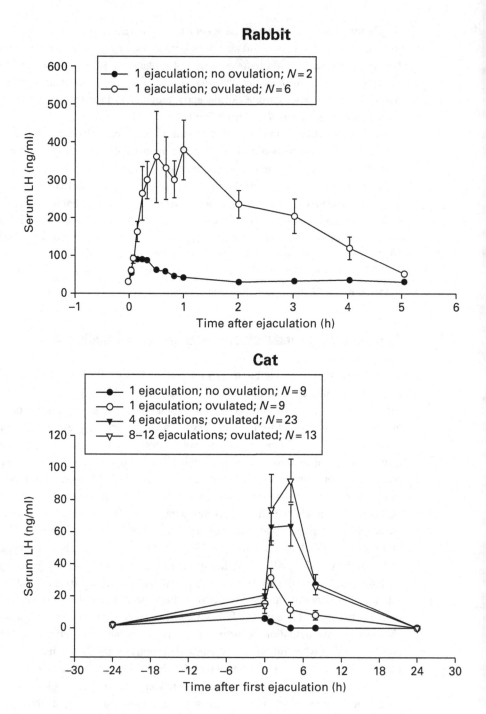

Figure 9.3 Effects of copulatory behaviour upon circulating concentrations of luteinizing hormone (LH) in two induced ovulators, the European rabbit and the domestic cat. (From Bakker and Baum, 2000; modified from Jones *et al.*, 1976 and Concannon *et al.*, 1980.)

in this species, as is the case in many other felids, and consists of a single deep thrust to bring about intromission and ejaculation. A single mating may induce ovulation, but repeated copulations are more effective, resulting in progressively greater LH responses and numbers of females that ovulate, as is shown in the lower section of Figure 9.3. Another example concerns the montane vole (*Microtus montanus*) in which males make a series of intromissions, with pelvic thrusting, to attain ejaculation. After a single ejaculatory series only 3 of 12 females (25 per cent) ovulated; this increased to 8 (66 per cent) after two ejaculatory series. When more than two series were completed, all 12 females ovulated (Davis *et al.*, 1974b).

Prolonged single intromission copulatory patterns, such as occur in the ferret and other mustelids, bring about a more sustained LH surge although, as Bakker and Baum (2000) point out, even when short copulations occur in some mustelids (e.g. in *Mustela nivalis*) they still result in ovulation. Copulation appears to exert an 'all or nothing' response in this group of carnivores. Eisenberg (1981) speculated that 'long intromission time might be a conservative pattern in the Mammalia, using vaginal stimulation to ensure that ovulation will occur'. There are problems with this hypothesis, however. For example, many marsupials have long intromission times, yet very few of them are induced ovulators. Nor are occurrences of induced ovulation in the various orders of placental mammals consistent with masculine copulatory patterns that involve prolonged intromission (Table 9.2). Prolonged intromission in association with induced ovulation is likely to represent an ancient trait for some carnivores (e.g. the mustelids and ursids), but not for the mammals as a whole.

Beta Nerve Growth Factor in Semen and Induced Ovulation

The first demonstration of the presence of an ovulation induction factor (OIF) in the semen of a mammalian species is due to Chen *et al.* (1985), who showed that seminal plasma (but not spermatozoa) triggers ovulation when administered intravaginally to bactrian camels. A minimum of 1.0 ml of seminal plasma was sufficient to induce ovulation, which occurred between 36 and 48 hours after treatment. This is similar to the time at which females ovulate after natural matings in bactrian camels. Induction of an LH surge and ovulation by seminal plasma was then identified in two more camelids (alpacas and llamas: Adams *et al.*, 2005). Further experiments revealed the OIF to be a 14 kilodalton protein that was subsequently identified as beta nerve growth factor (β-NGF: Kershaw-Young *et al.*, 2012; Ratto *et al.*, 2012). β-NGF also exerts a luteotrophic effect in llamas, resulting in increased vascularization of the corpus luteum during its early development (Ulloa-Leal *et al.*, 2014; but see also Stuart *et al.*, 2015). A similar luteotrophic effect of llama OIF had previously been reported when it was administered to cows (Tanco *et al.*, 2012).

Another insight arising from research on induced ovulation in camelids was the finding that penile stimulation of the vagina and cervix does not induce ovulation in the llama. Berland et al. (2016) mated female llamas with urethrostomized males, in which semen was diverted via an opening in the perianal region. This operation

Table 9.2 Masculine copulatory patterns and intromission durations in mammals that exhibit mating-induced ovulation

Species	Copulatory pattern no.	Prolonged intromission?
Marsupialia		
Phascolarctos cinereus	12	No
Placentalia		
Perissodactyla		
Dicerorhinus sumatrensis	11	Yes
Eulipotyphla		
Suncus murinus	10	No
Erinaceus europaeus	11?	Yes?
Rodentia		
Microtus montanus	10	No
Microtus pennsylvanicus	10	No
Microtus agrestis	10	No
Microtus californicus	12	No
Spermophilus tridecemlineatus	12	No
Chinchilla lanigera	12	No
Microcavia australis	10	No
Galea musteloides	12	No
Ctenomys talarum	10	No
Cryptomys hottentotus	10	No
Georychus capensis	10	No
Spalax ehrenbergi	10	No
Lagomorpha		
Oryctolagus cuniculus	16	No
Carnivora		
Felis catus	16	No
Panthera leo	16	No
Mustela putorius	15?	Yes
Mustela vison	11	Yes
Mustela nigripes	11?	Yes
Mephitis mephitis	11	Yes
Lontra canadensis	11	Yes
Ursus americanus	11	Yes

Copulatory patterns are classified using the scheme described in Chapter 3 and as listed in Appendix 1. Members of Family Camelidae have been omitted, as camelids ovulate in response to chemical cues in the semen.

prevented males from inseminating females, although they were otherwise able to mate normally (erection occurred and intromission lasted >20 minutes). No pre-ovulatory LH surges resulted from these matings, however, whereas intrauterine administration of seminal plasma or matings with non-operated males induced marked elevations of plasma LH (Figure 9.4). The physiological significance of prolonged intromission in camelids is likely to be that it facilitates the insemination of larger

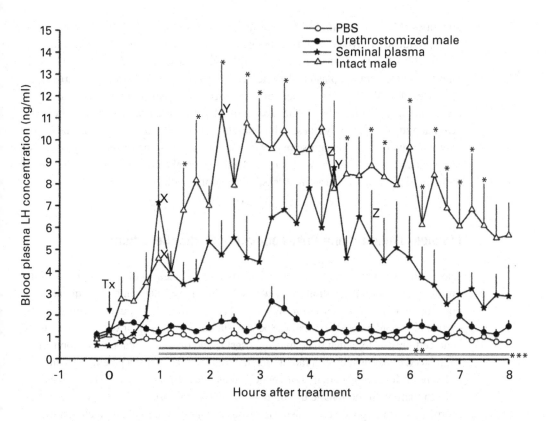

Figure 9.4 Plasma concentrations of LH in female llamas (*Lama glama*) measured under four conditions: mating by intact males (Δ) stimulates the pre-ovulatory LH surge. Intrauterine administration of seminal plasma (★) results in a surge of LH which is significantly lower. Urethrostomized males ● are unable to transfer semen during copulation and concentrations of LH in females remain unchanged, as is the case after intra-uterine administration of PBS (phosphate-buffered saline ○) as a control procedure. *P < 0.01; **P < 0.001. (From Berland *et al.*, 2016.)

volumes of semen and thus ensures a greater absorption of β-NGF by the lining of the uterus.

Nerve growth factor is transported in the bloodstream, and acts at the level of the brain to influence the release of GnRH and hence to trigger the pre-ovulatory surge of LH. However, current evidence indicates that β-NGF does not stimulate the GnRH neurons directly, acting instead via interneurons (for review, see Ratto *et al.*, 2019). Kisspeptin neurons interface with the GnRH system to control the LH surge in spontaneous ovulators, but whether this is the case in llamas is not known.

Nerve growth factor has been identified in the semen of several other mammals besides the camelids (e.g. in cattle, pigs and horses: Ratto *et al.*, 2019). Semen from several cetaceans has also been tested, but with negative results (in belugas and two dolphin species: Bergfelt *et al.*, 2018). Nerve growth factor is present at high concentrations in the semen of rabbits, in which the prostate gland secretes the largest quantities (Maranesi *et al.*, 2015). Attempts to implicate β-NGF as an OIF in rabbits have produced equivocal results, however. For example, intramuscular injection of murine β-NGF into six does resulted in only one ovulation. Treatment of does with rabbit or llama seminal plasma also yielded negative results (Silva *et al.*, 2011). The presence of β-NGF in the semen of some spontaneously ovulating mammals is, nonetheless, intriguing. Is β-NGF absent in the monotremes, given that the male echidna and platypus only possess bulbourethral glands? Does it occur in the accessory reproductive glands and semen of marsupials, or in some of the many orders of placental mammals that have still to be studied? Might β-NGF have subtle effects upon the timing of ovulation in at least some spontaneous ovulators?

Induced Ovulation and Post-copulatory Sexual Selection

The major differences between spontaneous and induced ovulators, as regards the timing of ovulation in relation to the act of mating, have interesting consequences for post-copulatory sexual selection. When a receptive female copulates with multiple partners in spontaneously ovulating species, such as rats, sheep or chimpanzees, there is no certainty as to which male mated closest to the time of ovulation. By contrast, in an induced ovulator such as a rabbit, the first male to mate gains a potential advantage, as his behaviour triggers ovulation, which takes place 10 hours later. Other males will have to mate with the female during that comparatively brief window of time if their sperm are to undergo the cascade of processes required to place them in contention for access to her ova. Table 9.3 provides examples of occurrences of single versus multiple paternities for litters of offspring in mammals that are induced ovulators. Soulsbury (2010), who compared the paternities of litters of offspring produced by spontaneous versus induced ovulators, concluded that 'ovulation mode alters the

Table 9.3 Paternity of litters in mammals that are induced ovulators

Species	Summary of findings	Sources
White-toothed shrew, *Crocidura russula*	72% of litters (*n* = 23) had one sire; 28% had multiple paternity	Lin *et al.*, 2009
European hedgehog, *Erinaceus europaeus*	60% of litters (*n* = 5) had one sire; 40% had multiple paternity	Moran *et al.*, 2009
Raccoon, *Procyon lotor*	7 of 8 litters (offspring ≥ 2) had multiple paternity	Nielsen and Nielsen 2007
Snowshoe hare, *Lepus americanus*	75% of litters (*n* = 16) had one sire; 25% had multiple paternity	Burton, 2002
European hare, *Lepus europaeus*	90% of pregnancies (*n* = 19*) had one sire; 10% had multiple sires	Suchentrunk and Hackländer, 2005
Pygmy rabbit, *Brachylagus idahoensis*	2 litters analysed: both had a minimum of 2 sires	Falćon *et al.*, 2011

* 67 foetuses were included in this study.

ability of males to monopolize paternity, with males of induced ovulators having higher single paternity and greater alpha paternity where male–female association is intermittent'.

The fact that multiple paternities occur in some litters of all the induced ovulators listed in Table 9.3 indicates that sperm competition takes place under these conditions. Just as important, however, is the influence of the female, because she may fail to ovulate unless a male provides sufficient stimulation. Cryptic female choice is therefore likely to occur in induced ovulators.

Summary and Conclusions

During the course of mammalian evolution, interactions between the sexes have resulted in a spectrum of effects involving female reproductive physiology and behaviour. The propensity for females to ovulate in response to copulatory (and associated) stimuli is but one example of such phenomena. Other examples include male effects upon the induction of ovarian activity and the onset of oestrus, the termination of female receptivity as a result of mating, and post-copulatory luteotrophic effects in some taxa. Induced ovulation is not an isolated phenomenon, therefore; indeed, it operates via many of the same underlying hypothalamic and pituitary mechanisms that result in spontaneous ovulation. The crucial difference is that in spontaneous ovulators the pre-ovulatory LH surge can occur in the absence of males and is controlled via positive feedback by ovarian steroids. Induced ovulation, by contrast, requires somatosensory stimulation by a male to trigger the LH surge. We have seen that males may gain advantages, in terms of paternity share, from inducing females to ovulate. Females may also benefit via cryptic choices for those males that provide the most effective types of stimulation. What constitutes the 'most effective' stimulation varies tremendously among taxa. Both prolonged and brief patterns of intromission are represented among induced ovulators, but in the latter case multiple copulations often occur so that a cumulative effect is produced. In the camelids, β-nerve growth factor in the male's semen triggers the pre-ovulatory LH surge, whereas in lagomorphs a variety of pre-copulatory and copulatory stimuli combine to induce ovulation.

The distinction between induced and spontaneous ovulatory mechanisms is not an absolute one. Spontaneous ovulators may sometimes ovulate in response to mating, as, for example, when female rats are maintained under a constant light regime. There are also cases where induced ovulators exhibit spontaneous ovulation, but it is often unclear whether females are switching to a steroid-sensitive mechanism to trigger the LH surge, or whether a lowered threshold of response to external cues is responsible (e.g. in the domestic cat: Gudermuth et al., 1997; Lawler et al., 1993).

Some researchers have proposed that induced ovulation represents the ancestral condition among mammals. Yet, an important negative piece of evidence is that induced ovulation has only rarely been identified in vertebrates other than mammals. Spontaneous ovulation appears to be the norm in fish, amphibians, reptiles and birds;

some of the few known exceptions to this rule were discussed earlier in this chapter. It seems likely, therefore, that the therapsids which gave rise to the earliest mammals would have been primarily spontaneous ovulators. Bakker and Baum (2000) have pointed out that 'There are numerous examples among mammals, birds, and reptiles in which the display of behaviors by a male stimulates gonadotropin secretion and consequent ovarian development and sexual behavior in female conspecifics.' These kinds of male-induced effects upon female reproductive physiology might have provided the basis for the later emergence of mating-induced ovulation in some mammals.

When one considers the distribution of induced ovulation among the 27 extant orders of the Mammalia (Table 9.1 and Figure 9.1), it is evident that adequate information concerning modes of ovulation is lacking for many of them, including the monotremes and many of the marsupials. One of the better-studied South American marsupials, the grey opossum, is an induced ovulator. However, there is very little information for most of the South American species. The reproductive biology of Australian marsupials has been much more extensively studied, but only two of them (the koala and the brush-tailed bettong) are currently known to exhibit mating-induced ovulation. Turning to the Placentalia, induced ovulation is likely to represent an ancient trait for some lineages of the Carnivora, Rodentia, Lagomorpha and Eulipotyphla, while spontaneous ovulation is the norm for most lineages of the Cetartiodactyla, Perissodactyla, Primates and Proboscidea. For the majority of the remaining 11 orders of placental mammals, there are not enough data to make firm judgements.

Gaps in the fossil record of mammalian evolution also constitute a challenge for potential phylogenetic analyses. In Chapter 2, it was noted that despite the fact that fossils of many small-bodied eutherian mammals are known from the Cretaceous Period, none of them can be assigned with certainty to the Subclass Placentalia. Clearly some connection must exist, but it remains elusive. The earliest known fossils of the various orders of placental mammals are from post K/T boundary sites, after the mass extinction event which occurred at the close of the Cretaceous Period, some 66 Mya. With the extinction of the non-avian dinosaurs, diversification of placental mammals took place rapidly during the Paleocene and Eocene Epochs (66–34 Mya), when 18 of the extant orders make their first appearance in the fossil record (Archibald, 2011). Which of the Cretaceous lineages survived to give rise to this diversity, and how did the current mix of induced and spontaneously ovulating taxa emerge from these early placentals? The honest answer, dear reader, is that we still do not know.

Part IV

Epilogue

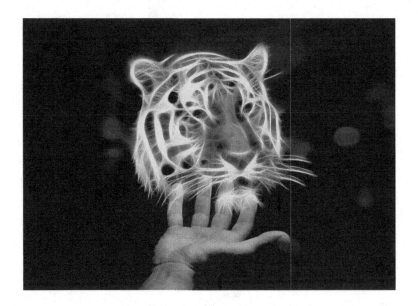

10 An End of Day Glass

Think of the whole of existence, of which you are the tiniest part; think of the whole of time, in which you have been assigned a brief and fleeting moment; think of destiny – what fraction of that are you?

Marcus Aurelius Antoninus, *Meditations*

The phrase 'an end of day glass' arises from an old custom among glassblowers, who used any remaining scraps of glass to make a final extra item at the close of work. End-of-day glass objects were often colourful mixtures of glass fragments.

This final chapter echoes this sentiment. First, it discusses insights and considers some of the many unresolved questions arising from the preceding chapters. Then, there is a discussion of how broad-based, comparative studies of mammals can inform debates concerning post-copulatory sexual selection and the evolution of human reproduction. Finally, some thoughts are offered concerning the consequences of uncontrolled human population growth and the ongoing extinction of our fellow mammals.

Conclusions and Unresolved Questions

Phylogeny, as well as modes of life, and post-copulatory sexual selection have influenced the evolution of mammalian copulatory behaviour, reproductive anatomy and physiology. Chapter 3 established that although 16 possible masculine copulatory patterns may be defined using current classification schemes, just five of them (pattern nos. 3, 10, 11, 12 and 16) are displayed by 92 per cent of all the mammals classified so far. The ancestral mammalian copulatory pattern most likely involved a single intromission and pelvic thrusting by the male partner. Intromission duration may have been brief (pattern no. 12) or prolonged, with repeated bouts of pelvic thrusting (pattern no. 11). In reality, a continuum of intromission durations, lasting from a few seconds up to 7 hours in various species, links these two copulatory patterns; they are not mutually exclusive.

The fact that so many of the marsupials (as well as the surviving monotremes) mate for long periods suggests that pattern no. 11 may be closest to the ancestral condition. Fossil evidence indicates that the metatherian and eutherian mammals of the Cretaceous Period were relatively small creatures; many of them no larger than rats or mice. They were probably nocturnal or crepuscular in their habits, just as the majority of marsupials and many placental mammals are today. In Chapter 3 an analysis of data on 170 genera, representing 19 orders of mammals, showed that intromission duration correlates inversely with body mass, so that, in general, small mammals tend to mate for longer periods of time than larger taxa. Given their small size, prolonged matings were also probably more common among mammals during the Cretaceous Period. Another factor which may have influenced the evolution of copulatory behaviour concerns the risk of predation experienced by different species. Almost 50 years ago, Ewer (1973) suggested that lengthy matings should occur more frequently in carnivorous mammals than in herbivores, given that the latter are subject to greater predation risks. The statistical comparisons of intromission durations in carnivorous vs herbivorous mammals presented in Chapter 3 support Ewer's hypothesis.

Evidence concerning the widespread occurrence of multiple-partner matings by female mammals, resulting in post-copulatory sexual selection, was reviewed in Chapter 4. Functional relationships between copulatory patterns and post-copulatory sexual selection are complex, however. There are taxa in which monogamous or polygynous species employ the same masculine copulatory patterns as polygynandrous species. This is the case, for example, among the African apes and humans, all of which display copulatory pattern no. 12. However, polygynandrous chimpanzees and bonobos copulate at much higher frequencies (as well as having much larger testes) and thus transfer greater numbers of spermatozoa to females than is possible for male gorillas or humans. Multiple rapid matings also occur in some mammals that are induced ovulators. This is the case in rabbits and hares (Family Leporidae) and in members of the cat family (Felidae). Males of these taxa make a single, very rapid copulatory thrust to achieve intromission and ejaculation (copulatory pattern no. 16). However, tom cats are reproductively more successful if they mate a number of times, thus increasing the level of stimulation provided to the female (see Figure 9.3).

Mating at high frequencies is thus one tactic by which males gain an advantage via sperm competition or cryptic female choice. Another strategy that may enable males to transfer greater numbers of sperm to the female is to make a series of mounts, and to move successive cohorts of sperm through the vasa deferentia prior to ejaculation (e.g. patterns nos. 10 and 14), or to prolong a single intromission and to ejaculate multiple times. Copulatory pattern no. 11 is of this latter type. It may have been the precursor of pattern no. 3, in which the prolonged intromission is combined with a genital lock between the sexes. This pattern occurs in at least 42 species scattered across 9 of the 27 orders of mammals, many of which are polygynandrous. Although foxes, dogs and wolves (Family Canidae) are usually considered to be monogamous, multiple-partner matings by females and multiple paternity of litters occurs in some species. Thus, it is likely that the genital lock in canids has evolved under sexual selection. With the exception of the domestic dog, very little is known about semen transfer in any of the mammals that copulate for extended periods. Nor are the functions of the diverse pelvic thrusting patterns exhibited by males during such lengthy intromissions understood (see Table 4.4).

The five major copulatory patterns discussed above, as well as six others that are represented in a minority of species, serve a dual purpose. They transfer sperm and secretions of the male accessory reproductive glands to the female, but they may also stimulate responses that increase the likelihood of reproductive success. The example of copulatory stimulation and induced ovulation has already been mentioned, but stimuli supplied during mounting and intromission also activate reflexes that result in females remaining immobile or adopting receptive postures (such as lordosis). Males may vary in their ability to elicit responses that constitute elements of cryptic female choice. Males may also engage in 'copulatory courtship', such as biting the skin of the female's neck, which serves to activate an immobilization reflex.

In Chapter 5, the huge diversity of phallic morphology displayed by mammals was scrutinized through the lens of copulatory and post-copulatory sexual selection. There is now ample evidence that complex penile morphologies have evolved as 'internal courtship devices' rather than as species isolating mechanisms (the 'lock and key' hypothesis), or the incidental targets of genes that have more important reproductive functions (the 'pleiotropism' hypothesis). Mammalian research in this field is still largely at the stage of establishing correlations. Thus, the penile morphologies of mammals in which females mate with multiple males tend to be morphologically complex (e.g. in primates, marsupial mice and hystricognath rodents). There is a positive correlation between the length of the baculum (penile bone) and the duration of intromission in carnivores and primates, but whether this correlation applies to rodents, bats and other taxa where a baculum occurs remains to be determined. From a biomechanical perspective it appears that the baculum, in conjunction with the corpora cavernosa, forms a functional unit that strengthens the erect penis and protects the urethra during extended matings. Its absence in mammals that have markedly fibroelastic penes may be due to the fact that erectile capacity is concentrated in the root of the penis, rather than in its shaft and distal region. However, the baculum has evolved independently a number of times and its functions must surely vary among the seven orders of placental mammals in which it occurs. Experiments have shown that the thickness of the baculum increases when mice reproduce under conditions where females mate with multiple partners, as compared to enforced monogamy. Mice do not exhibit prolonged intromission, however; instead, males make a series of brief intromissions with pelvic thrusting (pattern no. 10). This induces surges of prolactin which facilitate support of the corpus luteum and secretion of progesterone during early pregnancy. The increased thickness of the baculum may be adaptive in this context.

Androgen-dependent keratinized penile spines occur in the platypus, and in some marsupials and placental mammals. In the only experiment that has examined the behavioural effects of removing these spines in otherwise intact subjects, male marmosets took longer to achieve intromission and to ejaculate than sham-operated controls. One possibility is that small (Type 1) spines that enhance the tactile sensitivity of the penis represent the plesiomorphic condition among mammals. Penile spines are morphologically diverse, however, and their functions are still only partially understood. For example, in rats, one of their functions is to break up and remove copulatory plugs deposited by previous matings. Very large penile spines occur in some taxa in which there is a prolonged lock or tie during mating (copulatory pattern no. 3). This is the case in the Australian hopping mouse, the fossa and in the various galago species. Other specializations of penile morphology associated with this copulatory pattern include the erectile bulbus glandis in canids, and the peculiar 'S'-shaped glans of the shrew *Blarina brevicauda*. Such diverse traits have probably developed independently in different mammalian lineages.

The urethral meatus of the penis exhibits some unusual morphological specializations among mammals. For example, in goats and many other bovids, it is elongated to form a vermiform urethral process. The urethral process of the goat is erectile, and it probably functions to place the ejaculate as close as possible to the os cervix during the very brief intromission (copulatory pattern no. 16) that is typical of bovids. In some mammals the baculum extends beyond the tip of the penis and the urethra opens on its ventral side. This arrangement may function to place semen directly into the cervical canal at ejaculation (e.g. in the spring hare, *Pedetes surdaster*). In hystricognath rodents such as the agouti and guinea pig an intromittent sac is situated ventral to the opening of the urethra. This sac, which is everted during copulation, is clothed in robust spines, and bears two (or more) elongated spikes. It is probable that the backward-pointing penile spines might grip or otherwise stimulate the walls of the vagina during copulation, whilst the pair of large spikes might probe deeper to contact the cervix. In the guinea pig, vagino-cervical stimulation shortens the duration of female sexual receptivity. Intrauterine insemination also occurs in guinea pigs. It is possible that the intromittent sac is important in producing these effects, but experimental proof is lacking.

Intrauterine insemination occurs in a number of other taxa and, in these cases too, morphological specializations of the penis facilitate the process. In horses and asses (Family Equidae) the presence of a short urethral process and tumescence of the distal penis at ejaculation facilitate rapid transfer of semen through the cervical canal and into the uterine cavity. Pigs (Family Suidae) have a spiral penis, which engages with the cervix during a lengthy intromission. A large volume of semen is thus deposited into the uterus.

The striated penile muscles exert important effects during copulation. Their functions differ among taxa, and include the control of reflexive penile movements as well as the expulsion of semen during ejaculation. In the rat, for example, the ischiocavernosus (IC) muscles control penile responses ('flips') that are essential if the male is to attain intromission. By contrast, the bulbocavernosus (BC) muscles govern reflexes which pack and seal the copulatory plug against the cervix during the final mount of the series (Sachs, 1983). If the plug is positioned correctly, then sperm are transported rapidly into the uterus. As noted above, penile stimulation provided during preejaculatory intromissions serves to dislodge copulatory plugs deposited by previous males, and also to activate neuroendocrine responses in the female that are essential for pregnancy. The rat thus provides a powerful example of the penis acting as an internal courtship device that simultaneously promotes success in sperm competition, as well as being subject to cryptic female choice.

It is unlikely that such a dynamic mixture of copulatory interactions will be found to exist among the marsupials. I say this because there are major differences between marsupials and placentals in the functional anatomy of their striated penile muscles (Warburton *et al.*, 2019) as well as the anatomy of the female genitalia (as discussed in Chapter 8). These differences probably limit the expression of penile reflexes and penile/cervical interactions during copulation in marsupials. An effective test of this hypothesis will require much more detailed experimental investigations of copulatory mechanisms in marsupials.

Males that are able to produce and store larger numbers of sperm prior to mating may gain a reproductive advantage via post-copulatory sexual selection. Greater sperm production may be achieved by increasing the mass of gamete-producing (seminiferous) tissue in the testes, or by increasing the rate of spermatogenesis. Evidence regarding both these mechanisms was examined in Chapter 6, as well as discussing specializations of sperm morphology in some taxa that may increase their ability to survive the many challenges posed by the female reproductive tract.

More than 40 years ago Harcourt *et al.* reported in *Nature* that relative testes size in primates correlates with their mating systems, and with the likely greater occurrence of sperm competition in multimale–multifemale groups, such as those of macaques and chimpanzees. Since that time, relationships between sperm competition and relative testes size have been reported for monotremes and marsupials, as well bats, cetaceans, carnivores and rodents. Increases in testes size are usually due to larger volumes of sperm-producing tissue (seminiferous tubules), but a caveat concerns a minority of species in which the inter-tubular Leydig cells (which secrete testosterone) account for between 20 per cent and 60 per cent of testicular volume. This is the case, for example, in the capybara, naked mole-rat, warthog, European mole and some South American opossums.

Mammals that have larger relative testes sizes also tend to exhibit faster rates of spermatogenesis and thus to produce larger numbers of sperm per gram of testicular parenchyma. However, there is a 'trade-off' between sperm length and spermatogenesis (longer sperm take a longer time to produce) and also body weight (very large mammals tend to have slower rates of spermatogenesis; Ramm and Stockley, 2010). Larger mammals might also produce greater numbers of smaller sperm to combat dilution effects that occur due to the increased volume of the female reproductive tract (Lüpold and Fitzpatrick, 2015). Thus sexual selection has not always favoured the evolution of longer mammalian spermatozoa despite the potential advantages offered by their greater swimming velocity. This may explain why comparative studies have failed to reveal a simple correlation between relative testes sizes and sperm lengths in mammals (Anderson *et al.*, 2005; Gage and Freckleton, 2003).

Experiments by Holt *et al.* (2010) using the sperm of brown hares, pigs and cattle have shown that motility and success in 'swim-up' trials are greater in longer sperm (Figure 6.12). These authors noted, however, that linear swimming speeds of sperm are the result of the beat frequencies of their flagella as well as flagellar length. The mitochondria contained in the sperm midpiece provide an important source of energy for sperm motility, and in this case there is a positive correlation between sperm midpiece volume and relative testes size in mammals, as was discussed in Chapter 6.

Trivers (1985) pointed out that cooperation might be expected to occur between spermatozoa that are members of the same ejaculate, given that they are closely related. A possible example of such cooperative relationships concerns the sperm bundles of the short-beaked echidna, which contain up to 100 gametes joined at the tips of the sperm heads and swimming in unison. Johnston *et al.* (2007) suggest that sperm bundles might have evolved due to post-copulatory sexual selection, and also that storage of sperm may occur within the female reproductive tract. Further research on monotremes is required in order to resolve these questions.

In all the American marsupials, with the sole exception of *Dromiciops* (Order Microbiotheria), sperm become joined together in pairs (forming 'binary sperm') during their passage through the epididymis. Sperm pairing may serve to protect the acrosome of each partner, but there is also evidence that binary sperm are better at moving through viscous environments, such as the mucus of the female reproductive tract (Moore and Taggart, 1995). The Virginia opossum (*Didelphia virginiana*) releases only 3 million sperm during copulation, and its epididymal stores (13 miilion in each terminal segment) are likewise very modest. It would be interesting to know if the remarkable traits exhibited by binary sperm have reduced the need for polygynandrous taxa to invest in larger volumes of seminiferous tissue, and to develop larger relative testes sizes.

In many murid rodents there is an apical hook on the head of the sperm. Moore *et al.* (2002) reported that these hooks play an important role in the formation of 'trains' of spermatozoa (in the woodmouse: *Apodemus sylvaticus*). When woodmice sperm were observed *in vitro*, thousands of gametes sometimes formed trains, linked together by the hooks on their heads. In a sample of 37 murid species, the degree of curvature of their sperm hooks was positively correlated with relative testes sizes, leading to the conclusion that apical hooks are adaptations for sperm competition (Immler *et al.*, 2007). However, subsequent studies, by Firman and Simmons (2008) on mice and Touremente *et al.* (2016) on 25 species of rodents, have produced negative results. Thus, Touremente *et al.* found that, in most species, sperm did not form trains, woodmice being exceptional in this regard. Other theories have been advanced to account for the functions of hooked sperm. Might the shape of the hook enable the spermatozoon to swim faster (Montoto et al., 2011), or to penetrate the zona pellucida of the ovum (Flaherty *et al.*, 1983)? Do hooks assist sperm to attach to the epithelium in the isthmus of the oviduct (Smith and Yanagimachi, 1990; Suarez, 1987)?

Chapter 6 concluded with a discussion of testicular descent and the evolution of the scrotum in mammals. There it was noted that, during foetal development, the testes are initially situated close to the kidneys. In testicond mammals, such as the monotremes and afrotherians, the testes are retained deep within the body cavity throughout life. Partial descent of the testes occurs in some taxa, but in most placental mammals and marsupials the testes are fully descended and housed in an external pouch, the scrotum. Bedford (1978a, 1978b) proposed that the physiological requirement to store sperm in a cooler environment prior to copulation led to the evolution of the scrotum. In scrotal species, the terminal segment of each epididymis (which stores spermatozoa) forms a loop situated close to the exterior of the body, where lower temperatures occur. Moreover, in some species, loss of hair on the lower part of the scrotum may help to cool the underlying terminal segment. Bedford also reported results of experiments on rabbits and rats establishing that the negative effects of higher abdominal temperatures on the epididymis concern its storage functions, rather than its maturational functions.

The scrotum is situated cranially to the penis in marsupials, the reverse of its position in placental mammals. Kleisener *et al.* (2010) concluded that the scrotum has arisen twice during mammalian evolution: once in the marsupials, and once in placental mammals. Previously, however, Werdelin and Nilsonne (1999) had reached the opposite conclusion, arguing that the possession of a scrotum was the ancestral condition, and that it has undergone secondary loss in various groups of mammals. Most recently, a partial resolution to this debate has been provided by Sharma *et al.* (2018), who conducted a comparative study of two genes that play important roles in the development of the gubernaculum, the ligament which guides the testis during its descent. Results of their research indicate that testicular descent represents the ancestral condition among placental mammals (see Figure 6.17). However, no comparable data exist for marsupials.

In addition to spermatozoa, male mammals transfer the secretions of various accessory reproductive glands to females during copulation. The most phylogenetically ancient of these are the bulbourethral (Cowper's) glands, which occur in most orders of the Mammalia. Indeed, they are the only accessory reproductive glands present in monotremes, in which the ducts of a single pair of glands open into the penile canal. The echidna produces only a small volume of ejaculate, and the same may be said of the platypus. It is thought that in both these species, sperm are delivered directly to the oviductal ostia via specializations of distal penile morphology. The evolutionary origin of the bulbourethral glands in monotremes may thus reside in their ability to lubricate the penile canal and to assist sperm transport. Their functions in other mammals are obscure, however. Most of the placental mammals have one pair of bulbourethral glands, but in a few cases, such as in whales, dolphins and porpoises, they have been lost (for unknown reasons) during the course of evolution. In some rodents, the bulbourethral glands play a role in the coagulation of semen (Hart and Greenstein, 1968). In marsupials, 1–3 pairs of bulbourethral glands are present in various taxa, sometimes differing in their size and in histological structure. These variations hint at differences in function, yet very little is known about these matters. The same may also be said of the ampullary glands, which are present in some members of at least 11 orders of placental mammals (Figure 7.1). In most of these cases, nothing is known about the functions of the ampullary glands or the chemical composition of their secretions.

For the reasons outlined above, Chapter 7 focused on the prostate and vesicular glands, as much more is known about their physiology, particularly with regard to mechanisms of seminal coagulation and the formation of copulatory plugs. All the marsupials and placental mammals have a prostate gland, but only some placental mammals have vesicular glands. Coagulating glands (which derive from the prostate) occur in some rodents. The weights of the prostate gland and seminal vesicles are greater in those mammals where females mate with multiple partners, as compared with those that are monogamous or polygynous. Coagulation of semen and copulatory plug formation is also more typical of polygynandrous species. The most likely adaptive functions of copulatory plugs involve maintaining a sperm-rich fraction of the ejaculate in contact with the os cervix and facilitating sperm transport. The theory that plugs might block the sperm deposited by rival males or prevent females from re-mating (the 'chastity belt' hypothesis) is less likely to apply to mammals. The alkaline nature of semen, with pH values ranging from 7 to 8 in various species (see Table 8.4) may also be adaptive in counteracting acidic conditions in the vagina, thus assisting sperm survival.

The functions of most of the huge number of chemicals secreted by the accessory reproductive glands of males remain a mystery. In Chapter 8 it was noted that the spermatozoa and accessory glandular secretions are antigenic, so that they constitute a challenge to the female immune system. Post-copulatory interactions between the ejaculate and the female's genitalia are complex, and inevitably involve a degree of conflict as well as cooperation. Cooperation between the sexes is essential if fertiliza-tion is to occur; yet, from a female perspective, multiple-partner matings carry increased risks of contracting sexually transmitted infections as well as damage to the vagina and cervix by males that have complex, spiny genitalia. Males benefit by depositing their ejaculates as close as possible to the female's ova; hence the occur-rence of intrauterine insemination in mammals such as pigs, horses, camelids and some rodents. Intrauterine insemination is problematic for females, however, as it circumvents the protective functions of the vagina and cervix and directly exposes the uterine environment to risk.

As well as dealing with conflict and cooperation between the sexes, Chapter 8 discussed cryptic female choice. From the time that spermatozoa enter the female reproductive tract, until fertilization occurs in the oviduct, processes governed by the female's reproductive anatomy and physiology determine sperm survival, transport, temporary storage and their ability to locate and fuse with the ova. These processes were mapped out in Chapter 8 and need not be repeated here. Instead, it may be more productive to discuss at least a few of the many unanswered questions concerning mechanisms of cryptic female choice in mammals.

Theory posits that when a female mates with multiple partners, a variety of male traits (e.g. copulatory courtship, successful placement of ejaculates, sperm numbers and sperm quality) are subject to copulatory and post-copulatory sexual selection. The majority of sperm are winnowed out by phagocytosis and other processes in the vagina, cervix, uterus and uterotubal junction. Very few male gametes reach the oviduct. The 'raffle effect', which results when rival males maximize sperm numbers in the ejaculate, may result in a numerical advantage for some individuals whose gametes reach the oviduct. Cryptic female choice may thus have occurred at lower levels of the female tract, favouring the gametes of some males over others. However, it is likely that the oviduct plays a decisive role in post-copulatory selection, and especially so where cryptic female choice is concerned. A major problem in research on this topic is the inability to identify the gametes of individual males. Clearly, the sperm of a number of potential sires can access ova, as multiple paternity of litters occurs in many mammals. However, what is needed, from a research perspective, is the ability to identify the sperm of potential sires at various stages of their passage through the female tract. For example, which males are represented in the temporary sperm stores of the isthmus or in the oviductal crypts that occur in some marsupials and shrews? Which sperm successfully undergo capacitation, and exhibit hyperactivated motility? How do the sperm of rival males vary in their ability to ascend the oviduct and respond to the thermotactic and chemotactic cues that guide them to the ova? Artificial insemination studies have shown that when equal volumes of semen, or equal numbers of sperm, from two males are mixed together, then one male often sires a disproportionate number of the resulting offspring (rabbit: Beatty, 1960; mouse: Edwards, 1955; cattle: Beatty *et al.*, 1969). Might it be possible to employ markers that allow sperm of rival males to be tracked, in order to reveal the causative factors that underlie such effects?

It is now known that the oviduct expresses genetic mechanisms that may filter and screen spermatozoa. For example, when either X or Y chromosome-bearing sperm are inseminated into the oviducts of pigs, sex-specific genomic responses occur. Almiñana *et al.* (2014) suggest that such responses to spermatozoa might represent 'a gender biasing mechanism controlled by the female'. If this is correct, then could cryptic female choice for either X- or Y-bearing sperm explain how adaptive skewing of birth sex ratios is possible in some mammals?

Cryptic female choice is also likely to play a crucial role in those mammals in which mating-induced ovulation occurs. The first male to mate often secures a reproductive advantage in such circumstances because, once ovulation has been induced to occur, other males have a limited window of time in which to attempt copulation. Females of some induced ovulators certainly engage in multiple-partner matings, but the first male often achieves a larger paternity share. Females may also benefit via cryptic choices for males that provide the most effective types of stimulation. It is presumed that their male offspring are likely to inherit their sire's beneficial traits. What constitutes the 'most effective' stimulation varies tremendously among taxa. Both prolonged and brief patterns of intromission are represented among induced ovulators, but in the latter case multiple copulations often occur so that a cumulative effect is produced. In the camelids, β-nerve growth factor in the male's semen triggers the pre-ovulatory LH surge, whereas in lagomorphs a variety of pre-copulatory and copulatory stimuli combine to induce ovulation. The existence of such variability also indicates that induced ovulation has evolved independently a number of times in mammals.

Comparative approaches to unravelling the origins and evolution of induced ovulation remain problematic. A number of authors have proposed that induced ovulation represents the ancestral condition among mammals. Yet, an important negative piece of evidence is that induced ovulation has only rarely been identified in vertebrates other than mammals. Spontaneous ovulation appears to be the norm in fish, amphibians, reptiles and birds. Some of the few known exceptions to this rule were discussed in Chapter 9. It seems likely, therefore, that ancestral mammals were spontaneous ovulators.

Induced ovulation is likely to represent an ancient trait for some extant lineages of the Carnivora, Rodentia, Lagomorpha and Eulipotyphla, while spontaneous ovulation is the norm for most lineages of the Cetartiodactyla, Perissodactyla, Primates and Proboscidea. However, for many taxa there is insufficient information about their modes of ovulation to make firm judgements. We should also acknowledge that gaps in the fossil record of mammalian evolution during the late Cretaceous and the post K/T boundary phase currently limit the effectiveness of phylogenetic analyses.

Research into mechanisms of copulatory and post-copulatory sexual selection is gradually enlarging our understanding of the evolution of mammalian reproduction. However, there is a long road ahead for mammalogists and reproductive biologists if they are to emulate those workers who study post-copulatory sexual selection in insects and other invertebrates. Fortunately, many of the fundamental insights arising from the pioneering work of Geoffrey Parker, William Eberhard and other invertebrate biologists are directly applicable to research on mammals. Good progress has been made thus far, and I hope that this book may encourage more mammalian reproductive biologists to contribute to this field. Who knows?! Perhaps future editions of standard works, such as *Marshall's Physiology of Reproduction* and *Knobil and Neill's Physiology of Reproduction* may then include answers to some of the many unresolved questions concerning mammalian sperm competition and cryptic female choice.

Post-copulatory Sexual Selection and Human Evolution

They say that bears have love affairs, and even camels
We're merely mammals, let's misbehave!

                                        Cole Porter, 1928, from the musical *Paris*

Although direct information about the sexual behaviour of the earliest humans is unattainable, there are indirect sources of information that can throw some light upon this subject. Firstly, we may examine the types of mating systems that exist, or have existed until very recently, among human societies around the world. Secondly, the occurrence of various sexual dimorphic traits in modern humans may be useful in deciding to what extent polygyny might have played some role during our evolutionary past. Thirdly, the comparative data on mammalian reproduction reviewed in this book can be used to infer whether post-copulatory sexual selection might have played a significant role during human evolution.

Where human mating systems are concerned, anthropological studies indicate that most human societies are monogamous or polygynous. Almost 70 years ago, Ford and Beach (1952) noted that 'No human society condones promiscuous or indiscriminate mating. Every culture contains regulations that direct and restrict the individual's selection of a sexual partner or partners.' Their examination of 185 human societies led them to conclude that, in 84 per cent of cases, 'men are permitted by custom to have more than one mate at a time if they can arrange to do so'. However, many men are unable to arrange matters in this way, so that 'it is probable that at any given time less than half the adult males are in fact mated to more than one woman'.

A wide variety of sexually dimorphic traits occur in human beings. Women and men differ in body size (weight and height) and body composition (especially amounts of muscle and fat), as well as in the development of breasts, facial hair, the size of the larynx and other features listed in Figure 10.1. Comparative studies of sexually dimorphic traits in humans and in other primates support the conclusion that polygyny (as well as monogamy) has shaped human ancestry (Dixson, 2009; Dixson *et al.*, 2005; B.J. Dixson and Vasey, 2012).

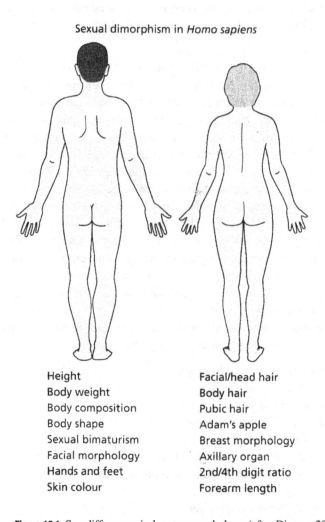

Sexual dimorphism in *Homo sapiens*

Height	Facial/head hair
Body weight	Body hair
Body composition	Pubic hair
Body shape	Adam's apple
Sexual bimaturism	Breast morphology
Facial morphology	Axillary organ
Hands and feet	2nd/4th digit ratio
Skin colour	Forearm length

Figure 10.1 Sex differences in human morphology (after Dixson, 2009).

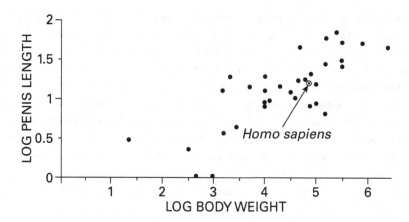

Figure 10.2 Relationship between body weight (g) and length of the erect penis (cm) in 34 species of mammals, including *H. sapiens*. Data on penile lengths are provided in Appendix 3.

The results of comparative studies of mammalian reproductive anatomy and physiology discussed in this book are also useful when deciding whether post-copulatory sexual selection might have affected the evolution of the human reproductive system. My own conclusion, having considered this question carefully (Dixson, 2009, 2012, 2018), is that sperm competition and cryptic female choice are unlikely to have played a significant role in this respect. However, one of the most persistent causes of confusion about the human genitalia concerns the size of the penis. Numerous authors have stated that the human penis is exceptionally large and morphologically complex. At least 11 books published between 1982 and 2010 include such statements (Dixson, 2012). Yet, as discussed in Chapter 5, human penile morphology is not unusual, except for its girth. Additional data listed in Appendix 3 made it possible to compare the length of the erect penis, in relation to body weight, in 34 mammals, including the human species. As Figure 10.2 makes clear, the data for *H. sapiens* are unremarkable, and fall within the range expected for mammals of similar body mass.

The 10 traits listed below are indicative of the effects of sperm competition and/or cryptic female choice in polygynandrous mammals:

1. Large testes relative to male body size
2. Faster rates of spermatogenesis
3. Greater capacity to sustain high sperm counts
4. Sperm with larger midpiece volumes
5. More muscular vasa deferentia
6. Large seminal vesicles and prostate glands relative to body size
7. More pronounced seminal coagulation/copulatory plug formation
8. Higher copulatory frequencies
9. Morphologically more complex penes
10. Longer oviducts in relation to female body size

Here is the situation concerning the same 10 traits in humans. It differs markedly from that described above for polygynandrous mammals:

1. Human testes are smaller than expected in relation to body weight, and especially so in some Asiatic populations (Dixson, 2009).
2. Men produce 4.4 million sperm each day per gram of testicular parenchyma; less than in any other mammal measured (Sharpe, 1994). Seminiferous epithelium cycle lengths are longer in men (16 days) and sperm production is slower than in other primates (Ramm and Stockley, 2010).
3. Men exhibit an 84 per cent decline in sperm counts during periods when they ejaculate three times per day (Freund, 1963).
4. Human sperm have very small midpiece volumes (Anderson et al., 2005). Morphological abnormalities commonly occur in 27 per cent of human sperm (Seuánez, 1980).
5. In polygynandrous mammals, the ratio of the vas deferens muscle wall thickness to lumen diameter averages 9.9 ± 0.7. The ratio in humans (6.31) is typical of other monogamous and polygynous taxa (Anderson et al., 2004a).
6. The human seminal vesicles are relatively small. Nor is the human prostate gland especially large (Anderson and Dixson, 2009; Dixson, 1998b).
7. Human semen exhibits a low level of coagulation post ejaculation. There is no distinct coagulum or copulatory plug (Dixson and Anderson, 2002).
8. Large-scale surveys of married couples (in the USA, UK and China) indicate that intercourse occurs 2–4 times per week on average (Kinsey et al., 1948; Liu et al., 1997; Wellings et al., 1994).
9. Human phallic morphology is not unusual, except for its girth, and even that is not unique among primates (Dixson, 2009, 2012, 2018).
10. Residuals of oviduct length correlate with residual testes sizes in mammals. However, women have comparatively short oviducts (Anderson et al., 2006; Dixson, 2009).

The Age of Mammals

Have pity on them all, for it is we who are the real monsters
Bernard Heuvelmans, 1958

There have been five major extinction events during the history of life on earth. The last of these occurred about 66 million years ago, at the close of the Cretaceous Period, when an enormous meteor collided with the planet. Catastrophic environmental changes resulting from the meteor strike led to the extinction of the non-avian dinosaurs and made possible the rise of various orders of mammals that are alive today. Indeed, as a member of the Order Primates, the human species is just one product of the flowering of biological diversity which constitutes 'The Age of Mammals'.

The diversity of behavioural and reproductive mechanisms displayed among the extant mammals is extraordinary, intellectually challenging and aesthetically satisfying. I have tried to convey some appreciation of these matters in this book, but I am also keenly aware that a great many of our fellow mammals are in rapid decline. Unfortunately, life on Earth now faces a sixth great extinction event, caused not by a meteor but by humanity itself. The human population of the world now exceeds 7.8 billion; our numbers are a nightmare. The total biomass of human beings, plus the biomass of our domesticated livestock (cattle, pigs, goats and sheep), vastly exceeds that of all the other mammals combined. Indeed, the other 6000+ species, from tiny shrews to gargantuan whales, represent just 5 per cent of total mammalian biomass. The requirement by an ever-expanding human population for access to land and to natural resources of all kinds is devastating the natural world.

The International Union for the Conservation of Nature (IUCN) maintains careful records of the status of the world's biodiversity. Currently, the IUCN Red List estimates that between 22 per cent and 37 per cent of all mammalian species are critically endangered, endangered or vulnerable to extinction. The list of extinctions grows longer every year. It includes the Yangtze River dolphin (*Lipotes vexillifer*), a victim of over-fishing and pollution, and Miss Waldron's red colobus monkey (*Piliocolobus waldronae*), killed off by forest destruction and hunting. Spare a thought also for the aptly named gloomy tube-nosed bat (*Munna tenebrosa*), which was discovered on the Japanese island of Tsushima in 1962. All attempts to find one since then have failed. Huge numbers of mammals are edging ever closer to extinction and, in virtually every case, habitat destruction and hunting by humans are the chief causes of their demise. Populations of all five rhinoceros species have plummeted during my own lifetime, and the same is true for all of the great apes, the asiatic elephant and the larger carnivores, including the tiger, snow leopard, cheetah and jaguar.

The close associations that have developed between humans and other mammals, via domestication of some species and the hunting and trafficking of wildlife, have sometimes produced catastrophic epidemics. A good many diseases that afflict humanity have been acquired from other mammals. An example of such a 'zoonotic infection' is the bubonic plague, a bacterial disease which is transmitted by the bite of the rat flea. The Black Death killed between 30 per cent and 50 per cent of the population of Europe during the fourteenth century (Cantor, 2001). Much more recently, the HIV/AIDS pandemic began in Africa in 1981; the source of HIV1 is the chimpanzee, while HIV2 derives from a monkey, the sooty mangabey. The history of its transmission to human beings in Africa and its spread to other countries has been documented in an excellent book by Jaques Pepin (2011). In 2018 the World Health Organization estimated that 75 million people had been infected since the pandemic began, and that 32 million of them had died.

During the time that I spent writing this book, countries around the world have struggled (and most have failed) to control another pandemic caused, this time, by a coronavirus that transferred from bats to humans. The first case of human infection with the coronavirus (COVID-19) occurred in an animal market in the Chinese city of Wuhan during December 2019. Seven months later, more than 7 million cases had been reported worldwide, and more than 400,000 people had died. 'Wet markets', such as the one in Wuhan, are common in China and in other Asian countries. They have been implicated in causing disease outbreaks in the past, most notably the severe acute respiratory syndrome (SARS) coronavirus outbreak of 2003. Some wet markets trade in living animals of all kinds, crowded together under insanitary conditions which have led to disasters such as SARS and COVID-19. The Wuhan market has been closed and one hopes that other such markets will also be shut down, otherwise it is only a matter of time until another pandemic arises. Some markets do not exist only to supply food; they also sell animals for use in traditional Chinese medicine. For example, hundreds of thousands of pangolins ('scaly anteaters') have been taken from the wild in Asia and Africa, not only for their flesh, but in order to strip off their scales for medical usage. Multiple body parts of tigers, as well as rhinoceros horns, and the gall bladders of bears also feature in Chinese traditional medicine. Of course, these practices are of no medical value and, given the increasing rarity of so many mammals, surely it is time not just to ban the trade in such things, but to ensure that such bans are enforced.

The types of activities discussed above may seem bizarre, given that modern medicine has eclipsed the need for such approaches to the treatment of human ailments. Tradition exerts a powerful effect upon human behaviour, however, and not so long ago western medicine included treatments that would be considered barbaric nowadays (Bryson, 2019). Although our species is now technologically highly sophisticated, this has occurred comparatively recently. The roots of our behavioural potential developed more than 200,000 years ago, in Africa, where the earliest fossils of anatomically modern humans have been discovered. Our ancestors were hunter-gatherers and their migrations reflected the necessity to search out new areas to exploit, whenever local resources had become depleted. Thus, by 100,000 years ago, *H. sapiens* had begun to explore the greater world; first in the Middle East, then Europe (40,000–45,000 years ago), China (60,000 years ago) and Australia by 50,000 years ago (Stringer and Andrews, 2005). Whenever our ancestors entered previously unoccupied areas of the globe, the devastation of the resident megafauna soon followed. This was the case in Australia, for example, with the demise of *Diprotodon* and most other large marsupials (Flannery, 1994), and in Madagascar where the largest and slowest lemur species became extinct soon after the advent of humans (Tattersall, 1982). In North America the disappearance of mammoths, dire wolves, sabre-toothed cats and ground sloths after the end of the last ice age was largely due to hunter-gatherers. In New Zealand, one of the last places on earth to be colonized, the giant moas along with many other flightless birds were hunted to extinction (Duff, 1977).

These earlier extinctions were thus driven by the human imperative to obtain sufficient food. Hunter-gatherer groups were small, however, and mortality rates, particularly among children, would have been high. Population growth has been constrained and gradual throughout most of the time our species has existed. It is estimated that 10,000 years ago there were only 8 million people, rising to 300 million during the first century AD. At that time it would take another 1600 years for the world's population to double in size (Raleigh, 1999). However, human numbers began to increase rapidly after the end of the Second World War. When I was born, in 1948, there were approximately two billion people in the world. Now, 72 years later, there are more than 7.8 billion of us, representing a 390 per cent increase in the population during my lifetime. Such huge increases in our numbers are disturbing; they remind me of the abnormal boom in mouse populations that sometimes afflicts the grain-producing areas of Australia.

Demographers have predicted that our population will 'plateau' by 2050, at somewhere between 7.7 and 11.2 billion. We may discount the lower estimate, as it was surpassed during 2020. The higher number thus seems more probable. How will 11.2 billion people obtain sufficient food? How will they gain access to clean water, medical care or a decent education? How will they cope with the havoc caused by climate change, pollution of the oceans and massive loss of the earth's biodiversity? In truth, nobody knows.

Appendix 1 Mammalian Copulatory Patterns

Taxa	Genital lock	Pelvic thrusts	Multiple intromissions	Prolonged intromission	Pattern number	Sources
Order Monotremata						
Family Ornithorynchidae						
Ornithorhynchus anatinus	Yes?	No?	No	Yes	7?	Hawkins and Battaglia, 2009
Family Tachyglossidae						
Tachyglossus aculeatus	?	Yes	No	Yes	. . .	Rissmiller and McKelvey, 2000
Order Diprotodontia						
Family Macropodidae						
Macropus giganteus	No	Yes	No	Yes	11	Sharman *et al.*, 1966
M. rufus	No	Yes	No	Yes	11	Sharman *et al.*, 1966
M. rufogriseous	No	Yes	No	Yes	11	Sharman *et al.*, 1966
M. robustus	No	Yes	No	Yes	11	Croft, 1981
M. eugenii	No	Yes	No	Yes	11	Rudd, 1994
M. parma	No	No	No	No	16	Tyndale-Biscoe and Renfree, 1987
Setonix brachyurus	No	?	No	Yes?	. . .	McClean and Schmitt, 1999
Family Potoroidae						
Potorous tridactylus	No	?	No	No	. . .	Tyndale-Biscoe and Renfree, 1987
Bettongia gaimardi	No	Yes	No	Yes	11	Rose, 1985
Family Vombatidae						
Vombatus ursinus	No	Yes	No	Yes	11	Hughes and Hughes, 2006; Marks, 1998
Lasiorhinus latifrons	No	Yes	No	Yes	11	Hogan *et al.*, 2010

283

(*cont.*)

Taxa	Genital lock	Pelvic thrusts	Multiple intromissions	Prolonged intromission	Pattern number	Sources
Family Phascolarctidae						
Phascolarctos cinereus	No	Yes	No	No	12	Smith, 1980
Family Phalangeridae						
Trichosurus vulpecula	No	Yes	No	No	12	Winter, 1976
Dactylopsila trivirgata	No?	...	...	No?	...	McKenna, 2005
Order Peramelemorphia						
Family Peramelidae						
Perameles nasuta	No	?	Yes	No	...	Stodart, 1966
P. gunnii	No	?	Yes	No	...	Dufty, 1994
Order Notoryctemorphia						
Order Dasyuromorphia						
Family Dasyuridae						
Antechinus stuartii	Yes	Yes	No	Yes	3	Woolley, 1966
A. agilis	Yes	Yes	No	Yes	3	Shimmin et al., 2002
A. swainsonii	?	?	No	Yes	...	Williams and Williams, 1982
A. flavipes	...	...	...	Yes	...	Strahan, 1995
A. leo	...	...	...	Yes	...	Strahan, 1995
Planigale gilesi	?	Yes	No	Yes	...	Whitford et al., 1982
Sminthopsis crassicaudata	?	Yes	No	Yes	...	Ewer, 1968
S. murina	?	Yes	No	Yes	...	Fox and Whitford, 1982
Ningua sp.	?	Yes	No	Yes	...	Fanning, 1982
Parantechinus apicalis	?	?	?	Yes	...	Wolfe et al., 2000
Dasycercus cristicauda	...	Yes	No	Yes	...	Michener, 1969; Sorenson, 1970
Dasyurus viverrinus	...	Yes	No	Yes	...	Eisenberg, 1977; Godsell, 1983

(*cont.*)

Taxa	Genital lock	Pelvic thrusts	Multiple intromissions	Prolonged intromission	Pattern number	Sources
D. maculatus	...	...	No	Yes	...	Strahan, 1995
Dasyuroides byrnei	...	...	...	Yes	...	Strahan, 1995
Sarcophilus harrisii	...	...	No	Yes	...	Eisenberg *et al.*, 1975
Order Didelphimorphia						
Family Marmosidae						
Monodelphis domestica	Yes	Yes	No	Yes	3	Trupin and Fadem, 1982
Marmosa robinsoni	?	Yes	No	Yes	...	Trupin and Fadem, 1982
Didelphis marsupialis	...	Yes	...	Yes	...	Dewsbury, 1972
D. virginiana	...	Yes	...	Yes	...	AFD
Orders Paucitubiculata and Microbiotheria	No data					
Placentalia						
Superorder Laurasiatheria						
Order Cetartiodactyla						
Family Hippopotamidae						
Hippopotamus amphibius	No	No	No	Yes	15	AFD
Choeropsis liberiensis	No	No	No	No	16	Flacke, personal communication; AFD
Family Suidae						
Sus scrofa	No	Yes	No	Yes	11	Dewsbury, 1972; AFD
Family Tayassuidae						
Phacochoerus africanus	No	Yes	No	No	12	AFD
Family Camelidae						
Camelus dromedarius	No	Yes	No	Yes	11	Mahla *et al.*, 2015
C. bactrianus	No	Yes	No	Yes	11	Vyas *et al.*, 2015

(cont.)

Taxa	Genital lock	Pelvic thrusts	Multiple intromissions	Prolonged intromission	Pattern number	Sources
Llama glama	No	Yes	No	Yes	11	England *et al.*, 1971
L. pacos	No	Yes	No	Yes	11	Vaughan *et al.*, 2003
L. guanicoe	No	Yes?	No	Yes?	11?	AFD
Vicugna vicugna	No	Yes	No	?	...	AFD
Family Tragulidae						
Moschiola indica	?	?	No	Yes	...	Parvathy *et al.*, 2014
Tragulus napa	No	Yes	?	Yes	...	Ralls *et al.*, 1975
Family Giraffidae						
Giraffa camelopardalis	No	No	No	No	16	Estes, 1991; AFD
Okapi johnstoni	No	No	No	No	16	AFD
Family Antilocapridae						
Antilocapra americana	No	No	No	No	16	Kitchen, 1974
Family Cervidae						
Hydropotes inermis	No	No	No	No	16	Sun and Dai, 1995
Muntiacus muntjak	No	No	No	No	16	Dubost, 1971; AFD
Muntiacus reevesi	No	No	No	No	16	Barrette, 1977; Yahner, 1979
Dama dama	No	No	No	No	16	Braza, 2011
Axis axis	No	No	No	No	16	AFD
Cervus elaphus	No	No	No	No	16	Asher *et al.*, 2007
C. eldi	No	No	No	No	16	Zeng *et al.*, 2011
C. canadensis	No	No	No	No	16	Dewsbury, 1972
C. nippon	No	No	No	No	16	Miura, 1984
C. albirostris	No	No	No	No	16	Miura *et al.*, 1993
Rusa unicolor	No	No	No	No	16	AFD
R. timorensis	No	No	No	No	16	Samsudewa *et al.*, 2013
Odocoileus virginianus	No	No	No	No	16	Warren *et al.*, 1978
O. hemionus	No	No	No	No	16	Dewsbury 1972
Ozotoceros bezoarticus	No	No	No	No	16	Morales-Pineyrua and Ungerfeld, 2012
Alces alces	No	No	No	No	16	Ballenberghe and Miquelle, 1993

(*cont.*)

Taxa	Genital lock	Pelvic thrusts	Multiple intromissions	Prolonged intromission	Pattern number	Sources
Family Bovidae						
Tragelaphus strepsiceros	No	No	No	No	16	Kingdon and Hoffmann, 2013a; AFD
T. imberbis	No	No	No	No	16	AFD
T. spekei	No	No	No	No	16	Popp, 1982
Taurotragus oryx	No	No	No	No	16	Kiley-Worthington, 1978
Syncerus caffer	No	No	No	No	16	AFD
Bos mutus	No	No	No	No	16	Leslie and Schaller, 2009
B. taurus	No	No	No	No	16	AFD
B. javanicus	No	No	No	No	16	AFD
Bison bison	No	No	No	No	16	Dewsbury, 1972
Sylvicapra grimmia	No	No	No	No	16	Kingdon and Hoffmann, 2013a
Cephalophus maxwelli	No	No	No	No	16	Kingdon and Hoffmann, 2013a
C. zebra	No	No	No	No	16	Kingdon and Hoffmann, 2013a
Kobus kob	No	No	No	No	16	Estes, 1991
K. leche	No	No	No	No	16	Estes, 1991
K. ellipsiprymnus	No	No	No	No	16	Estes, 1991
Redunca arundinum	No	No	No	No	16	Estes, 1991
R. redunca	No	No	No	No	16	Estes, 1991
Pelea capreolus	No	No	No	No	16	Estes, 1991
Hippotragus niger	No	No	No	No	16	Estes, 1991
H. equinus	No	No	No	No	16	AFD
Oryx gazella	No	No	No	No	16	Estes, 1991
O. beisa	No	No	No	No	16	Kingdon and Hoffmann, 2013a
Adax nasomaculatus	No	No	No	No	16	Estes, 1991
Damaliscus pygargus	No	No	No	No	16	David, 1975
D. lunatus	No	No	No	No	16	Joubert, 1975
Connochaetes taurinus	No	No	No	No	16	Kingdon and Hoffmann, 2013a
Raphicerus campestris	No	No	No	No	16	Kingdon and Hoffmann, 2013a

(cont.)

Taxa	Genital lock	Pelvic thrusts	Multiple intromissions	Prolonged intromission	Pattern number	Sources
Neotragus moschatus	No	No	No	No	16	Kingdon and Hoffmann, 2013a
Madoqua kirkii	No	No	No	No	16	Estes, 1991
Antilope cervicapra	No	No	No	No	16	Dubost and Feer, 1981
Litocranius walleri	No	No	No	No	16	Estes, 1991
Gazella granti	No	No	No	No	16	Estes, 1991
G. spekei	No	No	No	No	16	Kingdon and Hoffmann 2013a
G. thomsonii	No	No	No	No	16	AFD
G. gazella	No	No	No	No	16	Habibi *et al.*, 1993
G. subgutturosa	No	No	No	No	16	Habibi *et al.*, 1993
Antidorcus marsupialis	No	No	No	No	16	Estes, 1991
Pantholops hodgsoni	No	No	No	No	16	Schaller, 1998
Oreamnos americanus	No	No	No	No	16	AFD
Capra hircus	No	No	No	No	16	AFD
C. sibirica	No	No	No	No	16	Fedosenco and Orlov, 1977
Nemorhaedus caudatus	No	No	No	No	16	Myslenkov and Voloshina, 1998
Ovis aries	No	No	No	No	16	Bermant *et al.*, 1969
O. canadensis	No	No	No	No	16	AFD
Ammotragus lervia	No	...	No	No	...	Habibi, 1987
Family Planistidae						
Inia geoffrensis	No	No?	No?	No	16?	Best and Da Silva, 1993
Family Phocoenidae						
Phocoena phocoena	No	No	No	No	16	Keener *et al.*, 2018
Family Delphinidae						
Lagenorhynchus obscurus	No	No?	No	No	16?	Orbach *et al.*, 2014
Tursiops truncatus	No	No	...	No	...	AFD
Stenella rongirostris	No	No	...	No	...	AFD
Orca orca	No	No	No?	No	16?	AFD

(*cont.*)

Taxa	Genital lock	Pelvic thrusts	Multiple intromissions	Prolonged intromission	Pattern number	Sources
Family Balaenidae						
Eubalena glacialis	No	No	. . .	No	. . .	Mate *et al.*, 2015
Order Perissodactyla						
Family Equidae						
Equus caballus	No	Yes	No	No	12	AFD
E. quagga	No	Yes?	No	No	12	AFD
E. zebra	No	Yes	No	No	12	AFD
E. grevyi	No	Yes	No	No	12	AFD
E. asinus	No	Yes	No	No	12	Moehlman, 1974; AFD
Family Tapiridae						
Tapirus terrestris	No	Yes	No	. . .	. . .	AFD
T. indicus	No	Yes	No	No	12	AFD
Family Rhinocerotidae						
Diceros bicornis	No	Yes	No	Yes	11	Goddard, 1966
Ceratotherium simum	No	Yes	No	Yes	11	Kingdon and Hoffmann, 2013b; AFD
Rhinoceros unicornis	No	Yes	No	Yes	11	Laurie, 1982
Dicerorhinus sumatrensis	No	Yes	No	Yes	11	AFD
Order Carnivora						
Caniformia						
Family Canidae						
Vulpes vulpes	Yes	Yes?	No	Yes	3?	Pearson and Bassett, 1946
Fennecus zerda	Yes	. . .	No	Yes	. . .	Petter, 1957; Valdespino *et al.*, 2002
Nyctereutes procyonides	Yes	Yes?	No?	Yes?	3?	Dewsbury, 1972
Speothos venaticus	Yes	Yes?	No	Yes	3?	Dewsbury, 1972
Canis mesomelas	Yes	. . .	. . .	Yes?	. . .	Kingdon and Hoffmann, 2013b
C. aureus	Yes	Yes	No	Yes	3	Estes, 1991
C. simensis	Yes	?	No	Yes	. . .	Sillero-Zuberi *et al.*, 1996

(cont.)

Taxa	Genital lock	Pelvic thrusts	Multiple intromissions	Prolonged intromission	Pattern number	Sources
Canis latrans	Yes	Yes	No	Yes	3	Bekoff and Diamond, 1976
C. lupus	Yes	Yes	No	Yes	3	Gensch, 1968
C. familiaris	Yes	Yes	No	Yes	3	Hart, 1967
Lycaon pictus	Yes?	Yes	No	Yes	3?	Frame *et al.*, 1979
Chrysocyon brachyurus	Yes	Yes	No	Yes	3	Kleiman, 1968; Lippert, 1973
Octocyon megalotis	Yes	...	...	Yes	...	Kingdon and Hoffmann, 2013b
Cuon alpinus	Yes	Yes	No	Yes	3	Paulraj *et al.*, 1992
Family Ursidae						
Ursus americanus	No	Yes	No	Yes	11	Ludlow, 1976
U. arctos	No	Yes	No	Yes	11	Craighead *et al.*, 1969; Craighead and Mitchell, 1982
U. maritimus	No	Yes	No	Yes	11	Smith and Aars, 2015
Melursus ursinus	...	...	...	Yes	...	Joshi *et al.*, 1999
Ailuropoda melanoleuca	No	Yes	No	No	12	AFD
Family Procyonidae						
Ailurus fulgens	No	Yes	?	Yes	...	Roberts and Kessler, 1979
Bassariscus astutus	No	Yes	No?	No	12?	Bailey, 1974
Procyon lotor	No	?	No	Yes	...	AFD
Nasua narica	No	Yes	No	Yes	11	Hass and Roback, 2000
Potos flavus	...	...	...	Yes	...	Kays and Gittleman, 2001; Ewer, 1973
Family Mustelidae						
Mustela ermina	...	...	...	Yes	...	Larivière and Ferguson, 2002
M. nivalis	?	Yes	No	Yes	...	East and Lockie, 1965; Heidt *et al.*, 1968
M. frenata	...	...	No	Yes	...	Wright, 1948
M. vison	No	Yes	No	Yes	11	Enders, 1952
M. putorius	No?	No?	No	Yes	15?	Hammond and Walton, 1934
M. nigripes	No?	Yes	No?	Yes	11?	Williams *et al.*, 1991
Martes foina	...	...	...	Yes	...	Schmidt, 1934, 1943

(*cont.*)

Taxa	Genital lock	Pelvic thrusts	Multiple intromissions	Prolonged intromission	Pattern number	Sources
M. martes	No?	...	No?	Yes	...	Schmidt, 1934, 1943
M. americana	...	...	...	Yes	...	Larivière and Ferguson, 2002; Ruggiero and Henry, 1993
M. pennanti	...	...	...	Yes	...	Larivière and Ferguson, 2002
Ictonyx striatus	...	...	...	Yes	...	Kingdon and Hoffmann, 2013b
Poecilogale libya	?	...	...	Yes	...	Kingdon and Hoffmann, 2013b
Gulo gulo	No	Yes	No	Yes	11	Magoun and Volkanburg, 1983
Mellivora capensis	...	Yes	...	...	...	AFD
Meles meles	...	Yes	...	Yes	...	Neal, 1986; AFD
Spirogale pygmaea	...	Yes	No	Yes	...	Dewsbury, 1972; Teska et al., 1981
Mephitis mephitis	No?	Yes	No	Yes	11?	Wight, 1931
Lutra lutra	No	Yes	No	Yes	11	Laidler, 1982; AFD
Lontra canadensis	No?	Yes	No	Yes	11?	Liers, 1951
L. felina	...	...	...	Yes	...	Larivière, 1998
Pteronura brasiliensis	...	...	No	Yes	...	Londoño and Muñaz, 2006
Aonyx cinerea	No	Yes	No	Yes	11	AFD
Enhydra lutris	No?	Yes	...	Yes	...	Kenyon, 1969
Feliformia						
Family Viverridae						
Civettictis civetta	No	Yes	No	No	12	Ewer and Wemmer, 1974
Genetta genetta	...	...	...	No	...	Roeder, 1979
G. maculatta	No?	Yes	No	No?	12?	Dücker, 1965
Paguma larvata	No	Yes	Yes	Yes	9	Jia et al., 2001
Arctictis binturong	No	Yes	Yes?	No	10?	Wemmer and Murtaugh, 1981
Family Herpestidae						
Herpestes ichneumon	No	Yes	Yes	No	10	Kingdon and Hoffmann, 2013b
H. javanicus	No	Yes?	Yes	No	10?	Al-Razi et al., 2014
H. edwardsi	No	Yes?	Yes	No	10?	Murali et al., 2012

(*cont.*)

Taxa	Genital lock	Pelvic thrusts	Multiple intromissions	Prolonged intromission	Pattern number	Sources
Galerella sanguinea	No	...	...	No	...	Jacobsen, 1982
Crossarchus obscurus	No	Yes	Yes	No	10	Goldman, 1987
Helogale parvula	No	No	Yes	No	14	Rasa, 1977
Ichneumia albicauda	No	...	Yes	No	...	Waser and Waser, 1985
Cynictis penicillata	No	Yes	...	Yes	...	AFD
Suricata suricatta	No	No	...	...	...	Ewer, 1963; AFD
Family Eupleridae						
Cryptoprocta ferox	Yes	No	No	Yes	7	Hawkins and Racey, 2009
Family Hyaenidae						
Proteles cristatus	No	Yes	No	Yes	11	Koehler and Richardson, 1990
Parahyaena brunnea	...	No	...	Yes	...	Mills, 1983
Hyaena hyaena	...	No	No	Yes	...	Rieger, 1979
Crocuta crocuta	Yes?	Yes	No	Yes	3?	Szykman *et al.*, 2007
Family Felidae						
Felis catus	No	No	No	No	16	Dewsbury, 1972; Ewer, 1973
F. chaus	No	No	No	No	16	Mellen, 1993
F. margarita	No	No	No	No	16	Mellen, 1993
F. canadensis	No	No	No	No	16	Mellen, 1993
F. caracal	No	No	No	No	16	Mellen, 1993
F. rubiginosa	No	No	No	No	16	Mellen, 1993
F. geoffroyi	No	No	No	No	16	Mellen, 1993
F. pardalis	No	No	No	No	16	Mellen, 1993
Panthera uncia	No	No	No	No	16	Lanier and Dewsbury 1976
P. tigris	No	No	No	No	16	Lanier and Dewsbury, 1976
P. pardus	No	No	No	No	16	Lanier and Dewsbury, 1976
P. onca	No	No	No	No	16	Lanier and Dewsbury, 1976
P. leo	No	No	No	No	16	AFD
Acinomyx jubatus	No	No	No	No	16	AFD

(cont.)

Taxa	Genital lock	Pelvic thrusts	Multiple intromissions	Prolonged intromission	Pattern number	Sources
Pinnipedia						
Family Otariidae						
Callorhinus ursinus	...	Yes	...	Yes?	...	Baker, 1989; Bartholomew and Hoel, 1953
Arctocephalus forsteri	No	Yes	No	Yes	11	Stirling, 1971
Zalophus californicus	...	Yes?	...	...	...	Dewsbury, 1972
Otaria flavescens	...	...	No	Yes	...	Campagna and Le Boeuf, 1988
Eumetopias jubatus	...	...	...	Yes	...	Schusterman, 1968
Family Phocidae						
Hydrurga leptonyx	?	Yes	No	Yes	...	Marlow, 1967
Leptonychotes weddelli	...	Yes	...	Yes	...	Cline *et al.*, 1971
Mirounga angustirostis	No	No	No	Yes	15	Le Boeuf, 1972
M. leonina	No	No	No	Yes	15	Laws, 1956
Halichoerus grypus	No	No	No	Yes	15	Boness and James, 1979; Watkins, 1990
Phoca largha	No	Yes?	No	No	12?	Beier and Wartzok, 1979
P. vitulina	No?	No?	No	Yes?	15?	Allen, 1985; Venables and Venables, 1957, 1959
Order Pholidota						
Family Manidae						
Manis pentadactyla	...	...	...	Yes?	...	Fang and Wang, 1980
Manis javanica	No	Yes	No	Yes	11	Zhang *et al.*, 2020
Order Chiroptera						
Family Pteropodidae						
Pteropus giganteus	No	Yes	No	Yes	11	Koilraj *et al.*, 2001; Noureen *et al.*, 2014
P. alecto	No?	...	...	No	...	Markus, 2002
P. livingstonii	Yes	Yes	No	Yes?	3?	Smith and Leslie, 2006
Hipsignathus monstrosus	No	Yes	No	No	12	Bradbury, 1977
Cynopterus sphinx	No	Yes?	No	Yes?	11?	Tan *et al.*, 2009

(*cont.*)

Taxa	Genital lock	Pelvic thrusts	Multiple intromissions	Prolonged intromission	Pattern number	Sources
Family Vespertilionidae						
Myotis daubentonii	...	...	...	Yes?	...	Grimmberger *et al.*, 1987; Roer and Egsbaek, 1969
M. nigricans	Yes	Yes	No?	Yes?	3?	Wilson, 1971
M. subulatus	...	No	...	...	...	Wimsatt, 1945
M. myotis	...	Yes	No	Yes	...	Zahn and Dippel, 1997
M. lucifugus	Yes	...	...	yes	...	Wimsatt and Kalen, 1952
Eptesicus serotinus	...	...	No	Yes	...	Racey and Kleiman, 1970
E. fuscus	No?	Yes?	...	No?	...	Mendonça *et al.*, 1996
Scoteinus balstoni	No	No?	No	No	16?	Ryan, 1966
Nyctalus noctula	...	No?	No?	...	...	Kleiman and Racey, 1969
Family Phyllostomidae						
Carollia perspicillata	No	...	No?	No	...	Knörnschild *et al.*, 2014
Leptonycteris curasoae	No	Yes?	No	No	12?	Munoz-Romo and Kunz, 2009
Family Molossidae						
Tadarida brasiliensis	...	Yes	...	...	...	Keeley and Keeley, 2004
Order Eulipotyphla						
Family Erinaceidae						
Erinaceus europaeus	No	Yes	...	...	...	AFD
Atelerix albiventris	No	Yes	No	Yes?	11?	AFD
A. algirus	No	Yes	No	Yes	11	AFD
Family Soricidae						
Blarina brevicauda	Yes	No	no	Yes	3	Pearson, 1944
Suncus murinus	No	Yes	Yes	No	10	Eisenberg and Gould, 1970; Matsuzaki, 2002
Sorex araneus	No	Yes	No	No	12	Crowcroft, 1957

(cont.)

Taxa	Genital lock	Pelvic thrusts	Multiple intromissions	Prolonged intromission	Pattern number	Sources
S. isodon	No	...	...	No	...	Skarén, 1979
Neomys fodiens	Yes	...	...	...	...	Köhler, 2012
Cryptotis parva	Yes	No	...	Yes	...	Conaway, 1958; Pearson, 1944

Superorder Euarchontoglires

Order Rodentia

Family Cricetidae

Taxa	Genital lock	Pelvic thrusts	Multiple intromissions	Prolonged intromission	Pattern number	Sources
Microtus arvalis	No	Yes	Yes	No	10	De Jong and Ketel, 1981
M. pennsylvanicus	No	Yes	Yes	No	10	Gray and Dewsbury, 1975
M. montanus	No	Yes	Yes	No	10	Dewsbury, 1972
M. californicus	No	Yes	No	No	12	Kenney *et al.*, 1979
M. canicaudus	No	Yes	Yes	No	10	Dewsbury and Hartung, 1982
M. oeconomus	No	Yes	No	No	12	Dewsbury and Hartung, 1982
M. xanthognathus	No	Yes	No	No	12	Dewsbury and Hartung, 1982
M. agrestis	No	Yes	Yes	No	10	Milligan, 1975
M. ochrogaster	No	Yes	Yes	...	...	Dewsbury, 1978
M. pinetorum	No	Yes	No	...	...	Dewsbury, 1978
Peromyscus gossypinus	No	No	No	No	16	Lovecky *et al.*, 1979
P. polionotus	No	No	Yes	No	14	Dewsbury and Lovecky, 1974
P. leucopus	No	Yes	Yes	No	10	Dewsbury, 1975b
P. eremicus	No	Yes	Yes	...	...	Dewsbury and Estep, 1975
P. californicus	No	Yes	No	...	...	Dewsbury, 1978
P. crinitus	No	No	Yes	...	...	Dewsbury, 1978
P. floridanus	No	No	No	...	...	Dewsbury, 1978
P. melanophyrys	No	No	No	...	...	Dewsbury, 1978
P. maniculatus	No	No	Yes	...	...	Dewsbury, 1972
P. comanche	No	No	Yes?	...	...	Dewsbury, 1972
P. nasutus	No	No	Yes?	...	...	Dewsbury, 1972
P. truei	No	No	Yes?	...	...	Dewsbury, 1972

(*cont.*)

Taxa	Genital lock	Pelvic thrusts	Multiple intromissions	Prolonged intromission	Pattern number	Sources
Callomys callosus	No	Yes	Yes	No	10	Baumgardner and Dewsbury, 1979
Neotoma albigula	Yes	No	No	No	8	Dewsbury, 1974
N. lepida	No	No	No	No	16	Dewsbury, 1978; Fleming *et al.*, 1981
N. floridana	Yes	No	No	...	...	Dewsbury, 1978
Ochrotomys nuttalli	Yes	No	No	No	8	Dewsbury, 1974
O. torridus	Yes	No	No	No	8	Dewsbury and Jansen, 1972
Onychomys leucogaster	Yes	No	No	...	...	Dewsbury, 1978
Ototylomys phyllotis	Yes	Yes	No	...	...	Dewsbury, 1978
Clethrionomes glareolus	No	No	Yes	No	14	Milligan, 1979
Akodon molinae	Yes	No	Yes	No	6	Yunes and Castro-Vazquez, 1990
Baiomys taylori	Yes	No	No	No	8	Estep and Dewsbury, 1976
Mesocricetus auratus	No	No	Yes	No	14	AFD
Sigmodon hispidus	No	No	Yes	...	...	Dewsbury, 1978
Oryzomys palustris	No	No	Yes	...	...	Dewsbury, 1978
Reithrodontomys megalotis	No	No	Yes	...	...	Dewsbury, 1978
Nyctomys sumichrasti	...	Yes	...	...	...	Dewsbury, 1972
Tylomys nudicaudus	Yes	Yes	No	...	...	Dewsbury, 1978
Family Muridae						
Mus musculus	No	Yes	Yes	No	10	Dewsbury, 1972; AFD
Rattus norvegicus	No	No	Yes	No	14	Larsson, 1956; AFD
R. rattus	No	No	No?	...	...	Dewsbury, 1972
Gerbillus nanus	No	...	Yes	...	...	Dewsbury, 1972
Tatera indica	No	Yes	Yes	...	...	Thomas and Oommen, 1998
Meriones unguiculatus	No	No	Yes	No	14	Davis *et al.*, 1974a
Rhabdomys pumilio	No	No	Yes	No	14	Dewsbury and Dawson, 1979
Acomys cahirinus	No	No	Yes	No	14	Dewsbury and Hodges, 1987

(cont.)

Taxa	Genital lock	Pelvic thrusts	Multiple intromissions	Prolonged intromission	Pattern number	Sources
Otomys irroratus	No	Yes	Yes	No?	10?	Pitlay, 1997
Notomys alexis	Yes	No	No	Yes	7	Breed, 1990; Dewsbury and Hodges, 1987
Family Sciuridae						
Sciurus niger	No	Yes	Yes	No	10	McCloskey and Shaw, 1977
Xerus inauris	No	Yes	No	No	12	Waterman, 1998
Spermophilus richardsonii	No	Yes	No	No	12	Davis, 1982; Denniston, 1957
S. columbianus	No	Yes	No	No	12	Murie, 1995
S. tridecemlineatus	No	Yes	No	No	12	McCarley, 1966; Wistrand, 1974
S. beldingi	No	Yes	No	No	12	Sherman and Morton, 1979
Callosciurus notatus	...	...	...	No	...	Tamura, 1993
C. caniceps	...	...	...	No	...	Tamura, 1993
Tamias striatus	...	Yes	...	...	...	Smith and Smith, 1975
Glaucomys sabrinus	No?	Yes?	Yes?	...	...	Dewsbury, 1972
Family Echimyidae						
Proechimys semispinosus	No	Yes	No?	...	...	Maliniak and Eisenberg, 1971
Family Heteromyidae						
Dipodomys ordii	No	Yes	Yes?	No	10?	Engstrom and Dowler, 1981
D. microps	No	Yes	No	Yes	11	Behrends, 1981
D. deserti	No?	...	...	No	...	Butterworth, 1961
D. nitratoides	...	Yes	Yes?	...	...	Dewsbury, 1972
D. panamintinus	...	Yes	Yes?	...	...	Dewsbury, 1972
D. merriami	...	Yes?	Yes?	...	...	Dewsbury, 1972
Perognathus californicus	...	Yes	Yes?	...	...	Dewsbury, 1972
P. parvus	...	Yes	Yes?	...	...	Dewsbury, 1972
P. longimembris	...	Yes	Yes?	...	...	Dewsbury, 1972
Family Caviidae						
Microcavia australis	No	Yes	Yes	No	10	Rood, 1972
Galea musteloides	No	Yes	No	No	12	Rood, 1972

(*cont.*)

Taxa	Genital lock	Pelvic thrusts	Multiple intromissions	Prolonged intromission	Pattern number	Sources
Cavia aperea	No	Yes	Yes	No	10	Rood, 1972
C. porcellus	No	Yes	Yes	No	10	Young and Grunt, 1951
Family Bathyergidae						
Heliophobius argenteocinereus	No	Yes	No	No	12	Sumbera *et al.*, 1988
Georychus capensis	No	Yes	Yes	No	10	Bennett and Jarvis, 1988
Cryptomys hottentotus	No	Yes	Yes	No	10	Hickman, 1982
Family Heterocephalidae						
Heterocephalus glaber	No	Yes	No	No	12	Sherman *et al.*, 1991
Family Spalacidae						
Spalax ehrenbergi	No	Yes	Yes	No	10	Gazit and Terkel, 2000; Nevo, 1969
Family Geomyidae						
Thomomys talpoides	No	Yes	Yes?	No?	10?	Andersen, 1978; Schramm, 1961
T. bottae	No	Yes	Yes	No	10	Schramm, 1961
Family Hystricidae						
Hystrix cristata	No	Yes	Yes	No	10	Felicioli *et al.*, 1997
H. africaeaustralis	No	Yes	No	No	12	Morris and Van Arde, 1985
Family Erethizontidae						
Erethizon dorsatum	No	Yes	Yes?	No	10?	Shadle, 1946; AFD
Family Dasyproctidae						
Myoprocta pratti	No	Yes	Yes	No	10	Kleiman, 1971
Family Chinchillidae						
Chinchilla lanigera	No	Yes	No	No	12	Bignami and Beach, 1968
Family Ctenomyidae						
Ctenomys talarum	No	Yes	Yes	No	10	Fanjul and Zenuto, 2008
C. pearsoni	No	Yes	Yes	No	10	Altuna *et al.*, 1991; Kleiman, 1974

(*cont.*)

Taxa	Genital lock	Pelvic thrusts	Multiple intromissions	Prolonged intromission	Pattern number	Sources
Family Octodontidae						
Octodontomys gliroides	No	Yes	No	No	12	Kleiman, 1974
Order Lagomorpha						
Family Leporidae						
Oryctolagus cuniculus	No	No	No	No	16	Mollison, 1955
Lepus alleni	No	No	No	No	16	Vorhies and Taylor, 1933
L. californicus	No	No	No	No	16	Lechleitner, 1958
L. flavigularis	...	...	...	No	...	Rioja *et al.*, 2008
Romerolagus diazi	No	...	No	No	...	Cervantes and López-Forment, 1981
Brachylagus idahoensis	No	No	No	No	16	Scarlata *et al.*, 2012
Order Dermoptera						
Family Cynocephalidae						
Cynocephalus variegatus	No?	Yes	No	No?	12?	AFD
Order Scandentia						
Family Tupaiidae						
Tupaia glis	No	Yes	Yes?	No	10?	Kaufmann, 1965
T. belangeri	No	Yes	Yes?	No	10?	AFD
T. longipes	...	Yes	...	Yes	...	Conaway and Sorenson, 1966
Order Primates						
Family Cheirogaleidae						
Microcebus murinus	No	Yes	No	Yes	11	Dixson, 2012
Cheirogaleus major	No	Yes	No	No	12	Dixson, 2012
Family Lemuridae						
Lemur catta	No	Yes	No	No	12	Dixson, 2012
Varecia variegata	No	Yes	No	No	12	Dixson, 2012
Eulemur mongoz	No	Yes	Yes?	No?	10?	Perry *et al.*, 1992

(*cont.*)

Taxa	Genital lock	Pelvic thrusts	Multiple intromissions	Prolonged intromission	Pattern number	Sources
Family Daubentoniidae						
Daubentonia madagascariensis	Yes	Yes	No	Yes	3	Dixson, 2012
Family Lorisidae						
Otolemur garnettii	Yes	Yes	No	Yes	3	Dixson, 2012
O. crassicaudatus	Yes	Yes	No	Yes	3	Dixson, 2012
Galagoides demidoff	Yes	Yes	No	Yes	3	Dixson, 2012
Galago moholi	No	Yes	No	Yes	11	Dixson, 2012
Arctocebus calabarensis	No	Yes	No	Yes	11	Dixson, 2012
Loris tardigradus	No	Yes	No	Yes	11	Dixson, 2012
Nycticebus coucang	No	Yes	No	Yes	11	Dixson, 2012
Family Tarsiidae						
Tarsius bancanus	No	Yes	No	No	12	Dixson, 2012
T. spectrum	No	Yes	No	No	12	Hidayatik *et al.*, 2018
Family Cebidae						
Saimiri sciureus	No	Yes	Yes	No	10	Dixson, 2012
Cebus nigrivittatus	No	Yes	No	No	12	Dixson, 2012
Aotus lemurinus	No	Yes	No	No	12	Dixson, 2012
Callicebus molloch	No	Yes	No	No	12	Dixson, 2012
Alouatta palliata	No	Yes	No	No	12	Dixson, 2012
Ateles belzebuth	No	Yes	No	Yes	11	Dixson, 2012
A. geoffroyi	No	Yes	No	Yes	11	Dixson, 2012
A. fusciceps	No	Yes	No	Yes	11	Dixson, 2012
Brachyteles arachnoides	No	Yes	No	Yes	11	Dixson, 2012
Lagothrix lagotricha	No	Yes	No	Yes	11	Dixson, 2012
Cacajao calvus	No	Yes	Yes	No	10	Dixson, 2012
Family Callitrichidae						
Callimico goeldii	No	Yes	No	No	12	Dixson, 2012
Callithrix jacchus	No	Yes	No	No	12	Dixson, 2012

(*cont.*)

Taxa	Genital lock	Pelvic thrusts	Multiple intromissions	Prolonged intromission	Pattern number	Sources
Cebuella pygmaea	No	Yes	No	No	12	Dixson, 2012
Saguinus oedipus	No	Yes	No	No	12	Dixson, 2012
Leontopithecus rosalia	No	Yes	Yes	No	10	Dixson, 2012
Family Cercopithecinae						
Macaca silenus	No	Yes	Yes	No	10	Dixson, 2012
M. nemestrina	No	Yes	Yes	No	10	Dixson, 2012
M. nigra	No	Yes	Yes	No	10	Dixson, 2012
M. maurus	No	Yes	Yes	No	10	Dixson, 2012
M. radiata	No	Yes	No	No	12	Dixson, 2012
M. sylvanus	No	Yes	No	No	12	Dixson, 2012
M. fascicularis	No	Yes	Yes	No	10	Dixson, 2012
M. mulatta	No	Yes	Yes	No	10	Dixson, 2012
M. fuscata	No	Yes	Yes	No	10	Dixson, 2012
M. thibetana	No	Yes	Yes	No	10	Dixson, 2012
M. arctoides	Yes	Yes	No	Yes	3	Dixson, 2012
Papio hamadryas	No	Yes	Yes	No	10	Dixson, 2012
P. ursinus	No	Yes	Yes	No	10	Dixson, 2012
P. anubis	No	Yes	No	No	12	Dixson, 2012
Cercocebus sanjei	No	Yes	Yes?	No	10?	Ally-Mwamende, 2009
Lophocebus albigena	No	Yes	No	No	12	Dixson, 2012
Mandrillus sphinx	No	Yes	No	No	12	Dixson, 2012
M. leucophaeus	No	Yes	No	No	12	Dixson, 2012
Theropithecus gelada	No	Yes	No	No	12	Dixson, 2012
Chlorocebus aethiops	No	Yes	No	No	12	Dixson, 2012
Miopithecus talapoin	No	Yes	No	No	12	Dixson, 2012
Erythrocebus patas	No	Yes	No	No	12	Dixson, 2012
Family Colobinae						
Piliocolobus badius	No	Yes	Yes	No	10	Dixson, 2012
Nasalis larvatus	No	Yes	No	No	12	Dixson, 2012
Rhinopithecus roxellana	No	Yes	No	No	12	Li and Zhao, 2007
R. bieti	No	Yes	Yes	No	10	Cui and Xiao, 2004

(cont.)

Taxa	Genital lock	Pelvic thrusts	Multiple intromissions	Prolonged intromission	Pattern number	Sources
Superfamily Hominoidea						
Hylobates lar	No	Yes	No	No	12	Dixson, 2012
Pongo pygmaeus	No	Yes	No	Yes	11	Dixson, 2012
P. abelii	No	Yes	No	Yes	11	Dixson, 2012
Pan paniscus	No	Yes	No	No	12	Dixson, 2012
P. troglodytes	No	Yes	No	No	12	Dixson, 2012
Gorilla gorilla	No	Yes	No	No	12	Dixson, 2012
G. beringei	No	Yes	No	No	12	Dixson, 2012
Homo sapiens	No	Yes	No	No	12	Dixson, 2012
Superorder Xenarthra						
Order Pilosa						
Family Myrmecophagidae						
Tamandua mexicana	No	...	No	No	...	Matlaga, 2006
Family Bradipodidae						
Bradypus variegatus	...	...	...	Yes?	...	Bezerra *et al.*, 2008
B. tridactylus	No	...	No?	No?	...	Richard-Hansen and Taube, 1997
Family Megalonychidae						
Choloepus hoffmanni	No	Yes	No?	Yes?	11?	Hayssen, 2011
Order Cingulata						
Family Chlamyphoridae						
Euphractus sexcinctus	No	Yes	No	Yes?	11?	Tomas *et al.*, 2013
Superorder Afrotheria						
Order Afrosoricida						
Family Tenrecidae						
Geogale aurita	Yes	...	No	Yes	...	Stephenson, 1993
Microgale dobsoni	...	Yes	No?	Yes	...	Dewsbury, 1972; Eisenberg, 1975

(cont.)

Taxa	Genital lock	Pelvic thrusts	Multiple intromissions	Prolonged intromission	Pattern number	Sources
Tenrec ecaudatus	...	Yes	No?	Yes	...	Eisenberg, 1975; Stephenson, 1993
Setifer setosus	Yes	Yes?	No	Yes	3?	Eisenberg, 1975; Paduschka, 1974
Hemicentetes nigriceps	...	Yes	No?	Yes	...	Dewsbury, 1972; Eisenberg, 1975
Echinops telfairi	...	Yes	No?	Yes	...	Eisenberg, 1975, 1981
Order Macroscelididea						
Family Macroscelididae						
Elephantulus rufescens	No	Yes	No	No	12	Lumpkin and Koontz, 1986
Order Tubilidentata No Data						
Order Sirenia						
Family Trichechidae						
Trichechus manatus	No	?	No?	?	...	Hartman, 1979; AFD
Order Hyracoidea						
Family Procaviidae						
Procavia capensis	No	Yes	No	No	12	Olds and Shoshani, 1982
Heterohyrax brucei	No?	Yes?	No	Yes?	11?	Barry and Shoshani, 2000
Order Proboscidea						
Family Elephantidae						
Elephas maximus	No	Yes	No	No	12	Dewsbury, 1972; AFD
Loxodonta africana	No	Yes	No	No	12	AFD

AFD, author's observations; ..., insufficient information available.

Appendix 2 Intromission Durations of Mammals

Order and Genus	Mean intromission duration (min)	Mean body weight (g)
Monotremata		
Tachyglossus	105	4500
Ornithorhynchus	20	1700
Diprotodontia		
Macropus	17	24,014
Setonix	3	3600
Bettongia	4	1725
Potorous	2	1180
Lasiorhinus	64	25,500
Phascolarctos	33.9	12,000
Trichosurus	3	2900
Dactylopsila	1	423
Dasyuromorphia		
Antechinus	420	32.5
Ningaui	300	7.1
Planigale	135	11.5
Parantechinus	150	80
Dasycercus	150	122.5
Dasyurus	300	1300
Sarcophilus	360	9000
Didelphimorphia		
Monodelphis	5.5	117
Marmosa	42.5	57
Didelphis	22.75	2058
Cetartiodactyla		
Giraffa	0.05	1,190,000
Okapia	0.05	250,000
Madoqua	0.033	5000
Bison	0.033	949,000

(cont.)

Order and Genus	Mean intromission duration (min)	Mean body weight (g)
Bos	0.05	650,000
Gazella	0.166	23,400
Hydropotes	0.05	12,500
Dameliscus	0.046	137,000
Taurotragus	0.066	700,000
Tragulus	9.75	7500
Moschile	17.5	2450
Rusa	0.033	184,500
Cervus	0.056	166,000
Muntiacus	0.046	18,400
Alces	0.083	512,500
Tragelaphus	0.158	228,000
Ammotragus	0.066	122,500
Ovis	0.0125	108,000
Capra	0.016	140,000
Oreamnos	0.016	100,000
Nemorhaedus	0.068	28,500
Sus	4.25	170,000
Phacochoerus	1	66,120
Camelus	8.94	495,000
Llama	21.95	107,500
Hippopotamus	6.68	2,750,000
Choeropsis	0.416	215,000
Inia	0.416	160,000
Phocoena	0.033	48,900
Lagenorhynchus	0.081	110,000
Tursiops	0.025	199,000
Stenella	0.108	112,500
Orcinus	0.5	9,000,000
Perissodactyla		
Diceros	32.3	1,100,000
Ceratotherium	22.5	2,140,000
Dicerorhinus	5+	1,000,000

(*cont.*)

Order and Genus	Mean intromission duration (min)	Mean body weight (g)
Rhinoceros	46	1,410,000
Tapirus	1.28	296,000
Equus	0.488	354,750
Carnivora		
Vulpes	26	5330
Fennecus	120	1250
Nyctereutes	10	5000
Canis	36.4	20,000
Lycaon	6	26,500
Chrysocyon	14	23,000
Octocyon	4	4150
Cuon	14.7	18,000
Ursus	39.3	303,000
Melursus	18.5	100,000
Ailurus	23.3	5400
Bassariscus	1.5	1081
Procyon	4.77+	8500
Nasua	39	4750
Potos	68	3000
Mustela	125.9	709
Martes	131.2	1984
Poecilictis	70	225
Gulo	27	19,500
Meles	35	13,000
Spirogale	18	600
Mephitis	12.5	1600
Lutra	22.5	9500
Lontra	14.25	9000
Pteronura	57.5	30
Enhydra	14+	33,500
Civettictis	1	13,500
Cryptoprocta	32	9500
Proteles	150	11,500

(cont.)

Order and Genus	Mean intromission duration (min)	Mean body weight (g)
Hyaena	30	40,000
Crocuta	5	63,000
Felis	0.13	7426
Panthera	0.128	128,900
Acinomyx	0.066	46,500
Callorhinus	6.2	226,500
Arctocephalus	6.56	152,500
Otaria	10.8	275,000
Eumetopias	16.6	1,000,000
Hydrurga	10	327,500
Leptonychotes	5+	425,000
Mirounga	7.75	3,025,000
Halichoerus	20	240,000
Phoca	6.95	105,000
Pholidota		
Manis	4.15	4700
Chiroptera		
Pteropus	6.56	1125
Hipsignathus	0.75	420
Cynopterus	2.03	63
Myotis	27.5	11.4
Eptesicus	180	31.9
Scoteinus	2	9.3
Carollia	0.4	15
Eulipotyphla		
Ateles	5.38	468
Sorex	0.133	9
Blarina	4.7	162
Rodentia		
Neotoma	0.401	228
Ochrotomys	1.203	22.5
Dipodomys	4.5	56
Notomys	1.766	33.5

(cont.)

Order and Genus	Mean intromission duration (min)	Mean body weight (g)
Baiomys	0.591	9
Xerus	0.42	574
Spermophilus	2.35	228
Heliophobius	0.333	160
Callosciurus	1	240
Heterocephalus	0.566	35
Chinchilla	0.15	500
Octodontomys	0.833	150
Lagomorpha		
Oryctolagus	0.043	1530
Lepus	0.05	2250
Romerolagus	1.333	485
Brachylagus	0.016	354
Dermoptera		
Cynocephalus	0.75	1375
Primates		
Microcebus	3	80
Daubentonia	62	2800
Otolemur	247	1166
Galago	9.5	210
Galagoides	60	63
Arctocebus	4	207
Loris	13.5	294
Nycticebus	5	839
Eulemur	2.233	1800
Tarsius	1.25	123
Cebuella	0.116	122
Callithrix	0.091	310
Alouatta	0.533	7400
Saimiri	0.5	750
Brachyteles	4.966	10,200
Ateles	15.166	5872
Lagothrix	8.5	6800

(*cont.*)

Order and Genus	Mean intromission duration (min)	Mean body weight (g)
Nasalis	0.691	20,300
Rhinopithecus	0.278	16,400
Miopithecus	1	1400
Chlorocebus	1	4750
Lophocebus	0.231	9000
Macaca	1.791	8850
Mandrillus	1	32,500
Pongo	14	100,000
Gorilla	1.6	162,000
Pan	0.188	43,300
Homo	2	70,000
Pilosa		
Tamandua	0.333	4654
Bradypus	2.166	3930
Choloepus	3.833	6250
Afrosoricida		
Geogale	21	6.75
Microgale	7.5	36
Tenrec	8.25	1416
Setifer	74	236
Hemicentetes	15.5	145
Echinops	17	134
Macroscelidea		
Elephantulus	0.166	42.5
Proboscidea		
Elephas	0.333	4,210,000
Loxodonta	0.666	5,000,000

Appendix 3A Penile Lengths in Mammals

Species	Common name	Penile length (cm) E = erect	Source
Ornithorhynchus anatinus	Platypus	5–7	Griffiths, 1978
Phascolarctos cinereus	Koala	9–10 E	Smith, 1980
Inia geoffrensis	Boto	25–30 E	Layne and Caldwell, 1964
Megaptera nodosa	Humpback whale	141	Chittleborough, 1955
Physeter macrocephalus	Sperm whale	156	Bland and Kitchener, 2001
Delphinapterus leucas	Beluga	15–25	Guise *et al.*, 1994
Phocoena phocoena	Harbour porpoise	44.7 E	AFD
Phocoena phocoena	Harbour porpoise	22.1	Orbach *et al.*, 2017b
Tursiops truncatus	Bottlenose dolphin	12.1	Orbach *et al.*, 2017b
Delphinus delphis	Common dolphin	4.7	Orbach *et al.*, 2017b
Eschrichtius robustus	Grey whale	138	Brownell and Ralls, 1986
Balaenoptera acutorostrata	Minke whale	77	Brownell and Ralls, 1986
B. brydei	Bryde's whale	128	Brownell and Ralls, 1986
B. borealis	Sei whale	130	Brownell and Ralls, 1986
B. physalus	Fin whale	142	Brownell and Ralls, 1986
B. musculus	Blue whale	225	Brownell and Ralls, 1986
Caperea marginata	Pygmy right whale	56	Brownell and Ralls, 1986
Balaena mysticetus	Bowhead whale	200	Brownell and Ralls, 1986
Eubalaena glacialis	Right whale	233	Brownell and Ralls, 1986
Bos taurus	Bull	50 E	Seidel and Foote, 1969
Sus scrofa	Boar	60 E	Nickel *et al.*, 1979
Tragulus javanicus	Lesser mouse deer	4.87	Vidyadaran *et al.*, 1999
Camelus dromedarius	Dromedary	59.6	Mobarak *et al.*, 1972
Kobus ellipsiprymnus	Defassa waterbuck	15	Spinage, 1969
Ovis aries	Sheep	20 E	Lindsay, personal communication
Hippopotamus amphibius	Hippopotamus	45.4 E	AFD
Tapirus terrestris	Brazilian tapir	72 E	AFD
Tapirus indicus	Malayan tapir	48.6 E	AFD
Equus caballus	Horse	30 E	Nickel *et al.*, 1979
Crocuta crocuta	Spotted hyena	18 E	Glickman *et al.*, 1998
Helogale parvula	Dwarf mongoose	1 E	Rasa, 1977
Mephitis mephitis	Striped skunk	3.75 E	Wright, 1931
Cryptoprocta ferox	Fossa	>19.3 E?	AFD
Hydrurga leptonix	Leopard seal	25 E	Marlow, 1967
Phoca vitulina	Harbour seal	10.1	Orbach *et al.*, 2017b
Blarina brevicauda	Short-tailed shrew	3 E	Pearson, 1944
Talpa europaea	European mole	3.5–4	Matthews, 1935
Dasyprocta leporina	Red-rumped agouti	9.9	Mollineau *et al.*, 2005

(*cont.*)

Species	Common name	Penile length (cm) E = erect	Source
Tupaia belangeri	Treeshrew	1.2	Collins and Tsang, 1987
Lemur catta	Ring-tailed lemur	4.3 E	Dixson, 2012
Callithrix jacchus	Common marmoset	2.24 E	Dixson, 2012
Aotus griseimembra	Colombian owl monkey	1 E	Dixson, 2012
Lophocebus aterrimus	Black-crested mangabey	12.5 E	Dixson, 2012
Mandrillus sphinx	Mandrill	12.15 E	Dixson, 2012
Papio hamadryas	Hamadryas baboon	14	Dixson, 2012
Macaca mulatta	Rhesus macaque	9.3 E	Dixson, 2012
M. arctoides	Stump-tail macaque	8.26 E	Dixson, 2012
Pongo pygmaeus	Bornean orang-utan	8.5	Dixson, 2012
Pan paniscus	Bonobo	17	Dixson, 2012
Pan troglodytes	Chimpanzee	14.4 E	Dixson, 2012
Gorilla gorilla	Western lowland gorilla	6.5 E	Dixson, 2012
Homo sapiens	Human	16.5 E	Dixson, 2012
Euphractus sexcinctus	Six-banded armadillo	14.78 E	Tomas *et al.*, 2013; AFD
Chaetophractus villosus	Big hairy armadillo	19 E	Affanni *et al.*, 2001
Amblysomus hottentotus	Golden mole	0.17	Retief *et al.*, 2013
Tenrec ecaudatus	Tailless tenrec	13E	Bedford *et al.*, 2004
Elephas maximus	Indian elephant	50	Mariappa, 1986

AFD, author's data.

Appendix 3B Depth of Female Reproductive Tract to the point at which ejaculation occurs

Species	Common Name	Female Tract (cm)	Sources
Bos taurus	Cow	23.57	Drennan and MacPherson, 1966
Kobus ellipsiprymnus	Defassa waterbuck	14	Spinage, 1969
Ovis aries	Sheep	15	Lindsay, personal communication
Sus scrofa	Pig	40.31	Nickel *et al.*, 1979
Equus caballus	Horse	20	Brinsko *et al.*, 2011
Phocoena phocoena	Harbour porpoise	23	Orbach *et al.*, 2017b
Tursiops truncatus	Bottlenose dolphin	15	Orbach *et al.*, 2017b
Delphinus delphis	Common dolphin	8.1	Orbach *et al.*, 2017b
Phoca vitulina	Harbour seal	11.2	Orbach *et al.*, 2017b
Crocuta crocuta	Spotted hyaena	17	Matthews, 1939
Elephas maximus	Indian elephant	29.5	Mariappa, 1986
Lemur catta	Ring-tailed lemur	4.6	Dixson, 2012
Callithrix jacchus	Common marmoset	2.25	Dixson, 2012
Lophocebus aterrimus	Black-crested mangabey	7.3	Dixson, 2012
Mandrillus sphinx	Mandrill	13	Dixson, 2012
Macaca mulatta	Rhesus macaque	6.3	Dixson, 2012
M. arctoides	Stump-tail macaque	5.5	Dixson, 2012
Pan troglodytes	Chimpanzee	16.9	Dixson, 2012
Gorilla gorilla	Western lowland gorilla	9	Dixson, 2012
Homo sapiens	Human	11	Dixson, 2012

References

Abella, J., Valenciano, A., Perez-Ramos, A., Montoya, P. and Morales, J. (2013). On the socio-sexual behaviour of the extinct ursid *Indarctos arctoides*: an approach based on its baculum size and morphology. *PLoS ONE*, 8(9), e73711.

Adams, G.P., Ratto, M.H., Huanca, W. and Singh, J. (2005). Ovulation-inducing factor in the seminal plasma of alpacas and llamas. *Biology of Reproduction*, 73, 452–457.

Adler, N.T. (1978). On the mechanisms of sexual behaviour and their evolutionary constraints. In *Biological Determinants of Sexual Behaviour*, ed. J.B. Hutchison. Chichester: John Wiley and Sons, pp. 657–695.

Adler, N.T. and Toner, J.P. (1986). The effects of copulatory behavior on sperm transport and fertility in rats. *Annals of the New York Academy of Sciences*, 474, 21–32.

Affanni, J.M., Cervino, C.O. and Marcos, H.J.A. (2001). Absence of penile erections during paradoxical sleep. Peculiar penile events during wakefulness and slow wave sleep in the armadillo. *Journal of Sleep Research*, 10, 219–228.

Aisenberg, A. and Eberhard, W.G. (2009). Possible cryptic female choice in a spider: female cooperation in making a copulatory plug depends upon male copulatory courtship. *Behavioral Ecology*, 20, 1236–1241.

Akbari, G., Babaei, M., Kianifard, D. and Mohebi, D. (2018). The gross anatomy of the male reproductive system of the European hedgehog (*Erinaceous europaeus*). *Folia Morphologica*, 77(1), 36–43.

Al-Eknah, M., Hemeida, N. and Al-Haider, A. (2001). A new approach to collect semen by artificial vagina from the dromedary camel. *Journal of Camel Practice and Research*, 8, 127–130.

Al-Razi, H., Alam, S.H.I., Baki, M.A. and Parves, N. (2014). Notes on mating behaviour of two small carnivores in Bangladesh. *Small Carnivore Conservation*, 50, 78–80.

Alcock, J. (2013). *Animal Behavior*. Tenth edn. Sunderland, MA: Sinauer Associates Inc.

Allen, S.G. (1985). Mating behavior in the harbor seal. *Marine Mammal Science*, 1(1), 84–87.

Allen, T.O. and Adler, N.T. (1985). Neuroendocrine consequences of sexual behavior. In *Handbook of Behavioral Neurobiology, Vol. 7*, eds. N. Adler, D. Pfaff and R.W. Goy. New York: Plenum Press, pp. 725–766.

Ally-Mwamende, K. (2009). Social Organization, Ecology and Reproduction in the Sanje Mangabey (*Cercocebus sanjei*) in the Udzungwa Mountains National Park, Tanzania. MSc Thesis, Victoria University of Wellington, New Zealand.

Almiñana, C., Caballero, I., Heath, P.R., Maleki-Dizaji, S., Parrilla, I., *et al.* (2014). The battle of the sexes starts in the oviduct: modulation of oviductal transcriptome by X and Y-bearing spermatozoa. *BMC Genomics*, 15, 293–303.

Altringham, J.D. (1996). *Bats: Biology and Behaviour*. Oxford: Oxford University Press.

Altuna, C.A., Francescoli, G. and Izquierdo, G. (1991). Copulatory pattern of *Ctenomys pearsoni* (Rodentia, Octodontidae) from Balneario Solis, Uruguay. *Mammalia*, 55(3), 440–442.

Amann, R.P. (1981). A critical review of methods for evaluation of spermatogenesis from seminal characteristics. *Journal of Andrology*, 2, 37–58.

Andersen, D.C. (1978). Observations on reproduction, growth, and behaviour of the northern pocket gopher (*Thomomys talpoides*). *Journal of Mammalogy*, 59, 418–422.

Anderson, M.J. and Dixson A.F. (2002). Sperm competition: mobility and the midpiece in primates. *Nature*, 416, 496.

Anderson, M.J. and Dixson, A.F. (2009). Sexual selection affects the sizes of the mammalian prostate gland and seminal vesicles. *Current Zoology*, 55, 1–8.

Anderson, M.J., Nyholt, J. and Dixson, A.F. (2004a). Sperm competition affects the structure of the mammalian vas deferens. *Journal of Zoology, London*, 264, 97–103.

Anderson, M.J., Hessel, J.K. and Dixson, A.F. (2004b). Primate mating systems and the evolution of immune response. *Journal of Reproductive Immunology*, 61, 31–38.

Anderson M.J., Nyholt J. and Dixson A.F. (2005). Sperm competition and the evolution of sperm midpiece volume in mammals. *Journal of Zoology, London*, 267, 135–142.

Anderson, M.J., Dixson, A.S. and Dixson, A.F. (2006). Mammalian sperm and oviducts are sexually selected: evidence for coevolution. *Journal of Zoology, London*, 270, 682–686.

Anderson, M.J., Chapman, S.J., Videan, E.N., Evans, E., Fritz, J., *et al.* (2007). Functional evidence for differences in sperm competition in humans and chimpanzees. *American Journal of Physical Anthropology*, 134, 274–280.

Anderson, P.K. (1997). Shark bay dugongs in summer. 1. Lek mating. *Behaviour*, 134, 433–462.

Anderson, R.P. and Handley, C.O. (2001). A new species of three-toed sloth (Mammalia: Xenarthra) from Panamá, with a review of the genus *Bradypus*. *Proceedings of the Biological Society of Washington*, 114(1), 1–33.

Anyonge, W. and Roman, C. (2006). New body mass estimates for *Canis dirus*, the extinct Pleistocene dire wolf. *Journal of Vertebrate Paleontology*, 26(1), 209–212.

Arakaki, P.R., Salgado, P. A. B., Teixeira, R.H.F., Rassy, F.B., Guimãres, M.A., *et al.* (2019). Testicular volume and semen characteristics in the endangered southern muriqui (*Brachyteles arachnoides*). *Journal of Medical Primatology*, 48(4), 244–250.

Archibald, J.D. (2011). *Extinction and Radiation: How the Fall of Dinosaurs Led to the Rise of Mammals*. Baltimore, MD: Johns Hopkins University Press.

Archie, E.A., Morrison, T.A., Foley, C.A.H., Moss, C.J. and Alberts, S.C. (2006). Dominance rank relationships among wild female African elephants, *Loxodonta africana*. *Animal Behaviour*, 71, 117–127.

Arnqvist, G. and Rowe, I. (2005). *Sexual Conflict. Monographs in Behavior and Ecology*. Princeton, NJ: Princeton University Press.

Aronson, L.R. and Cooper, M.L. (1967). Penile spines of the domestic cat: their endocrine-behavior relations. *Anatomical Record*, 157, 71–78.

Asa, C.S., Bauman, J.E., Coonan, T.J. and Gray, M.M. (2007). Evidence for induced estrus or ovulation in a canid, the island fox (*Urocyon littoralis*). *Journal of Mammalogy*, 88(2), 436–440.

Ashdown, R.R. and Smith, J.A. (1969). The anatomy of the corpus cavernosum penis of the bull and its relationship to spiral deviation of the penis. *Journal of Anatomy*, 104, 153–159.

Asher, G.W., Haigh, J.C. and Wilson, P.R. (2007). Reproductive behavior of red deer and wapiti. In *Large Animal Theriogenology*. Second edn, eds. R.S. Youngquist and W.R. Threlfall. St. Louis, MO: Saunders Press, pp. 937–942.

Asher, R.J., McKenna, M.C., Emry, R.J., Tabrum, A.R. and Kron, D.G. (2002). Morphology and relationships of *Apternodus* and other extinct, zalambdodont, placental mammals. *Bulletin of the American Museum of Natural History*, 273, 1–117.

Asher, R.J., Bennett, N. and Lehmann, T. (2009). The new framework for understanding placental mammal evolution. *BioEssays*, 31, 853–864.

Austin, C.R. (1951). Observations on the penetration of sperm into the mammalian egg. *Australian Journal of Scientific Research, B*, 4, 581–596.

Austin, C.R. (1976). Specialization of gametes. In *Reproduction in Mammals, Vol. 6, The Evolution of Reproduction*, eds. C.R. Austin and R.V. Short. Cambridge: Cambridge University Press, pp. 149–182.

Bahat, A., Tur-Kaspa, I., Gakamsky, A. and Giojalas, L.C. (2003). Thermotaxis of mammalian sperm cells: a potential navigation mechanism in the female genital tract. *Nature Medicine*, 9, 149–150.

Bahat, A., Eisenbach, M. and Tur-Kaspa, I. (2005). Periovulatory increase in temperature difference within the rabbit oviduct. *Human Reproduction*, 20, 2118–2121.

Bailey, E.P. (1974). Notes on the development, mating behavior, and vocalization of captive ringtails. *The Southwestern Naturalist*, 19(1), 117–119.

Baker, J.D. (1989). Aquatic copulation in the northern fur seal, *Callorhinus ursinus*. *Northwestern Naturalist*, 70(2), 33–36.

Baker, P.J., Funk, S.M., Bruford, M.W. and Harris, S. (2004). Polygynandry in a red fox population: implications for the evolution of group living in canids? *Behavioral Ecology*, 15(5), 766–778.

Baker, R.R. and Bellis, M.A. (1993). Human sperm competition: ejaculate manipulation by females and a function for the female orgasm. *Animal Behaviour*, 46, 887–909.

Baker, R.R. and Bellis, M.A. (1995). *Human Sperm Competition*. London: Chapman and Hall.

Bakker, C.M., Hollmann, M., Mehlis, M. and Zbinden, M. (2014). Functional variation of sperm morphology in sticklebacks. *Behavioral Ecology and Sociobiology*, 68, 617–627.

Bakker, J. and Baum, M.J. (2000). Neuroendocrine regulation of GnRH release in induced ovulators. *Frontiers in Neuroendocrinology*, 21, 220–262.

Ballenberghe, V.V. and Miquelle, D.G. (1993). Mating in moose: timing, behavior, and male access patterns. *Canadian Journal of Zoology*, 71, 1687–1690.

Bancroft, J. (2009). *Human Sexuality and its Problems*. Third edn. Edinburgh: Churchill Livingstone.

Barclay, R.M.R. and Thomas, D.W. (1979). Copulation call of *Myotis lucifugus*: a discrete situation-specific communication signal. *Journal of Mammalogy*, 60(3), 632–634.

Barklow, W.E. (2004). Low-frequency sounds and amphibious communication in *Hippopotamus amphibius*. *Journal of the Acoustical Society of America*, 115, 2555A.

Barratt, E.M., Deaville, R., Burland, T.M., Bruford, M.W., Jones, G., *et al.* (1997). DNA answers the call of pipistrelle bat species. *Nature*, 387, 138–139.

Barrette, C. (1977). The social behaviour of captive muntjacs *Muntiacus reevesi* (Ogilby 1939). *Zeitschrift für Tierpsychologie*, 48, 188–213.

Barros, F.F.P.C., Queiroz, J.P.A.F., Filho, A.C.M., Santos, E.A.A., Paula, V.V., *et al.* (2009). Use of two anesthetic combinations for semen collection by electroejaculation from captive coatis (*Nasua nasua*). *Theriogenology*, 71, 1261–1266.

Barry, R. and Shoshani, J. (2000). *Heterohyrax brucei. Mammalian Species*, 645, 1–7.

Bartholomew, G.A. and Hoel, P.G. (1953). Reproductive behavior of the Alaska fur seal, *Callorhinus ursinus. Journal of Mammalogy*, 34(4), 417–436.

Bartosiewicz, L. (2000). Baculum fracture in carnivores: osteological, behavioural and cultural implications. *International Journal of Osteoarchaeology*, 10, 447–450.

Bar Ziv, E., Ilany, A., Demartsev, V., Barocas, A., Geffen, E., *et al.* (2016). Individual, social and sexual niche traits affect copulation success in a polygynandrous mating system. *Behavioral Ecology and Sociobiology*, 70, 901–912.

Batra, S.K. (1974). Sperm transport through vas deferens: review of hypotheses and suggestions for a quantitative model. *Fertility and Sterility*, 25, 186–202.

Baumgardner, D.J. and Dewsbury, D.A. (1979). Copulatory behavior of *Calomys callosus. Bulletin of the Psychonomic Society*, 14(2), 127–128.

Baumgardner, D.J., Hartung, T.C., Sawrey, K., Webster, D.G., Dewsbury, D.A., *et al.* (1982). Muroid copulatory plugs and female reproductive tracts: a comparative investigation. *Journal of Mammalogy*, 63(1), 110–117.

Beach, F.A. (1967). Cerebral and hormonal control of reflexive mechanisms involved in copulatory behaviour. *Physiological Reviews*, 47, 289–316.

Beach, F.A. (1976). Sexual attractivity, proceptivity and receptivity in female mammals. *Hormones and Behavior*, 7, 105–138.

Beach, F.A. and Levinson, G. (1950). Effects of androgen on the glans penis and mating behavior of castrated rats. *Journal of Experimental Zoology*, 114, 159–171.

Bearder, S.K., Oates, J.F., Dowsett-Lemaire, F. and Dowsett, R. (2015). Evidence of an undescribed form of tree hyrax in the forests of western Nigeria and the Dahomey Gap. *Afrotherian Conservation*, 11, 2–5.

Beasely, J.C., Beatty, W.S., Olson, Z.H. and Rhodes, O.E. (2010). A genetic analysis of the Virginia opossum mating system: evidence for multiple paternity in a highly fragmented landscape. *Journal of Heredity*, 101(3), 368–373.

Beatty, R.A. (1960). Fertility of mixed semen from different rabbits. *Journal of Reproduction and Fertility*, 19, 52–60.

Beatty, R.A., Bennett, G.H., Hall, J.G., Hancock, J.L. and Stewart, D.L. (1969). An experiment with heterospermic insemination in cattle. *Journal of Reproduction and Fertility*, 19, 491–501.

Beck, R.M.D. (2008). A dated phylogeny of marsupials using a molecular supermatrix and multiple fossil constraints. *Journal of Mammalogy*, 89(1), 175–189.

Beck, R.M.D., Godthelp, H., Weisbecker, V., Archer, M. and Hand, S.J. (2008). Australia's oldest marsupial fossils and their biogeographical implications. *PLoS ONE*, 3(3), e1858.

Beckett, S.D., Hudson, R.S., Walker, D.F., Vachon, R.I. and Reynolds, T. M. (1972). Corpus cavernosum penis pressure and external penile muscle activity during erection in the goat. *Biology of Reproduction*, 7, 359–364.

Beckett, S.D., Hudson, R.S., Walker, D.F., Reynolds, T.M. and Vachon R.I. (1973). Blood pressures and penile muscle activity in the stallion during coitus. *American Journal of Physiology*, 225(5), 1072–1075.

Bedford, J.M. (1978a). Anatomical evidence for the epididymis as the prime mover in the evolution of the scrotum. *American Journal of Anatomy*, 152, 483–507.

Bedford, J.M. (1978b). Influence of abdominal temperature on epididymal function in the rat and rabbit. *American Journal of Anatomy*, 152, 509–521.

Bedford, J.M. (1982). Fertilization. In *Reproduction in Mammals, Vol. 1*. Second edn, eds. C.R. Austin and R.V. Short. Cambridge: Cambridge University Press, pp. 128–163.

Bedford, J.M. (2008). Puzzles of mammalian fertilization and beyond. *International Journal of Developmental Biology*, 52, 415–426.

Bedford, J.M. (2015). The epididymis re-visited: a personal view. *Asian Journal of Andrology*, 17, 693–698.

Bedford, J.M. and Breed, W.G. (1994). Regulated storage and subsequent transformation of spermatozoa in the fallopian tube of an Australian marsupial, *Sminthopsis crassicaudata*. *Biology of Reproduction*, 50, 845–854.

Bedford, J.M. and Hoskins D.D. (1990). The mammalian spermatozoon: morphology, biochemistry and physiology. In *Marshall's Physiology of Reproduction. Vol. 2, Reproduction in the Male*, ed. G.E. Lamming. Edinburgh: Churchill Livingstone, pp. 379–568.

Bedford, J.M., Rodger, J.C. and Breed, W.G. (1984). Why so many mammalian spermatozoa – a clue from marsupials? *Proceedings of the Royal Society of London, B*, 221, 221–233.

Bedford, J.M., Mock, O.B. and Goodman, S.M. (2004). Novelties of conception in insectivorous mammals (Lipotyphla), particularly shrews. *Biological Reviews*, 79, 891–909.

Behrends, P.R. (1981). Copulatory behavior of *Dipodomys microps* (Heteromyidae). *The Southwestern Naturalist*, 25, 562–563.

Beier, J.C. and Wartzok, D. (1979). Mating behavior of captive spotted seals (*Phoca largha*). *Animal Behaviour*, 27, 772-781.

Bekoff, M. and Diamond, J. (1976). Precopulatory and copulatory behavior in coyotes. *Journal of Mammalogy*, 57(2), 372–375.

Bennett, N.C. and Jarvis, J.U.M. (1988). The reproductive biology of the Cape mole rat, *Georychus capensis* (Rodentia, Bathyergidae). *Journal of Zoology, London*, 214, 95–106.

Benshemesh, J. and Johnson. K. (2003). Biology and conservation of marsupial moles: unique Aussie diggers. In *Predators with Pouches: The Biology of Carnivorous Marsupials*, eds. M. Jones, C.R. Dickman and M. Archer. Melbourne: CSIRO Publishing, pp. 464–474.

Bercovitch, F.B. and Nürnberg, P. (1996). Socioendocrine and morphological correlates of paternity in rhesus macaques. *Journal of Reproduction and Fertility*, 107, 59–68.

Bercovitch, F.B., Berry, P.S.M., Dagg, A., Deacon, F., Doherty, J.B., *et al.* (2017). How many species of giraffe are there? *Current Biology*, 27, R123–R138.

Bergfelt, D.R., Blum, J.I., Ratner, J.R., Ratto, M.H., O'Brien, J.K., *et al.* (2018). Preliminary evaluation of seminal plasma proteins and immunoreactivity of nerve growth factor as indicative of an ovulation inducing factor in odontocetes. *Journal of Zoo Biology*, 2(1), 21–29.

Berland, M.A., Ulloa-Leal, C., Barria, M., Wright, H., Dissen, G.A., *et al.* (2016). Seminal plasma induces ovulation in llamas in the absence of a copulatory stimulus: role of nerve growth factor as an ovulation-inducing factor. *Endocrinology*, 15(8), 3224–3232.

Bermant, G. (1964). Effects of single and multiple enforced intercopulatory intervals on the sexual behavior of male rats. *Journal of Comparative and Physiological Psychology*, 57, 398–403.

Bermant, G. and Westbrook, W.H. (1966). Peripheral factors in the regulation of sexual contact by female rats. *Journal of Comparative and Physiological Psychology*, 61(2), 244–250.

Bermant, G., Clegg, M.T. and Beamer, W. (1969). Copulatory behavior of the ram, *Ovis aries*. 1: A normative study. *Animal Behaviour*, 17, 700–705.

Berta, A., and Ray, C.E. (1990). Skeletal morphology and locomotor capabilities of the archaic pinniped *Enaliarctos mealsi*. *Journal of Vertebrate Paleontology*, 10(2), 141–157.

Best, R.C. and Da Silva, V.M.F. (1993). *Inia geoffrensis. Mammalian Species*, 426, 1–8.

Beyer, C., Contreras, J. L., Larsson, K., Olmedo, M. and Morali, G. (1982). Pattern of motor and seminal vesicle activities during copulation in the male rat. *Physiology and Behavior*, 29, 495–500.

Bezerra, B.M., Souto, A.S., Halsey, L.G. and Schiel, N. (2008). Observation of brown-throated three-toed sloths: mating behaviour and the simultaneous nurturing of two young. *Journal of Ethology*, 26, 175–178.

Biewener, A.A. and Baudinette, R.V. (1995). *In vivo* muscle force and elastic energy storage during steady-speed hopping of tammar wallabies (*Macropus eugenii*). *Journal of Experimental Biology*, 198, 1829–1841.

Biggers, J.D. (1966). Reproduction in male marsupials. In *Comparative Biology of Reproduction in Mammals*, ed. I.W. Rowlands. *Symposia of the Zoological Society of London*, 15, 251–280.

Bignami, G. and Beach, F.A. (1968). Mating behaviour in the chinchilla. *Animal Behaviour*, 16, 45–53.

Bingham, H.C. (1928). Sex development in apes. *Comparative Psychology Monograph*, 5, 1–165.

Bininda-Emonds, O.R.P., Cardillo, M., Jones, K.E., MacPhee, R.D.E., Beck, R.M.D., *et al.* (2007). The delayed rise of present-day mammals. *Nature*, 446, 507–512.

Birkhead, T.R. and Møller, A.P. (1992). *Sperm Competition in Birds*. London: Academic Press.

Birkhead, T.R. and Møller, A.P. (1993). Sexual selection and the temporal separation of reproductive events: sperm storage data from reptiles, birds and mammals. *Biological Journal of the Linnean Society*, 50, 295–311.

Birney, E.C. and Baird, D.D. (1985). Why do some mammals polyovulate to produce a litter of two? *The American Naturalist*, 126(1), 136–140.

Bland, K.B. and Kitchener, A.C. (2001). The anatomy of the penis of a sperm whale (*Physeter catodon* L., 1758). *Mammal Review*, 31(3), 239–244.

Blandau, R.J. (1945). On factors involved in sperm transport through the cervix uteri of the albino rat. *American Journal of Anatomy*, 73, 253–272.

Blandau, R.J., Boling, J.L. and Young, W.C. (1941). The length of heat in the albino rat as determined by the copulatory response. *Anatomical Record*, 79, 453–463.

Bland-Sutton, J. (1905). Fracture of the os penis in otters. *The Lancet*, July 1st 1905, 23–24.

Bloom, W. and Fawcett, D.W. (1962). *A Textbook of Histology*. Eighth edn. Philadelphia, PA: W.B. Saunders.

Boellsstorff, D.E., Qwings, D.H., Penedo, M.C.T. and Hersek, M.J. (1994). Reproductive behaviour and multiple paternity of California ground squirrels. *Animal Behaviour*, 47, 1057–1064.

Boness, D.J. and James, H. (1979). Reproductive behaviour of the grey seal (*Halichoerus grypus*) on Sable Island, Nova Scotia. *Journal of Zoology, London*, 188, 477–500.

Boone, W.R., Catlin, J.C., Casey, K.T., Boone, E.T., Dye, P.S., *et al.* (1998). Bears as induced ovulators: a preliminary study. *Ursus*, 10, 503–505.

Bradbury, J.W. (1977). Lek mating behavior in the hammer-headed bat. *Zeitschrift für Tierpsychologie*, 45, 225–255.

Bradley, A.J., McDonald, I.R. and Lee, A.K. (1980). Stress and mortality in a small marsupial (*Antechinus stuartii*). *General and Comparative Endocrinology*, 40, 188–200.

Bradley, B.J., Robbins, M.M., Williamson, E.E., Steklis, N.G. Eckhardt, N., *et al.* (2005). Mountain gorilla tug-of-war: silverbacks have limited control over reproduction in multimale groups. *Proceedings of the National Academy of Sciences USA*, 102, 9418–9423.

Braithwaite, R.W. and Lee, A.K. (1979). A mammalian example of semelparity. *American Naturalist*, 113, 151–155.

Brassey, C.A., Gardiner, J.D. and Kitchener, A.C. (2018). Testing hypotheses for the function of the carnivoran baculum using finite-element analysis. *Proceedings of the Royal Society of London, B*, 285, 20181473.

Bravo, P.W., Moscoso, J., Ordoñez, C. and Alarcon, V. (1996). Transport of spermatozoa and ova in female alpaca. *Animal Reproduction Science*, 43(2–3), 173–179.

Braza, F. (2011). *Dama dama*. In *Virtual Encyclopedia of Spanish Vertebrates*, eds. L.M. Carrascal and L.M. Salvador. Madrid: Museo National de Ciencias Naturales, pp. 1–14. www.vertebradosibericos.org/mamiferos/damdam.html

Breed, W.G. (1990). Copulatory behavior and coagulum formation in the female reproductive tract of the Australian hopping mouse, *Notomys alexis*. *Journal of Reproduction and Fertility*, 88, 17–24.

Breed, W.G. and Taylor, J. (2000). Body mass, testes mass, and sperm size in murine rodents. *Journal of Mammalogy*, 81, 758–768.

Breed, W.G., Leigh, C.M and Speight, N. (2013). Coevolution of the male and female reproductive tracts in an old endemic murine rodent of Australia. *Journal of Zoology, London*, 289, 94–100.

Brennan, P.L. and Prum, R.O. (2012). The erection mechanism of the ratite penis. *Journal of Zoology, London*, 286, 140–144.

Briceño, R.D. and Eberhard, W.G. (2009). Experimental demonstration of possible cryptic female choice on male tsetse fly genitalia. *Journal of Insect Physiology*, 55, 989–996.

Brindle, M. and Opie, C. (2016). Postcopulatory sexual selection influences baculum evolution in primates and carnivores. *Proceedings of the Royal Society of London, B*, 283, 20161736.

Brinsko, S.P., Blanchard, T.L., Varner, D.D., Schumacher, J., Love, C.C., *et al.* (2011). *Manual of Equine Reproduction*. Third edn. Maryland Heights, MO: Mosby Inc.

Bronner, G. (2013). Family Chrysochloridae: golden moles. In *Mammals of Africa. Volume I: Introductory Chapters and Afrotheria*, eds. J. Kingdon, D. Happold, M. Hoffman, T. Butynski, M. Happold and J. Kalina. London: Bloomsbury Publishing, pp. 223–225.

Bronson, R. (1998). Is the oocyte a non-professional phagocyte? *Human Reproduction Update*, 4(6), 763–775.

Brooks, C.M. (1937). The role of the cerebral cortex and of various sense organs in the excitation and execution of mating activity in the rabbit. *American Journal of Physiology*, 120(3), 544–553.

Brooks, D.E. (1973). Epididymal and testicular temperature in the unrestrained conscious rat. *Journal of Reproduction and Fertility*, 35, 157–160.

Broom, L.S. and Geiser, F. (1995). Hibernation in free-living mountain pygmy-possums, *Burramys parvus* (Marsupialia, Burramyidae). *Australian Journal of Zoology*, 43(4), 373–379.

Brown, G.R. and Silk, J.B. (2002). Reconsidering the null hypothesis: is maternal rank associated with birth sex ratios in primate groups? *Proceedings of the National Academy of Sciences USA*, 99, 11252–11255.

Brown-Grant, K., Davidson, J.M. and Greig, F. (1973). Induced ovulation in albino rats exposed to constant light. *Journal of Endocrinology*, 57, 7–22.

Brownell, R.L. and Ralls, K. (1986). Potential for sperm competition in baleen whales. *Report of the International Whaling Commission*, 8, 97–112.

Bryant, K.A. (2004). The Mating System and Reproduction in the Honey Possum, *Tarsipes rostratus*: A Life-History and Genetic Perspective. PhD Thesis, Murdoch University, School of Biological Sciences and Biotechnology.

Bryson, B. (2019). *The Body: A Guide for Occupants*. London: Doubleday.

Burgin, C.J., Colella, J.P., Kahn, P.L. and Upham, N.S. (2018). How many species of mammals are there? *Journal of Mammalogy*, 99(1), 1–14.

Burrell, H. (1927). *The Platypus*. Sydney: Rigby Ltd.

Burton, C. (2002). Microsatellite analysis of multiple paternity and male reproductive success in the promiscuous snowshoe hare. *Canadian Journal of Zoology*, 80, 1948–1956.

Busso, J.M., Ponzio, M.F., de Cuneo, M.F. and Ruiz, R.D. (2005). Year-round testicular volume and semen quality evaluations in captive *Chinchilla lanigera*. *Animal Reproduction Science*, 90, 127–134.

Butterworth, B.B. (1961). The breeding of *Dipodomys deserti* in the laboratory. *Journal of Mammalogy*, 42(3), 413–414.

Byers, J.A., Moodie, J.D. and Hall, N. (1994). Pronghorn females choose vigorous males. *Animal Behaviour*, 47, 33–43.

Byrnes, G., Lim, N. T.-L., Yeong, C. and Spence, A. J. (2011). Sex differences in the locomotor ecology of a gliding mammal, the Malayan colugo (*Galeopterus variegatus*). *Journal of Mammalogy*, 92(2), 444–451.

Cade, C.E. (1967). Notes on breeding the cape hunting dog, *Lycaon pictus*, at Nairobi Zoo. *International Zoo Yearbook*, 7, 722–733.

Callahan, J.R. and Davis, R. (1982). Reproductive tract and evolutionary relationships of the Chinese rock squirrel, *Sciurotamias davidianus*. *Journal of Mammalogy*, 63(1), 42–47.

Cameron, E.Z. (2004). Facultative adjustment of mammalian sex ratios in support of the Trivers–Willard hypothesis: evidence for a mechanism. *Proceedings of the Royal Society, B*, 271, 1723–1728.

Cameron, E.Z., Linklater, W.L., Stafford, K.J. and Veltman, C.J. (1999). Birth sex ratios relate to mare condition in Kaimanawa horses. *Behavioral Ecology*, 10(5), 472–475.

Campagna, C. and Le Boeuf, B.J. (1988). Reproductive behaviour of southern sea lions. *Behaviour*, 104(3–4), 233–261.

Campbell, C.J. (2007). Primate sexuality and reproduction. In *Primates in Perspective*, eds. C.J. Campbell, A. Fuentes, K.C. Mackinnon, M. Panger, and S.K. Bearder. New York: Oxford University Press, pp. 423–437.

Cantor, N.F. (2001). *In the Wake of the Plague*. London: Simon and Schuster.

Carayon, J. (1966). Traumatic insemination and the paragenital system. In *Monograph of Cimicidae*, ed. R. Usinger. Philadelphia, PA: Thomas Say Foundation 7, Entomological Society of America.

Carleton, M.D., Hooper, E.T. and Honacki, J. (1975). Karyotypes and accessory reproductive glands in the rodent genus *Scotinomys*. *Journal of Mammalogy*, 56, 916–921.

Carling, M.D., Wiseman, P.A. and Byers, J.A. (2003). Analysis reveals multiple paternity in a population of wild pronghorn antelopes (*Antilocapra americana*). *Journal of Mammalogy*, 84(4), 1237–1243.

Carmichael, L.E., Szor, G., Berteaux, D., Giroux, M.A., Cameron, C., *et al.* (2007). Free love in the far north: plural breeding and polyandry of arctic foxes (*Alopex lagopus*) on Bylot Island, Nunavut. *Canadian Journal of Zoology*, 85(3), 338–343.

Carmichael, M.S., Humbert, R., Dixen, J., Palmisano, G., Greenleaf, W., *et al.* (1987). Plasma oxytocin increases in the human sexual response. *Journal of Clinical Endocrinology and Metabolism*, 64, 27–31.

Carraway, L.N. and Verts, B.J. (1993). *Aplodontia rufa. Mammalian Species*, No. 431, 1–10.

Carrick, F.N. and Setchell, B.P. (1977). The evolution of the scrotum. In *Reproduction and Evolution*, ed. B.P. Setchell. London: Paul Elek, pp. 90–108.

Carter, C.S. (1973). Stimuli contributing to the decrement in sexual receptivity of female golden hamsters (*Mesocricetus auratus*). *Animal Behaviour*, 21, 827–834.

Carter, C.S. and Getz, L.L. (1985). Social and hormonal determinants of reproductive patterns in the prairie vole. In *Neurobiology*, eds. R. Gilles and J. Balthazart. Berlin: Springer-Verlag, pp. 18–36.

Carter, C.S., Witt, D.M., Manock, S.R., Adams, K.A., Bahr, J.M., *et al.* (1989). Hormonal correlates of sexual behavior and ovulation in male-induced and post-partum estrus in female prairie voles. *Physiology and Behavior*, 46, 941–948.

Ceballos, G. and Ehrlich, P.R. (2009). Discoveries of new mammal species and their implications for conservation and ecosystem services. *Proceedings of the National Academy of Sciences USA*, 106(10), 3841–3846.

Cervantes, R.F. and López-Forment, C.W. (1981). Observations on the sexual behavior, gestation period, and young of captive Mexican volcano rabbits, *Romerolagus diazi. Journal of Mammalogy*, 62(3), 634–635.

Chamberlin, R.V. and Ivie, W. (1943). A new genus of Theridiid spiders in which the male develops only one palpus. *Bulletin of the University of Utah*, 24, 190–220.

Chang, M.C. (1951). Fertilizing capacity of spermatozoa deposited into the fallopian tubes. *Nature*, 168, 697–698.

Chapman, T. (2018). Sexual conflict: mechanisms and emerging themes in resistance biology. *The American Naturalist*, 192(2), 217–229.

Chapman, T., Liddle, L. F., Kalb, J. M., Wolfner, M. F. and Partridge, L. (1995). Cost of mating in *Drosophila melanogaster* females is mediated by male accessory gland products. *Nature*, 373, 241–244.

Charles-Dominique, P. (1977). *Ecology and Behaviour of Nocturnal Primates*. London: Duckworth.

Chen, B.X., Yuen, Z.X. and Pan, G.W. (1985). Semen-induced ovulation in the bactrian camel (*Camelus bactrianus*). *Journal of Reproduction and Fertility*, 74, 335–339.

Cheng, M.-F., Peng, J.P. and Johnson, P. (1998). Hypothalamic neurons preferentially respond to female nest coo stimulation: demonstration of direct acoustic stimulation of luteinizing hormone release. *The Journal of Neuroscience*, 18(14), 5477–5489.

Chittleborough, R.G. (1955). Aspects of reproduction in the male humpback whale, *Megaptera nodosa* (Bonnaterre). *Australian Journal of Marine and Freshwater Research*, 9, 1–20.

Christian, J.J., Steinberger, E. and McKinney, T.D. (1972). Annual cycle of spermatogenesis and testis morphology in woodchucks. *Journal of Mammalogy*, 53, 708–716.

Cifelli, R.L., and Davis, B.M. (2003). Marsupial origins. *Science*, 302, 1899–1900.

Clapham, P.J. (1996). The social and reproductive biology of humpback whales: an ecological perspective. *Mammal Review*, 26(1), 27–49.

Clark, W.E. Le Gros (1962). *The Antecedents of Man*. Second edn. Edinburgh: Edinburgh University Press.

Claus, R. and Schams, D. (1990). Influence of mating and and intra-uterine oestradiol infusion on peripheral oxytocin concentrations in the sow. *Journal of Endocrinology*, 126, 361–365.

Clinchy, M., Taylor, A.C., Zanette, Y., Krebs, J. and Jarman, P.J. (2004). Body size, age and paternity in common brushtail possums (*Trichosurus vulpecula*). *Molecular Ecology*, 13, 195–202.

Cline, D.R., Siniff, D.B. and Erickson, A.W. (1971). Copulation of the Weddell seal. *Journal of Mammalogy*, 52(1), 216–218.

Clutton-Brock, T. (2016). *Mammal Societies*. Chichester: Wiley-Blackwell.

Clutton-Brock, T.H. and Iason, G.R. (1986). Sex ratio variation in mammals. *Quarterly Review of Biology*, 61(3), 339–374.

Clutton-Brock, T.H., Albon, S.D. and Guinness, F.E. (1984). Maternal dominance, breeding success and birth sex ratios in red deer. *Nature*, 308, 358–360.

Coe, M.J. (1969). The anatomy of the reproductive tract and breeding in the spring haas, *Pedetes surdaster larvalis* Hollister. *Journal of Reproduction and Fertility, Supplement*, 6, 159–174.

Cole, F.J. (1897). On the structure and morphology of the intromittent sac of the male guinea-pig (*Cavia cobaya*). *Journal of Anatomy and Physiology*, 32, 141–152.

Collins, P.M. and Tsang, W.M. (1987). Growth and reproductive development in the male tree shrew (*Tupaia belangeri*) from birth to sexual maturity. *Biology of Reproduction*, 37, 261–267.

Coltman, D.W., Bancroft, D.R., Robertson, A., Smith, A., Clutton-Brock, T.H., *et al.* (1999). Male reproductive success in a promiscuous mammal: behavioural estimates compared with genetic paternity. *Molecular Ecology*, 8, 1199–1209.

Conaway, C.H. (1958). Maintenance, reproduction and growth of the least shrew in captivity. *Journal of Mammalogy*, 39(4), 507–512.

Conaway, C.H. (1971). Ecological adaptation and mammalian reproduction. *Biology of Reproduction*, 4, 239–241.

Conaway, C.H. and Sorenson, M.W. (1966). Reproduction in tree shrews. In *Comparative Biology of Reproduction in Mammals*, ed. I.W. Rowlands. Symposia of the Zoological Society of London, 15, 471–492.

Concannon, P., Hodgson, B. and Lein, D. (1980). Reflex LH release in estrous cats following single and multiple copulations. *Biology of Reproduction*, 23, 111–117.

Connor, R.C., Read, A.J. and Wrangham, R. (2000). Male reproductive strategies and social bonds. In *Cetacean Societies*, eds. J. Mann, R.C. Connor, P.L. Tyack and H. Whitehead. Chicago: The University of Chicago Press, pp. 247–269.

Contreras, J.L. and Beyer, C. (1979). A polygraphic analysis of mounting and ejaculation in the New Zealand white rabbit. *Physiology and Behavior*, 23, 939–943.

Contreras, L.C., Torres-Mura, J., Spotorno, A.E. and Catzeflis, F.M. (1993). Morphological variation of the glans penis of South American octodontid and abrocomid rodents. *Journal of Mammalogy*, 74(4), 926–935.

Cooper, J.D., Waser, P.M., Hellgren, E.C., Gabor, T.M. and DeWoody, J.A. (2011). Is sexual monomorphism a predictor of polygynandry? Evidence from a social mammal, the collared peccary. *Behavioral Ecology and Sociobiology*, 65, 775–785.

Cooper, K.K. (1972). Cutaneous mechanoreceptors of the glans penis of the cat. *Physiology and Behavior*, 8, 793–796.

Courts, S.E. (1996). An ethogram of captive Livingstone's fruit bats, *Pteropus livingstonii*, in a new enclosure at Jersey Wildlife Preservation Trust. *Dodo: Jersey Wildlife Preservation Trust*, 32, 15–37.

Coutinho da Silva, M.A., Ferreira, H.N. and Johnson, A.E.M. (2008). Effects of tempol and L-ergothioneine on motility parameters of cryopreserved stallion sperm. *Animal Reproduction Science*, 107(3–4), 177–360. doi:10.1016/j.anireprosci.2008.05.094.

Cowper, W. (1704). A letter to Dr Edward Tyson. Giving an account of the anatomy of those parts of a male opossum that differ from the female. *Philosophical Transactions of the Royal Society*, 24, 1576–1590.

Craighead, J.J. and Mitchell, J.A. (1982). Grizzly bear. In *Wild Mammals of North America*, eds. J.A. Chapman and G.A. Feldhamer. Baltimore, MD: Johns Hopkins University Press, pp. 515–556.

Craighead, J.J., Hornocker, M.G. and Craighead, F.C. (1969). Reproductive biology of young female grizzly bears. *Journal of Reproduction and Fertility, Supplement*, 6, 447–475.

Crawford, J.L., McLeod, B.J., Thompson, E.G. and Hurst, P.R. (1998). Presence of males affects incidence of ovulation after pouch young removal in brushtail possums (*Trichosurus vulpecula*). *Animal Reproduction Science*, 51, 45–55.

Crews, D. and Silver, R. (1985). Reproductive physiology and behavior interactions in non-mammalian vertebrates. In *Handbook of Behavioral Neurobiology, Vol. 7*, eds. N. Adler, D. Pfaff and R.W. Goy. New York: Plenum Press, pp. 101–182.

Croft, D.B. (1981). Social behaviour of the euro, *Macropus robustus* (Gould), in the Australian arid zone. *Australian Wildlife Research*, 8, 13–49.

Cronin, J.E., Cann, R. and Sarich, V.M. (1980). Molecular evolution and systematics of the Genus *Macaca*. In *The Macaques: Studies in Ecology, Behavior and Evolution*, ed. D.G. Lindburg. New York: Van Nostrand Reinhold, pp. 31–51.

Crowcroft, P. (1957). *The Life of the Shrew*. London: Max Reinhardt.

Cruz, Y., Rodríguez-Antolin, J., Nicolás, L., Martínez-Gómez, M. and Lucio, R.A. (2010). Components of the neural circuitry of the vaginocavernosus reflex in rabbits. *Journal of Comparative Neurology*, 518, 199–210.

Cryan, P.M., Jameson, J.W., Baerwald, E.F., Willis, C.K.R., Barclay, R.M.R., et al. (2012). Evidence of late-summer mating readiness and early sexual maturation in migratory tree-roosting bats found dead at wind turbines. *PLoS ONE*, 7(10), e47586.

Cui, L.-W. and Xiao, W. (2004). Sexual behavior in a one-male unit of *Rhinopithecus bieti* in captivity. *Zoo Biology*, 23, 545–550.

Cukierski, M.A., Sina, J.L., Prahalada, S. and Robertson, R.T. (1991). Effects of seminal vesicle and coagulating gland ablation on fertility in rats. *Reproductive Toxicology*, 5, 347–352.

Cummins, J. (2010). Sperm motility and energetics. In *Sperm Biology: An Evolutionary Perspective*, eds. T.R. Birkhead, D.J. Hosken, S. Pitnik. San Diego, CA: Elsevier/ Academic Press, pp. 185–206.

Cummins, J.M. and Woodall, P. F. (1985). On mammalian sperm dimensions. *Journal of Reproduction and Fertility*, 75, 153–175.

Cummins, J.M., Temple-Smith, P.D. and Renfree, M.D. (1986). Reproduction in the male honey possum (*Tarsipes rostratus*: Marsupialia): the epididymis. *The American Journal of Anatomy*, 177, 385–401.

Cuzzuol, M.A., Clozato, C.L., Holanda, E.C., Rodrigues, F.H.G., Nienow, S., et al. (2013). A new species of tapir from the Amazon. *Journal of Mammalogy*, 94(6), 1331–1345.

Darwin, C. (1859). *On the Origin of Species by Means of Natural Selection or the Preservation of Favoured Races in the Struggle for Life*. London: John Murray.

Darwin, C. (1871). *The Descent of Man and Selection in Relation to Sex*. London: John Murray.

David, A., Vilenski, A. and Nathan, H. (1972). Temperature changes in the different parts of the rabbit's oviduct. *International Journal of Gynaecology and Obstetrics*, 10, 52–56.

David, J.H.M. (1975). Observations on mating behaviour, parturition, suckling and the mother–young bond in the bontebok (*Damaliscus dorcas dorcas*). *Journal of Zoology, London*, 177, 203–223.

Davies, N.B., Krebs, J.R. and West, S.A. (2012). *An Introduction to Behavioural Ecology*. Fourth edn. Chichester: Wiley-Blackwell.

Davis, H.N., Estep, D.Q. and Dewsbury, D.A. (1974a). Copulatory behavior of Mongolian gerbils. *Animal Learning and Behavior*, 2(1), 69–73.

Davis, H.N., Gray, G.D., Zerylnick, M. and Dewsbury, D.A. (1974b). Ovulation and implantation in montane voles (*Microtus montanus*) as a function of varying amounts of copulatory stimulation. *Hormones and Behavior*, 5, 383–388.

Davis, H.N., Gray, J.D. and Dewsbury, D.A. (1977). Maternal age and male behavior in relation to successful reproduction by female rats (*Rattus norvegicus*). *Journal of Comparative and Physiological Psychology*, 91(2), 281–289.

Davis, L.S. (1982). Copulatory behaviour of Richardson's ground squirrels (*Spermophilus richardsonii*) in the wild. *Canadian Journal of Zoology*, 60, 2953–2955.

Dawson, T.J. (1995). *Kangaroos. Biology of the Largest Marsupials*. Sydney: University of New South Wales Press.

De Jong, G. and Ketel, N.A.J. (1981). An analysis of copulatory behaviour of *Microtus agrestis* and *M. arvalis* in relation to reproductive isolation. *Behaviour*, 78(3/4), 227-259.

Dean, M.D. (2013). Genetic disruption of the copulatory plug in mice leads to severely reduced fertility. *PLOS Genetics*, 9(1), e1003185.

Delgado, R., Fernández-Llario, P., Azevedo, M., Beja-Pereira, A. and Santos, P. (2008). Paternity assessment in free-ranging wild boar (*Sus scrofa*). Are littermates full-sibs? *Mammalian Biology*, 73, 169–176.

Delson, E. (1980). Fossil macaques, phyletic relationships and a scenario of deployment. In *The Macaques: Studies in Ecology, Behavior and Evolution*, ed. D.G. Lindburg. New York: Van Nostrand Reinhold, pp. 10–30.

Delsuc, F., Catzeflis, F.M, Stanhope, M.J. and Douzery, E.J.P. (2001). The evolution of armadillos, anteaters and sloths depicted by nuclear mitochondrial phylogenies: implications for the status of the enigmatic fossil *Eurotamandua*. *Proceedings of the Royal Society of London, B*, 268, 1605–1615.

Dempsey, E.W. and Searles, H.F. (1943). Environmental modification of certain endocrine phenomena. *Endocrinology*, 32, 119–128.

Denniston, R.H. (1957). Notes on breeding and size of young in the Richardson's ground squirrel. *Journal of Mammalogy*, 38, 414–416.

Desbiez, A.L.J., Massocato, G.F., Kluyber, D. and Santos, R.C.F. (2018). Unraveling the cryptic life of the southern naked-tailed armadillo, *Cabassous unicinctus squamicaudis* (Lund, 1845), in a Neotropical wetland: home range, activity pattern, burrow use and reproductive behaviour. *Mammalian Biology*, 91, 95–103.

Dewsbury, D.A. (1972). Patterns of copulatory behavior in male mammals. *Quarterly Review of Biology*, 47, 1–33.

Dewsbury, D.A. (1974). Copulatory behaviour of white-throated wood rats (*Neotoma albigulara*) and golden mice (*Ochrotomys nuttalli*). *Animal Behaviour*, 22, 601–610.

Dewsbury, D.A. (1975a). Diversity and adaptation in rodent copulatory behavior. *Science*, 190, 947–954.

Dewsbury, D.A. (1975b). Copulatory behavior of white-footed mice (*Peromyscus leucopus*). *Journal of Mammalogy*, 56, 420–428.

Dewsbury, D. A. (1978). The comparative method in studies of reproductive behavior. In *Sex and Behavior: Status and Prospectus*, eds. T.E. McGill, D.A. Dewsbury and B.D. Sachs. New York: Plenum Press, pp. 83–112.

Dewsbury, D.A. (1988). Copulatory behavior as courtship communication. *Ethology*, 79, 218–234.

Dewsbury, D.A. and Dawson, W.W. (1979). African four-striped grass mice (*Rhabdomys pumilio*), a diurnal–crepuscular muroid rodent, in the behavioral laboratory. *Behavior Research Methods and Instrumentation*, 11(3), 329–333.

Dewsbury, D.A. and Estep, D.Q. (1975). Pregnancy in cactus mice: effects of prolonged copulation. *Science*, 187, 552–553.

Dewsbury, D.A. and Hartung, T.G. (1982). Behavior of three species of *Microtus*. *Journal of Mammalogy*, 63(2), 306–309.

Dewsbury, D.A. and Hodges, A.W. (1987). Copulatory behavior and related phenomena in spiny mice (*Acomys cahirinus*) and hopping mice (*Notomys alexis*). *Journal of Mammalogy*, 69, 49–57.

Dewsbury, D.A. and Jansen, P.E. (1972). Copulatory behavior of southern grasshopper mice (*Onychomys torridus*). *Journal of Mammalogy*, 53, 267–278.

Dewsbury, D.A. and Lovecky, D.V. (1974). Copulatory behavior of old field mice (*Peromyscus polionotus*) from different natural populations. *Behavioral Genetics*, 4, 347–355.

De Young, R.W., Demarais, S., Gonzales, R.A., Honeycutt, R.L. and Gee, K.L. (2002). Multiple paternity in white-tailed deer (*Odocoileus virginianus*) revealed by DNA microsatellites. *Journal of Mammalogy*, 83(3), 884–892.

Diakow, C. (1971). Effects of genital desensitization on mating behavior and ovulation in the female cat. *Physiology and Behavior*, 7, 47–54.

Dines J.P. (2014). The Evolution and Functional Significance of Cetacean Pelvic Bones. PhD Thesis, University of Southern California.

Dines, J.P., Otárola-Castillo, E., Ralph, P., Alas, J., Daley, T., *et al.* (2014). Sexual selection targets cetacean pelvic bones. *Evolution*, 68, 3296–3306.

Dines, J.P., Mesnick, S.L., Ralls, K., May-Collado, L., Agnarsson, I., *et al.* (2015). A trade-off between precopulatory and postcopulatory trait investment in male cetaceans. *Evolution*, 69(6), 1560–1572.

Dixson, A.F. (1976). Effects of testosterone on the sternal cutaneous glands and genitalia of the male greater galago (*Galago crassicaudatus crassicaudatus*). *Folia Primatologica*, 26, 207–213.

Dixson, A.F. (1983a). The hormonal control of sexual behaviour in primates. *Oxford Reviews of Reproductive Biology*, 5, 131–218.

Dixson, A.F. (1983b). Observations on the evolution and behavioral significance of 'sexual skin' in female primates. *Advances in the Study of Behavior*, 13, 63–106.

Dixson, A.F. (1986). Genital sensory feedback and sexual behaviour in male and female marmosets (*Callithrix jacchus*). *Physiology and Behavior*, 37, 447–450.

Dixson, A.F. (1987a). Observations on the evolution of the genitalia and copulatory behaviour in male primates. *Journal of Zoology, London*, 213, 423–443.

Dixson, A.F. (1987b). Baculum length and copulatory behavior in primates. *American Journal of Primatology*, 13, 51–60.

Dixson, A.F. (1989). Sexual selection, genital morphology and copulatory behaviour in male galagos. *International Journal of Primatolology*, 10, 47–55.

Dixson, A.F. (1991). Penile spines affect copulatory behaviour in a primate (*Callithrix jacchus*). *Physiology and Behavior*, 49, 557–562.

Dixson, A.F. (1995a). Sexual selection and the evolution of copulatory behaviour in nocturnal prosimians. In *Creatures of the Dark: The Nocturnal Prosimians*, eds. L. Alterman, G.A. Doyle and M.K. Izard. New York: Plenum, pp. 93–118.

Dixson, A.F. (1995b). Sexual selection and ejaculatory frequencies in primates. *Folia Primatologica*, 64, 146–152.

Dixson, A.F. (1995c). Baculum length and copulatory behaviour in carnivores and pinnipeds (Grand Order Ferae). *Journal of Zoology, London*, 235, 67–76.

Dixson, A.F. (1998a). *Primate Sexuality: Comparative Studies of the Prosimians, Monkeys, Apes, and Human Beings*. First edn. Oxford: Oxford University Press.

Dixson, A.F. (1998b). Sexual selection and evolution of the seminal vesicles in primates. *Folia Primatologica*, 69, 300–306.

Dixson, A.F. (2009). *Sexual Selection and the Origins of Human Mating Systems*. Oxford: Oxford University Press.

Dixson, A.F. (2012). *Primate Sexuality: Comparative Studies of the Prosimians, Monkeys, Apes, and Humans*. Second edn. Oxford: Oxford University Press.

Dixson, A.F. (2015a). Primate sexuality. In *The International Encyclopedia of Human Sexuality, Vol. 2*, eds. P. Whelehan and A. Bolin. Chichester: Wiley Blackwell, pp. 988–996.

Dixson, A.F. (2015b). *The Mandrill: A Case of Extreme Sexual Selection*. Cambridge: Cambridge University Press.

Dixson, A.F. (2018). Copulatory and postcopulatory sexual selection in primates. *Folia Primatologica*, 89, 258–286.

Dixson, A.F. and Anderson, M.J. (2002). Sexual selection, seminal coagulation and copulatory plug formation in primates. *Folia Primatologica*, 73, 63–69.

Dixson, A.F. and Herbert, J. (1974). The effects of testosterone on the sexual skin and genitalia of the male talapoin monkey. *Journal of Reproduction and Fertility*, 38, 217–219.

Dixson, A.F. and Mundy, N.I. (1994). Sexual behavior, sexual swelling and penile evolution in chimpanzees (*Pan troglodytes*). *Archives of Sexual Behavior*, 23, 267–280.

Dixson, A.F. and Nevison, C.M. (1997). The socioendocrinology of adolescent development in male rhesus monkeys (*Macaca mulatta*). *Hormones and Behavior*, 31, 126–135.

Dixson, A.F., Pissinatti, A. and Anderson, M. J. (2004a). Observations on genital morphology and anatomy of a hybrid male muriqui (genus *Brachyteles*). *Folia Primatologica*, 75, 61–69.

Dixson, A.F., Nyholt, J. and Anderson, M. J. (2004b). A positive relationship between baculum length and prolonged intromission patterns in mammals. *Acta Zoologica Sinica*, 50, 490–503.

Dixson, A.F., Dixson, B.J. and Anderson, M. (2005). Sexual selection and the evolution of visually conspicuous sexually dimorphic traits in male monkeys, apes, and human beings. *Annual Reviews of Sex Research*, 15, 1–19.

Dixson, B.J. and Vasey, P.L. (2012). Beards augment perceptions of men's age, social status, and aggressiveness, but not attractiveness. *Behavioral Ecology*, 23(3), 481–490.

Djakiew, D. (1982). Reproduction in the Male Echidna (*Tachyglossus aculateus*) with Particular Emphasis on the Epididymis. Thesis, Department of Biological Sciences, University of Newcastle, Australia.

Djakiew, D. and Jones, R.C. (1981). Structural differentiation of the male genital ducts of the echidna (*Tachyglossus aculeatus*). *Journal of Anatomy*, 132(2), 187–202.

Djakiew, D. and Jones, R.C. (1983). Sperm maturation, fluid transport, and secretion and absorption of protein in the epididymis of the echidna, *Tachyglossus aculeatus*. *Journal of Reproduction and Fertility*, 68, 445–456.

Doak, R.L., Hall, A. and Dale, H.E. (1967). Longevity of spermatozoa in the reproductive tract of the bitch. *Journal of Reproduction and Fertility*, 13, 51–58.

Domning, D.P. (2001). The earliest known fully quadrupedal sirenian. *Nature*, 413, 625–627.

Dorus, S., Evans, P.D., Wyckoff, G.J., Choi, S.S. and Lahn, B.T. (2004). Rate of molecular evolution of the seminal gene SEMG2 correlates with levels of female promiscuity. *Nature Genetics*, 36, 1326–1329.

Douady, C.J., Chatelier, P.I., Madsen, O., de Jong, W.W., Catzeflis, F., *et al.* (2002a). Molecular phylogenetic evidence confirming the Eulipotyphla concept and in support of hedgehogs as the sister group to shrews. *Molecular Phylogenetics and Evolution*, 25, 200–209.

Douady, C.J, Catzeflis, F., Kao, D.J., Springer, M.S. and Stanhope, M.J. (2002b). Molecular evidence for the monophyly of Tenrecidae (Mammalia) and the timing of the colonization of Madagascar by Malagasy tenrecs. *Molecular Phylogenetics and Evolution*, 22(3), 357–363.

Dowsett, K.F. and Knott, L.M. (1996). The influence of age and breed on stallion semen. *Theriogenology*, 48, 397–412.

Drea, C.M. and Weil, A. (2008). External genitalia of the ring-tailed lemur (*Lemur catta*): females are naturally 'masculinized'. *Journal of Morphology*, 269, 451–463.

Drea, C.M., Coscia, E.M. and Glickman, S.E. (1999). Hyenas. In *Encyclopedia of Reproduction, Vol. 2*, eds. E. Knobil, J. Neill and P. Licht. San Diego, CA: Academic Press, pp. 718–725.

Drea, C.M., Place, N.J., Weldele, M.L., Coscia, E.M., Licht, P., *et al.* (2002). Exposure to naturally circulating androgens during fetal life incurs direct reproductive costs in female spotted hyenas, but is prerequisite for male mating. *Proceedings of the Royal Society of London, B*, 269, 1981–1987.

Drennan, W.G. and MacPherson, J.W. (1966). The reproductive tract of bovine slaughter heifers (a biometrical study). *Canadian Journal of Comparative Veterinary Medical Science*, 30, 224–227.

Drobnis, E.Z. and Overstreet, J.W. (1992). Natural history of mammalian spermatozoa in the female reproductive tract. In *Oxford Reviews of Reproductive Biology, Vol. 14*, ed. S.R. Milligan. Oxford: Oxford University Press, pp. 1–45.

Dubost, G. and Feer, F. (1981). The behaviour of the male *Antilope cervicapra* L., its development according to age and social rank. *Behaviour*, 76(1–2), 62–127.

Dubost, P.G. (1971). Observations éthologiques sur le muntjak (*Muntiacus muntjac*, Zimmermann 1780 et *M. reevesi* Ogilby 1839) en captivité et semi-liberté. *Zeitschrift für Tierpsychologie*, 28, 387–427.

Dücker, G. (1965). Das verhalten der schleichkatzen (Viverridae). *Berlin: Handbuch der Zoologie*, 8, 1–48.

Ducrocq, S., Buffetaut, E., Buffetaut-Tong, H., Jaeger, J.-J., *et al.* (1992). First fossil flying lemur: a dermopteran from the late Eocene of Thailand. *Palaeontology*, 35, 373–380.

Duff, R.S. (1977). *The Moa Hunter Period of Maori Culture*. Third edn. Wellington, New Zealand: Government Printer.

Dufour, C.M.-S., Pillay, N. and Ganem, G. (2015). Ventro-ventral copulation in a rodent: a female initiative? *Journal of Mammalogy*, 96(5), 1017–1023.

Dufty, A.C. (1994). Field observations of the behaviour of free-ranging eastern barred bandi-coots, *Perameles gunnii*, at Hamilton, Victoria. *The Victorian Naturalist*, 111, 54–59.

Dunham, A.E. and Rudolf, V.H.W. (2009). Evolution of sexual size monomorphism: the influence of passive mate guarding. *Journal of Evolutionary Biology*, 22, 1376–1386.

East, K. and Lockie, J.D. (1965). Further observations on weasels (*Mustela nivalis*) and stoats (*Mustela ermina*) born in captivity. *Proceedings of the Zoological Society of London*, 147, 234–238.

Eaton, G.G., Slob, A.K. and Resko, J.A. (1973). Cycles of mating behaviour, oestrogen and progesterone in the thick-tailed bushbaby, *Galago crassicaudatus crassicaudatus*, under laboratory conditions. *Animal Behaviour*, 21, 309–315.

Eberhard, W.G. (1985). *Sexual Selection and Animal Genitalia*. Cambridge, MA and London: Harvard University Press.

Eberhard, W.G. (1990). Animal genitalia and female choice. *American Scientist*, 78, 134–141.

Eberhard, W.G. (1991). Copulatory courtship in insects. *Biological Reviews*, 66, 1–31.

Eberhard, W.G. (1994). Evidence for widespread courtship during copulation in 131 species of insects and spiders, and implications for cryptic female choice. *Evolution*, 48, 711–733.

Eberhard, W.G. (1996). *Female Control: Sexual Selection by Cryptic Female Choice*. Princeton, NJ: Princeton University Press.

Eberhard, W.G. (2004). Rapid divergent evolution of sexual morphology: comparative tests of antagonistic coevolution and traditional female choice. *Evolution*, 58(9), 1947–1970.

Eberhard, W.G. (2011). Experiments with genitalia; a commentary. *Trends in Ecology and Evolution*, 26(1), 16–21.

Eberhard, W.G. and Huber, B.A. (2010). Spider genitalia: precise maneuvers with a numb structure in a complex lock. In *The Evolution of Primary Sex Characters in Animals*, eds. J.L. Leonard and A. Córdoba-Aguilar. New York: Oxford University Press, pp. 249–284.

Eberle, M. and Kappeler, P.M. (2004). Selected polyandry, female choice and inter-sexual conflict in a small nocturnal solitary primate (*Microcebus murinus*). *Behavioral Ecology and Sociobiology*, 57, 91–100.

Edwards, R.G. (1955). Selective fertilization following the use of sperm mixtures in the mouse. *Nature*, 175, 215–223.

Egerbacher, M., Weber, H. and Hauer, S. (2000). Bones in the heart skeleton of the otter (*Lutra lutra*). *Journal of Anatomy*, 196, 485–491.

Eisenbach, M. and Giojalas, L. (2006). Sperm guidance in mammals: an unpaved road to the egg. *Nature*, 7, 275–284.

Eisenberg, J.F. (1975). Tenrecs and solenodons in captivity. *International Zoo Yearbook*, 15, 6–12.

Eisenberg, J.F. (1977). The evolution of the reproductive unit in the Class Mammalia. In *Reproductive Behavior and Evolution*, eds. E.S. Rosenblatt and S. Komisaruk. New York: Plenum Press, pp. 39–71.

Eisenberg, J.F. (1981). *The Mammalian Radiations: An Analysis of Trends in Evolution, Adaptation and Behaviour*. London: Athlone Press.

Eisenberg, J.F. and Gould, E. (1970). The tenrecs: a study in mammalian behavior and evolution. *Smithsonian Contributions to Zoology*, 27, 1–127.

Eisenberg, J.F., Collins, L.R. and Wemmer, C. (1975). Communication in the Tasmanian devil (*Sarcophilus harrisii*) and a survey of auditory communication in the the the Marsupialia. *Zeitschrift für Tierpsychologie*, 37, 379–399.

Enders, A.C. (2002). Implantation in the nine-banded armadillo: how does a single blastocyst form four embryos? *Placenta*, 23, 71–85.

Enders, R.K. (1952). Reproduction in the mink (*Mustela vison*). *Proceedings of the American Philosophical Society*, 96(6), 691–755.

England, B.G., Foote, W.C., Cardozo, A.G., Matthews, D.H. and Riera, S. (1971). Oestrus and mating behaviour in the llama (*Llama glama*). *Animal Behaviour*, 19, 722–726.

England, G.C.W., Burgess, C.M., Freeman, S.L., Smith, S.C. and Pacey, A.A. (2006). Relationship between the fertile period and sperm transport in the bitch. *Theriogenology*, 66, 1410–1418.

Engstrom, M.D. and Dowler, R.C. (1981). Field observations of mating behavior in *Dipodomys ordii*. *Journal of Mammalogy*, 62(2), 384–386.

Erbajeva, M.A., Mead, J.I., Alexeeva, N.V., Angelone, C. and Swift, S.L. (2011). Taxonomic diversity of late Cenozoic Asian and North American ochotonids (an overview). *Paleontologica Electronica*, 14, 1–9.

Erickson, C.J. and Lehrman, D.S. (1964). Effects of castration of male ring doves upon ovarian activity of females. *Journal of Comparative and Physiological Psychology*, 58, 164–166.

Estep, D.Q. and Dewsbury, D.A. (1976). Copulatory behavior of *Neotoma lepida* and *Baiomys taylori*: relationships between penile morphology and behavior. *Journal of Mammalogy*, 57 (3), 570–573.

Estes, R.D. (1991). *The Behavior Guide to African Mammals*. Berkeley, CA: University of California Press.

Eudy, A.A. (1980). Pleistocene glacial phenomena and the evolution of Asian macaques. In *The Macaques: Studies in Ecology, Behavior and Evolution*, ed. D.G. Lindburg. New York: Van Nostrand Reinhold, pp. 52–83.

Ewer, R.F. (1963). The behaviour of the meercat, *Suricata suricatta* (Schreber). *Zeitschrift für Tierpsychologie*, 20, 570–607.

Ewer, R.F. (1968). *Ethology of Mammals*. London: Logos Press.

Ewer, R.F. (1973). *The Carnivores*. New York: Cornell University Press.

Ewer, R.F. and Wemmer, C. (1974). The behaviour in captivity of the African civet, *Civettictis civetta* (Schreber). *Zeitschrift für Tierpsychologie*, 34, 359–394.

Fadel, H.E., Berns, D., Zaneveld, L.J.D., Wilbanks, G.D. and Brueschke, E.E. (1976). The human uterotubal junction: a scanning electron microscope study during different phases of the menstrual cycle. *Fertility and Sterility*, 27(10), 1176–1186.

Fadem, B.H. and Rayve, R.S. (1985). Characteristics of the oestrous cycle and influence of social factors in grey short-tailed opossums (*Monodelphis domestica*). *Journal of Reproduction and Fertility*, 73, 337–342.

Fair, S., Meade, K.G., Reynaud, K., Druart, X. and de Graaf, S.P. (2019). The biological mechanisms mediating sperm selection by the ovine cervix. *Reproduction*, 158, R1–R13.

Falcón, W., Goldberg, C.S., Waits, L.P., Estes-Zumpf, W.A. and Rachlow, J.L. (2011). First record of multiple paternity in the pygmy rabbit (*Brachylagus idahoensis*): evidence from analysis of 16 microsatellite loci. *Western North American Naturalist*, 71(2), 271–275.

Fallas-López, M., De Lara, R.R., Gama, R.B., Esqueda, M.T. and Romero, O.A. (2011). Rabbit sexual behavior, semen and semen characteristics when supplemented with sprouted wheat. *Animal Reproduction Science*, 129, 221–228.

Fang, L.X. and Wang, S. 1980. A preliminary survey on the habits of pangolins. *Memoirs of Beijing Natural History Museum*, 7, 1–6.

Fanjul, M.S. and Zenuto, R.R. (2008). Copulatory pattern of the subterranean rodent *Ctenomys talarum*. *Mammalia*, 72, 102–108.

Fanning, F.D. (1982). Reproduction, growth and development in *Ningaui* sp. (Dasyuridae, Marsupialia) from the Northern Territory. In *Carnivorous Marsupials, Vol. 1*, ed. M. Archer. Sydney: Royal Society of New South Wales, pp. 23–37.

Fasel, N.J., Mamba, M.L. and Monadjem, A. (2020). Penis morphology facilitates identification of cryptic African bat species. *Journal of Mammalogy*, DOI: 10.1093/jmammal/gyaa073.

Faulkes, C.G., Sichilima, A.M., van Sandwyk, J., Lutermann, H. and Bennett, N.C. (2010). Control of ovulation in female giant mole-rats *Fukomys mechowii* (Rodentia: Bathyergidae), and phylogenetic trends within the family. *Journal of Zoology London*, 282, 64–74.

Fawcett, D.W., Neaves, W.B. and Flores, M.N. (1973). Comparative observations on inter-tubular lymphatics and the organization of the interstitial tissue of the mammalian testis. *Biology of Reproduction*, 9, 500–532.

Fazeli, A., Affara, N.A., Hubank M. and Holt, W.V. (2004). Sperm-induced modification of the oviductal gene expression profile after natural insemination in mice. *Biology of Reproduction*, 71(1), 60–65.

Fedosenko, A.K. and Orlov, G.I. (1977). On the sexual behavior of the wild sheep and the Siberian ibex. In *The Group Behavior of Animals. Reports of the Participants of the Second All-Union Conference on Animal Behavior*, ed. B.P. Manteifel. Moscow: Nauka, pp. 402–404.

Fee, A.R. and Parkes, A.S. (1930). Studies on ovulation. 111. Effect of vaginal anaesthesia on ovulation in the rabbit. *Journal of Physiology*, 70, 385–388.

Felicioli, A., Grazzini, A. and Santini, L. (1997). The mounting and copulation behaviour of the crested porcupine *Hystrix cristata*. *Italian Journal of Zoology*, 64(2), 155–161.

Fennessy, J., Bidon, T., Reuss, F., Kumar, V., Elkan, P., *et al.* (2016). Multi-locus analyses reveal four giraffe species instead of one. *Current Biology*, 26, 1–7.

Fenton, M.B. and Simmons, N.B. (2014). *Bats: A World of Science and Mystery*. Chicago: University of Chicago Press.

Fietz, J., Zischler, H., Schwiegk. C., Tomiuk, J., Dausmann, K.H., *et al.* (2000). High rates of extra-pair young in the pair-living fat-tailed dwarf lemur, *Cheirogaleus medius*. *Behavioral Ecology and Sociobiology*, 49, 8–17.

Firman, R.C. and Simmons, L.W. (2008). The frequency of multiple paternity predicts variation in testes size among island populations of house mice. *Journal of Evolutionary Biology*, 21, 1524–1533.

Firman, R.C. and Simmons, L.W. (2009). Sperm competition and the evolution of the sperm hook in house mice. *Journal of Evolutionary Biology*, 22, 2505–2511.

Firman, R.C. and Simmons, L.W. (2010). Sperm midpiece length predicts sperm swimming velocity in house mice. *Biology Letters*, 6, 513–516.

Firman, R.C., Cheam, L.Y. and Simmons, L.W. (2011). Sperm competition does not influence sperm hook morphology in selection lines of house mice. *Journal of Evolutionary Biology*, 24, 856–862.

FitzGibbon, C.D. (1997). The adaptive significance of monogamy in the golden-rumped elephant-shrew. *Journal of Zoology, London*, 242, 167–177.

Fitzpatrick, J.L., Almbro, M., Gonzalez-Voyer, A., Kolm, N. and Simmons, L.W. (2012). Male contest competition and the coevolution of weaponry and testes in pinnipeds. *Evolution*, 66, 3595–3604.

Flaherty, S.P., Breed, W.G. and Sarafis, V. (1983). Localization of actin in the sperm head of the plains mouse, *Pseudomys australis*. *Journal of Experimental Zoology*, 225, 497–500.

Flamini, M.A., Barreto, R.S.N., Matias, G.S.S., Birbrair, A., de Castro, T.H., *et al.* (2020). Key characteristics of the ovary and uterus for reproduction with particular reference to poly-ovulation in the plains viscacha (*Lagostomus maximus*, Chinchillidae). *Theriogenology*, 142, 184–195.

Flannery, T. (1994). *The Future Eaters: An Ecological History of the Australasian Lands and People*. Sydney: New Holland Publishers.

Fleming, A.S., Chee, P. and Vaccarino, F. (1981). Sexual behaviour and its olfactory control in the desert wood rat (*Neotoma lepida lepida*). *Animal Behaviour*, 29, 727–745.

Flynn, J.J. and Nedbal, M.A. (1998). Phylogeny of the Carnivora (Mammalia): congruence vs incompatibility among multiple data sets. *Molecular Phylogenetics and Evolution*, 9, 414–426.

Fontaine, P.M. and Barrette, C. (1997). Megatestes: anatomical evidence for sperm competition in the harbor porpoise. *Mammalia*, 61(1), 65–71.

Fontaine, R. (1981). The uakaris, genus *Cacajao*. In *Ecology and Behavior of Neotropical Primates, Vol. 1*, eds. A.F. Coimbra-Filho and R.A. Mittermeier. Rio de Janeiro: Academia Brasileira de Ciências, pp. 443–493.

Fooden, J. (1967). Complementary specialization of male and female reproductive structures in the bear macaque, *Macaca arctoides*. *Nature*, 214, 939–941.

Fooden, J. (1971). Female genitalia and taxonomic relationships of *Macaca assamensis*. *Primates*, 12(1), 63–73.

Fooden, J. (1975). Taxonomy and evolution of liontail and pigtail macaques (Primates: Cercopithecidae). *Fieldiana Zoology*, 67, 1–169.

Fooden, J. (1991). New perspectives on macaque evolution. In *Primatology Today*, eds. A. Ehara, T. Kimura, O. Takenaka and M. Iwamoto. Amsterdam: Elsevier, pp. 1–7.

Ford, C.S. and Beach, F.A. (1952). *Patterns of Sexual Behaviour*. London: Eyre and Spottiswoode Ltd.

Fox, B.J. and Whitford, D. (1982). Polyoestry in a predictable coastal environment: reproduction, growth and development in *Sminthopsis murina* (Dasyuridae, Marsupialia). In *Carnivorous Marsupials, Vol. 1*, ed. M. Archer. Sydney: Royal Society of New South Wales, pp. 39–48.

Frädrick, H. (1974). A comparison of behavior. In *Behavior of Ungulates and its Relation to Management*, eds. V. Geist and F.R. Walther. IUCN Publication No. 24. Morges: IUCN, pp. 133–143.

Frame, L.H., Malcolm, J.R., Frame, G.W. and Van Lawick, H. (1979). Social organization of African wild dogs (*Lycaon pictus*) on the Serengeti Plains, Tanzania, 1967–1978. *Zeitschrift für Tierpsychologie*, 50, 225–249.

França, L.R., Avelar, G.F. and Almeida F.F. (2005). Spermatogenesis and sperm transit through the epididymis in mammals with emphasis on pigs. *Theriogenology*, 63(2), 300–318.

Frasier, T.R., Hamilton, P.K., Brown, M.W., Conger, L.A., Knowlton, A.R., *et al.* (2007). Patterns of male reproductive success in a highly promiscuous whale species: the endangered North Atlantic right whale. *Molecular Ecology*, 16, 5277–5293.

Frederick, H. and Johnson, C.N. (1996). Social organization in the rufous bettong, *Aepyprymnus rufescens*. *Australian Journal of Zoology*, 44, 9–17.

Freund, M. (1963). The effect of frequency of emission on semen output and an estimate of daily sperm production in man. *Journal of Reproduction and Fertility*, 6, 269–286.

Frey, R. (1994). Der Zusammenhang zwischen Lokomotionsweise, begattungsstellung und penislänge bei säugetieren. 1. Testiconda (Mammalia mit intraabdominaler hodenlage). *Journal of Zoological Systems and Evolutionary Research*, 32, 137–155.

Friesen, C.R., Uhrig, E.J., Squire, M.K., Mason, R.T. and Brennan, P.L. (2014). Sexual conflict over mating in red-sided garter snakes (*Thamnophis sirtalis*) as indicated by experimental manipulation of genitalia. *Proceedings of the Royal Society of London, B*, 281, 20132694.

Frink, R.J. and Merrick, B. (1974). The sheep heart: coronary and conduction system anatomy with special reference to an *os cordis*. *Anatomical Record*, 179, 189–200.

Gaddum-Rosse, P. (1981). Some observations on sperm transport through the uterotubal junction of the rat. *American Journal of Anatomy*, 160, 333–341.

Gage, M.J.G. and Freckleton, R. (2003). Relative testis size and sperm morphometry across mammals: no evidence for an association between sperm competition and sperm length. *Proceedings of the Royal Society of London, B*, 270, 625–632.

Galbreath, G.J. (1985). The evolution of monozygotic polyembryony in *Dasypus*. In *The Evolution and Ecology of Armadillos, Sloths, and Vermilinguas*, ed. G.G. Montgomery. Washington, DC: Smithsonian Institution Press.

Gallup, G.G. Jr., Burch, R.L., Zappieri, M.L., Parvez, R.A., Stockwell, M.L., et al. (2003). The human penis as a semen displacement device. *Evolution and Human Behavior*, 24, 277–289.

Gañán, N., Gonzalez, R., Garde, J.J., Martinez, F., Vargas, A., et al. (2009). Assessment of semen quality, sperm cryopreservation and heterologous IVF in the critically endangered Iberian lynx. *Reproduction, Fertility and Development*, 21, 848–859.

Garcés-Restrepo, M.F., Peery, M.Z., Reid, G. and Pauli, J.N. (2017). Individual reproductive strategies shape the mating system of tree sloths. *Journal of Mammalogy*, 98(5), 1417–1425.

Gazit, I. and Terkel, J. (2000). Reproductive behavior of the blind mole-rat (*Spalax ehrenbergi*) in a seminatural burrow system. *Canadian Journal of Zoology*, 78, 570–577.

Gebhard, J. (1995). Observations on the mating behaviour of *Nyctalus noctula* (Schreber, 1774) in the hibernaculum. *Myotis*, 32, 123–129.

Gensch, W. (1968). Notes on breeding timber wolves, *Canis lupus occidentalis*, at Dresden Zoo. *International Zoo Yearbook*, 8, 15–16.

Gillan, P. and Brindley, G.S. (1979). Vaginal and pelvic floor responses to sexual stimulation. *Psychophysiology*, 16, 471–481.

Gizjewski, Z. (2004). Effect of season on characteristics of red deer, *Cervus elaphus* L. semen collected using modified artificial vagina. *Reproductive Biology*, 4(1), 51–66.

Glickman, S.E., Coscia, E.M., Frank, L.G., Licht, P., Weldele, M.L., et al. (1998). Androgens and masculinization of genitalia in the spotted hyaena (*Crocuta crocuta*). 3. Effects of juvenile gonadectomy. *Journal of Reproduction and Fertility*, 113, 129–135.

Glover, T. (2012). *Mating Males: An Evolutionary Perspective on Mammalian Reproduction*. Cambridge: Cambridge University Press.

Glover, T.D. and Sale, J.B. (1968). The reproductive system of the male rock hyrax (*Procavia* and *Heterohyrax*). *Journal of Zoology, London*, 156, 351–362.

Glucksmann, A., Ooka-Souda, S., Miura-Yasugi, E. and Mizuno, T. (1976). The effect of neonatal treatment of male mice with antiandrogens and of females with androgens on the development of the *os penis* and *os clitoridis*. *Journal of Anatomy*, 121(2), 363–370.

Goblet, C., West, G., Campos-Krauer, J.M. and Newell-Fugate, A.E. (2018). Semen analysis parameters from a captive population of the endangered Chacoan peccary (*Catagonus wagneri*) in Paraguay. *Animal Reproduction Science*, 195, 162–167.

Goddard, J. (1966). Mating and courtship of the black rhinoceros (*Diceros bicornis* L.). *East African Wildlife Journal*, 4, 69–75.

Godsell, J. (1983). Ecology of the Eastern Quoll, *Dasyurus viverrinus* (Dasyuridae: Marsupialia). PhD Dissertation, Australian National University, Canberra, pp. 1–422.

Godthelp, H., Archer, M., Cifelli, R.L., Hand, S.J. and Gilkeson, C.F. (1992). Earliest known Australian Tertiary mammal fauna. *Nature*, 356, 514–516.

Goldfoot, D.A. and Goy, R.W. (1970). Abbreviation of behavioral estrus in guinea pigs by coital and vagino-cervical stimulation. *Journal of Comparative and Physiological Psychology*, 72, 426–434.

Goldman, C. (1987). *Crossarchus obscurus. Mammalian Species*, No. 290, 1–5.

Gomendio, M. and Roldan, E.R.S. (1991). Sperm size and sperm competition in mammals. *Proceedings of the Royal Society of London, B*, 243, 181–185.

Gomendio, M. and Roldan, E.R.S. (2008). Implications of diversity in sperm size and function for sperm competition and fertility. *International Journal of Developmental Biology*, 52, 439–447.

Goodall, J. (1986). *The Chimpanzees of Gombe: Patterns of Behavior*. Cambridge, MA: Belknap Press of Harvard University Press.

Goossens, B., Graziani, L., Waits, L.P., Farand, E., Magnolon, S., *et al.* (1998). Extra-pair paternity in the monogamous alpine marmot revealed by nuclear DNA microsatellite analysis. *Behavioral Ecology and Sociobiology*, 43(4–5), 281–288.

Goshal, N.G. and Bal, H.S. (1976). Histomorphology of the urethral process of the goat (*Capra hircus*). *Acta Anatomica*, 94, 567–573.

Goswami, A. and Friscia, A. (2010). *Carnivoran Evolution: New Views on Phylogeny, Form and Function*. Cambridge: Cambridge University Press.

Gould, E. and Eisenberg, J.F. (1966). Notes on the biology of the Tenrecidae. *Journal of Mammalogy*, 47(4), 660–686.

Gould, J.E., Overstreet, J.W. and Hanson, F.W. (1984). Assessment of human sperm function after recovery from the female reproductive tract. *Biology of Reproduction*, 31, 888–894.

Gowans, S., Würsig, B. and Karczmarski, L. (2008). The social structure and strategies of delphinids: predictions based on an ecological framework. *Advances in Marine Biology*, 53, 195–294.

Grant, J. and Hawley, A. (1991). Some observations on the mating behaviour of captive American pine martens *Martes americana. Acta Theriologica*, 41(4), 439–442.

Grant, T.R. and Temple-Smith, P.D. (1998). Field biology of the platypus (*Ornithorhynchus anatinus*): historical and current perspectives. *Philosophical Transactions of the Royal Society of London, B: Biological Sciences*, 353, 1081–1091.

Gray, G.D. and Dewsbury, D.A. (1975). A quantitative description of the copulatory behaviour of meadow voles (*Microtus pennsylvanicus*). *Animal Behaviour*, 23, 261–267.

Gredler, M.L., Larkins, C.E., Leal, F., Lewis, A.K., Herrera, A.M., *et al.* (2014). Evolution of external genitalia: insights from reptilian development. *Sexual Development*, 8, 311–326.

Greer, W.E., Roussel, J.D. and Austin, C.R. (1968). Prevention of coagulation in monkey semen by surgery. *Journal of Reproduction and Fertility*, 15, 153–155.

Griffiths, M. (1978). *The Biology of the Monotremes*. New York: Academic Press.

Griffiths, M. (1998). Monotremes. In *Encyclopedia of Reproduction Vol. 3*, eds. E. Knobil and J.D. Neill. New York: Academic Press, pp. 295–302.

Grimmberger, E., Hackethal, H. and Urbanczyk, Z. (1987). Beitrag zum Paarungsverhalten der Wasserfledermaus, *Myotis daubentonii* (Kuhl, 1819), im Winterquartier. *Zeitschrift für Saugetierkunde*, 52, 133–140.

Gudermuth, D.F., Newton, L., Daels, P. and Concannon, P. (1997). Incidence of spontaneous ovulation in young, group-housed cats based on serum and faecal concentrations of progesterone. *Journal of Reproduction and Fertility, Supplement*, 51, 177–184.

Guise, S.D., Bisaillon, A., Séguin, B. and Lagacé, A. (1994). The anatomy of the male genital system of the beluga whale, *Delphinapterus leucas*, with special reference to the penis. *Anatomia, Histologia, Embryologia*, 23, 207–216.

Habibi, K. (1987). Behavior of aoudad (*Ammotragus lervia*). *Mammalia*, 51(4), 497–513.

Habibi, K., Thouless, C.R. and Lindsay, N. (1993). Comparative behaviour of sand and mountain gazelles. *Journal of Zoology, London*, 229, 41–53.

Hafez, E.S.E., ed. (1968). *Reproduction in Farm Animals*. Second edn. Philadelphia, PA: Lea and Febiger.

Hafez, E.S.E. (1973). The comparative anatomy of the mammalian cervix. In *The Biology of the Cervix*, eds. R.J. Blandau and K. Moghissi. Chicago: The University of Chicago Press, pp. 23–56.

Haight, J.R. and Nelson, J.E. (1987). A brain that doesn't fit its skull: a comparative study of the brain and endocranium of the koala *Phascolarctos cinereus* (Marsupialia, Phascolarctidae). In *Possums and Opossums: Studies in Evolution*, ed. M. Archer. Sydney: Surrey Beatty and Sons/Royal Zoological Society of New South Wales, pp. 331–352.

Hall, K.R.L. and DeVore, I. (1965). Baboon social behavior. In *Primate Behaviour: Field Studies of Monkeys and Apes*, ed. I. DeVore. New York: Holt, Rinehart and Winston, pp. 53–110.

Hamede, R.K., Bashford, J., McCallum, H. and Jones, M. (2009). Contact networks in a wild Tasmanian devil (*Sarcophilus harissii*) population: using social network analysis to reveal seasonal variability in social behaviour and its implications for transmission of devil facial tumour disease. *Journal of Animal Ecology*, 82, 182–190.

Hamilton, D.W. (1990). Anatomy of mammalian male accessory reproductive organs. In *Marshall's Physiology of Reproduction, Vol. 2*. Fourth edn, ed. G.E. Lamming. Edinburgh: Churchill Livingstone, pp. 691–746.

Hamilton, D.W. and Cooper, T.G. (1978). Gross and histological variations along the length of the rat vas deferens. *Anatomical Record*, 190, 795.

Hammond, J. and Marshall, F.H.A. (1925). *Reproduction in the Rabbit*. Edinburgh: Oliver and Boyd.

Hammond, J. and Walton, A. (1934). Notes on ovulation and fertilization in the ferret. *Journal of Experimental Biology*, 11, 307–319.

Handasyde, K., Coulson, G., Martin, J. and Taylor, A. (2007). Long-term pair-bonds without mating fidelity in a mammal. *Behaviour*, 144(11), 1419–1455.

Hanken, J. and Sherman, P. W. (1981). Multiple paternity in Belding's ground squirrels. *Science*, 212, 351–353.

Harcourt, A.H. and Gardiner, J. (1994). Sexual selection and genital anatomy of male primates. *Proceedings of the Royal Society of London, B*, 255, 47–53.

Harcourt, A.H., Harvey, P.H., Larson, S.G. and Short, R.V. (1981). Testis weight, body weight and breeding system in primates. *Nature*, 293, 55–57.

Harcourt, A.H., Purvis, A. and Liles, L. (1995). Sperm competition: mating system, not breeding season, affects testes size of primates. *Functional Ecology*, 9, 468–476.

Hardy, D.F. and DeBold, J.F. (1972). Effects of coital stimulation upon behavior of the female rat. *Journal of Comparative and Physiological Psychology*, 78(3), 400–408.

Harper, M.J.K. (1982). Sperm and egg transport. In *Reproduction in Mammals. Vol. 1*. Second edn, eds. C.R. Austin and R.V. Short. Cambridge: Cambridge University Press, pp. 102–127.

Harper, M.J.K. (1994). Gamete and zygote transport. In *The Physiology of Reproduction, Vol. 1*. Second edn, eds. E. Knobil and J.D. Neill. New York: Raven Press, pp. 123–187.

Harrison, J.A. (1981). The baculum of *Plesiogulo* (Carnivora: Mustelidae). *Journal of Paleontology*, 56(5), 1266–1273.

Harrison, R.J. (1949). Observations on the female reproductive organs of the ca'aing whale *Globiocephala melaena* Traill. *Journal of Anatomy*, 83(3), 238–252.

Hart, B.L. (1967). Sexual reflexes and mating behavior in the male dog. *Journal of Comparative and Physiological Psychology*, 64, 388–399.

Hart, B.L. (1970). Mating behavior in the female dog and the effects of estrogen on sexual reflexes. *Hormones and Behavior*, 2, 93–104.

Hart, B.L. (1971). Facilitation by estrogen of sexual reflexes in female cats. *Physiology and Behavior*, 7, 675–678.

Hart, B.L. (1978). Hormones, spinal reflexes and sexual behaviour. In *Biological Determinants of Sexual Behaviour*, ed. J. B. Hutchison. Chichester: John Wiley, pp. 319–347.

Hart, B.L. and Kitchell, R.L. (1965). External morphology of the erect glans penis of the dog. *Anatomical Record*, 152, 193–198.

Hart, B.L. and Kitchell, R.L. (1966). Penile erection and contraction of penile muscles in the spinal and intact dog. *American Journal of Physiology*, 210, 257–261.

Hart, J.A., Detwiler, K., Gilbert, C.C., Burrell, A.S., Fuller, J.L., *et al.* (2012). *Lesula*: a new species of *Cercopithecus* monkey endemic to the Democratic Republic of Congo and implications for conservation of Congo's central basin. *PLoS ONE*, 7(9), e44271.

Hart, R.G. and Greenstein, J.S. (1968). A newly discovered role for Cowper's gland secretion in rodent semen coagulation. *Journal of Reproduction and Fertility*, 17, 87–94.

Hartman, D.S. (1979). Ecology and behavior of the manatee (*Trichecus manatus*) in Florida. *Special Publication: American Society of Mammalogists*, 5, 1–153.

Hartstone-Rose, A., Dundas, R.G., Boyde, B., Long, R.C., Farrell, A.B., *et al.* (2015). The bacula of Rancho La Brea. *Natural History Museum of Los Angeles County, Science Series*, 42, 53–63.

Hartung, T.G. and Dewsbury, D.A. (1978). A comparative analysis of copulatory plugs in muroid rodents and their relationship to copulatory behavior. *Journal of Mammalogy*, 59, 717–723.

Hass, C. and Roback, J.F. (2000). Copulatory behavior of white-nosed coatis. *The Southwestern Naturalist*, 45(3), 329–331.

Hawkins, C.E. and Racey, P.A. (2009). A novel mating system in a solitary carnivore: the fossa. *Journal of Zoology, London*, 277, 196–204.

Hawkins, C.E., Dallas, J.F., Fowler, P.A., Woodroffe R. and Racey, P.A. (2002). Transient masculinization in the fossa, *Cryptoprocta ferox* (Carnivora, Viverridae). *Biology of Reproduction*, 66, 610–615.

Hawkins, C.E., Baars, C., Hesterman, H., Hocking, G.J., Jones, M.E., *et al.* (2006). Emerging disease and population decline of an island endemic, the Tasmanian devil *Sarcophilus harissii*. *Biological Conservation*, 13i, 307–324.

Hawkins, M. and Battaglia, A. (2009) Breeding behaviour of the platypus (*Ornithorhynchus anatinus*) in captivity. *Australian Journal of Zoology*, 57, 283–293.

Hawkins, W.E., and Geuze, J.J. (1977). Secretion in the rat coagulating gland (anterior prostate) after copulation. *Cell and Tissue Research*, 181, 519–529.

Hayssen, V. (2011). *Choloepus hoffmanni* (Pilosa: Megalonychidae). *Mammalian Species*, 43 (1), 37–55.

Heath, E., Schaeffer, N., Meritt, D.A. and Jeyendran, R.S (1987). Rouleaux formation by spermatozoa in the naked-tail armadillo, *Cabassous unicinctus*. *Journal of Reproduction and Fertility*, 79, 153–158.

Heidt, G.A., Petersen, M.K. and Kirkland, G.L. (1968). Mating behavior and development of least weasels (*Mustela nivalis*) in captivity. *Journal of Mammalogy*, 49(3), 413–419.

Helgen, K.M. and Flannery, T.F. (2004). A new species of bandicoot, *Microperoryctes aplini*, from western New Guinea. *Journal of Zoology, London*, 264, 117–124.

Helgen, K.M., Miguez, R.P., Kohen, J.L. and Helgen, L.E. (2012). Twentieth century occurrence of the long-beaked echidna *Zaglossus bruijnii* in the Kimberley region of Australia. *ZooKeys*, 255, 103–132.

Herbert, J. (1972). Behavioural patterns. In *Reproduction in Mammals, Vol. 4*, eds. C.R. Austin and R.V. Short. Cambridge: Cambridge University Press, pp. 34–68.

Herbert, J. (1974). Some functions of hormones and the hypothalamus in the sexual activity of primates. *Progress in Brain Research*, 41, 331–348.

Herdina, A.N., Kelly, D.A., Jahelková, H., Lina, P.H.C. Horáček, I., *et al.* (2015). Testing hypotheses of bat baculum function with 3D models derived from microCT. *Journal of Anatomy*, 226, 229–235.

Hernández-López, L., Cerda-Molina, A.L., Páez-Ponce, D.L. and Mondragón-Ceballos, R. (2008). The seminal coagulum favours passage of fast-moving sperm into the uterus in the black-handed spider monkey. *Reproduction*, 136, 411–421.

Hershkovitz, P. (1992). The South American gracile mouse opossums, Genus *Gracilianus* Gardner and Creighton, 1989 (Marmosidae, Marsupialia): a taxonomic review with notes on general morphology and relationships. *Fieldiana Zoology*, 70, 1–56.

Hershkovitz, P. (1993). Male external genitalia of the non-prehensile tailed South American Monkeys. Part 1: Subfamily Pithecinae, Family Cebidae. *Fieldiana Zoology*, 73, 1–17.

Hershkovitz, P. (1999). *Dromiciops gliroides* Thomas, 1894, last of the Microbiotheria (Marsupialia), with a review of the Family Microbiotheriidae. *Fieldiana Zoology*, 98, 1–56.

Heuvelmans, B. (1958). *On the Track of Unknown Animals*. London: Rupert Hart-Davis.

Hickman, G.C. (1982). Copulation of *Cryptomys hottentotus* (Bathyergidae), a fossorial rodent. *Mammalia*, 46, 293–298.

Hidayatik, N., Yusuf, T.L., Agil, M., Iskandar, E. and Sajuthi, D. (2018). Sexual behaviour of the spectral tarsier (*Tarsius spectrum*) in captivity. *Folia Primatologica*, 89, 157–164.

Higdon, J.W., Bininda-Emonds, O.R.P., Beck, R.M.D. and Ferguson, S.H. (2007). Phylogeny and divergence of the pinnipeds (Carnivora: Mammalia) assessed using a multigene dataset. *BMC Evolutionary Biology*, 7, 216–225.

Hill, W.C.O. (1945). Notes on the dissection of two dugongs. *Journal of Mammalogy*, 26(2), 153–175.

Hill, W.C.O. (1953). *Primates, Comparative Anatomy and Taxonomy, Vol. 1. Strepsirhini*. Edinburgh: Edinburgh University Press.

Hill, W.C.O. (1966). *Primates, Comparative Anatomy and Taxonomy, Vol. 6. Catarrhini, Cercopithecoidea, Cercopithecinae*. Edinburgh: Edinburgh University Press.

Hill, W.C.O. (1972). *Evolutionary Biology of the Primates*. London: Academic Press.

Hinds, L.A. and Smith, M.J. (1992). Evidence from plasma progesterone concentrations for male-induced ovulation in the brush-tailed bettong, *Bettongia penicillata*. *Journal of Reproduction and Fertility*, 95, 291–302.

Hoeck, H.N., Klein, H. and Hoeck, P. (1982). Flexible social organization in a hyrax. *Zeitschrift für Tierpsychologie*, 59, 265–298.

Hogan, L.A., Janssen, T. and Johnston, S.D. (2013). Wombat reproduction (Marsupialia; Vombatidae): an update and future directions for the development of artificial breeding technology. *Reproduction*, 145, R157–R173.

Hogan, L.A., Phillips, C.J.C., Lisle, A.T. and Johnston, S.D. (2010). Reproductive behaviour of the southern hairy-nosed wombat (*Lasiorhinus latifrons*). *Australian Journal of Zoology*, 58 (6), 350–361.

Hogarth, P.J. (1982). *Immunological Aspects of Mammalian Reproduction*. Glasgow: Blackie.

Hogg, J.T. (1984). Mating in bighorn sheep: multiple creative male strategies. *Science*, 225, 526–529.

Hogg, J.T. (1988). Copulatory tactics in relation to sperm competition in Rocky Mountain bighorn sheep. *Behavioral Ecology and Sociobiology*, 22(1), 49–59.

Hohoff, C., Franzen, K. and Sachser, N. (2003). Female choice in a promiscuous wild guinea pig, the yellow-toothed cavy (*Galea musteloides*). *Behavioral Ecology and Sociobiology*, 53, 341–349.

Holleley, C.E., Dickman, C.R., Crowther, M.S. and Oldroyd, B.P. (2006). Size breeds success: multiple paternity, multivariate selection and male semelparity in a small marsupial, *Antechinus stuartii*. *Molecular Ecology* 15, 3439–3448.

Hollister-Smith, J.A., Poole, J.H., Archie, E.A., Vance, E.A., Georgiadis, N.J., *et al.* (2007). Age, musth and paternity success in wild male African elephants, *Loxodonta africana*. *Animal Behaviour*, 74(2), 287–296.

Holroyd, P.A. and Mussell, J.C. (2005). Macroscelidea and Tubilidentata. In *The Rise of Placental Mammals: Origins and Relationships of the Major Extant Clades*, eds. K.D. Rose and J.D. Archibald. Baltimore, MD: Johns Hopkins University Press, pp. 71–83.

Holstein, A.F. (1969). Morphologische studien an nebenhoden des menschen. In *Zwanglose Abbandlungen aus dem Gebiet der Normal und Pathologischen Anatomie, Vol. 20*. Fourth edn, eds. W. Bargmann and W. Doeu. Stuttgart: George Thiem, pp. 1–91.

Holt, W.V. (2011). Mechanisms of sperm storage in the female reproductive tract: an inter-species comparison. *Reproduction in Domestic Animals*, (Supplement 2), 68–74.

Holt, W.V. and Fazeli, A. (2016). Sperm selection in the female mammalian reproductive tract. Focus on the oviduct: hypotheses, mechanisms, and new opportunities. *Theriogenology*, 85, 105–112.

Holt, W.V., Hernandez, M., Warrell, L. and Sakate, N. (2010). The long and the short of sperm selection *in vitro* and *in vivo*: swim-up techniques select for the longer and faster swimming mammalian sperm. *Journal of Evolutionary Biology*, 23, 598–608.

Hoogland, J.L. (1995). *The Black-Tailed Prairie Dog*. Chicago: The University of Chicago Press.

Hook, S.J. and Hafez, E.S.E. (1968). A comparative anatomical study of the mammalian uterotubal junction. *Journal of Morphology*, 125, 159–184.

Hosken, D.J. (1997). Sperm competition in bats. *Proceedings of the Royal Society of London, B*, 264, 385–392.

Howard, J.G., Bush, M. and Wildt, D.E. (1984). Electroejaculation, semen characteristics and serum testosterone concentrations of free-ranging African elephants (*Loxodonta africana*). *Journal of Reproduction and Fertility*, 72(1), 187–195.

Hrbek, T., da Silva, V.M.F., Dutra, N., Gravena, W., Martin, A.R., *et al.* (2014). A new species of river dolphin from Brazil or: how little do we know our biodiversity. *PLoS ONE*, 9(1), e83623.

Huck, U.W. and Lisk, R.D. (1986). Mating-induced inhibition of receptivity in the female golden hamster. 1. Short-term and long-term effects. *Behavioral and Neural Biology*, 45, 107–119.

Huck, U.W., Lisk, R.D. and Thierjung, C. (1987a). Mating-induced inhibition of receptivity in the female golden hamster (*Mesocricetus auratus*): II. Stimuli mediating short-term effects. *Journal of Comparative Psychology*, 101(1), 33–39.

Huck U.W., Lisk, R.D., Parente, E.J. and Guyton, C.L. (1987b). Mating-induced inhibition of receptivity in the female golden hamster (*Mesocricetus auratus*): III. Stimuli mediating long-term effects. *Physiology and Behavior*, 39, 421–428.

Hughes, M.A. and Hughes, R.D. (2006). Field observation of daytime courtship and mating of the common wombat, *Vombatus ursinus*. *Australian Mammalogy*, 28, 115–116.

Hughes, R.L. (1982). Reproduction in the Tasmanian devil, *Sarcophilus harissii* (Dasyuridae, Marsupialia). In *Carnivorous Marsupials, Vol. 1*, ed. M. Archer. Sydney: Royal Zoological Society of New South Wales, pp. 49–63.

Hunter, R.H. and Nicol, R. (1986). A preovulatory temperature gradient between the isthmus and the ampulla of pig oviducts during the phase of sperm storage. *Journal of Reproduction and Fertility*, 77, 599–606.

Hunter, R.H.F. (1988). *The Fallopian Tubes: Their Role in Fertility and Infertility*. Berlin: Springer-Verlag.

Hunter, R.H.F. (1995). Ovarian endocrine control of sperm progression in the fallopian tubes. *Oxford Reviews of Reproductive Biology*, 17, 85–124.

Hunter, R.H.F. and Rodriguez-Martinez, H. (2004). Capacitation of mammalian spermatozoa in vivo, with a specific focus on events in the fallopian tubes. *Molecular Reproduction and Development*, 67, 243–250.

Hussain, Y.H., Guasto, J.S., Zimmer, R.K., Stocker, R. and Riffell, J.A. (2016). Sperm chemotaxis promotes individual fertilization success in sea urchins. *Journal of Experimental Biology*, 219, 1458–1466.

Hutchinson, E., Atkinson, S. and Huntington, K. B. (2015). Growth and sexual maturation in male northern sea otters (*Enhydra lutris kenyoni*) from Gustavus, Alaska. *Journal of Mammalogy*, 96(5), 1045–1054.

Huynh, H.K., Willemsen, T.M., Lovick, T.A. and Holstege, G. (2013). Pontine control of ejaculation and female orgasm. *Journal of Sexual Medicine*, 10, 3038–3048.

Hynes, E.F., Rudd, C.D., Temple-Smith, P.D., Sofronidis, G., Paris, D., *et al.* (2005). Mating sequence, dominance and paternity success in captive male tammar wallabies. *Reproduction*, 130, 123–130.

Ignotz, G.G., Cho, M.Y. and Suarez, S.S. (2007). Annexins are candidate oviductal receptors for bovine sperm surface proteins and thus may serve to hold bovine sperm in the oviductal reservoir. *Biology of Reproduction*, 77(6), 906–913.

Immler, S. and Birkhead, T.R. (2007). Sperm competition and sperm midpiece size: no consistent pattern in passerine birds. *Proceedings of the Royal Society of London, B*, 274, 561–568.

Immler, S., Moore, H.D.M., Breed, W.G. and Birkhead, T.R. (2007). By hook or by crook? Competition and cooperation in rodent sperm. *PLoS ONE*, 2(1), e170.

Imrat, P., Suthanmapinanth, P., Saikhun, K., Mahasawangkul, S., Sostaric, E., *et al.* (2013). Effect of pre-freeze semen quality, extender and cryoprotectant on the post-thaw quality of Asian elephant (*Elephas maximus indicus*) semen. *Cryobiology*, 66, 52–59.

Inoue, N., Sasagawa, K., Ikai, K., Sasaki, Y., Tomikawa, J., *et al.* (2011). Kisspeptin neurons mediate reflex ovulation in the musk shrew (*Suncus murinus*). *Proceedings of the National Academy of Sciences USA*, 108(42), 17527–17532.

Insler, V., Glezerman, M., Zeidel, L., Bernstein, D. and Misgav, N. (1980). Sperm storage in the human cervix: a quantitative study. *Fertility and Sterility*, 33(3), 288–293.

Iossa, G., Soulsbury, C.G., Baker, P.G. and Harris, S. (2008). Sperm competition and the evolution of testes size in terrestrial mammalian carnivores. *Functional Ecology*, 22, 655–662.

Isawa-Arai, T., Serejo, C.S., Siciliano, S., Ott, P.H., Freire, A.S., *et al.* (2018). The host-specific whale louse (*Cyamus boopis*) as a potential for interpreting humpback whale (*Megaptera novaeangliae*) migratory routes. *Journal of Experimental Marine Biology and Ecology*, 505, 45–51.

Jacobsen, N.H.G. (1982). Observations on the behaviour of slender mongooses *Herpestes sanguineus*, in captivity. *Saugetierkundliche Mitteilungen*, 30, 168–183.

Janeca, J.E., Helgen, K.M., Lim, N.T.-L., Baba, M., Izawa, M., *et al.* (2008). Evidence for multiple species of Sunda colugo. *Current Biology*, 18(21), R1001–1002.

Janson, C. (1984). Female choice and the mating system of the brown capuchin monkey, *Cebus apella* (Primates: Cebidae). *Zeitschrift für Tierpsychologie*, 65, 177–200.

Jarman, P J. (1983). Mating system and sexual dimorphism in large, terrestrial, mammalian herbivores. *Biological Reviews*, 58, 485–520.

Jarvis, J.U.M. (1991). Reproduction of naked mole-rats. In *The Biology of the Naked Mole-Rat*, eds. P.W Sherman, J.U.M. Jarvis and R.D. Alexander. Princeton, NJ: Princeton University Press, pp. 384–425.

Jasczak, S. and Hafez, E.S.E. (1972). The cervix uteri and sperm transport in female macaques. In *Medical Primatology, Proceedings of the 3rd Conference on Experimental Medicine and Surgery*, eds. E.I. Goldsmith and J. Moor-Jankowski. Basel: Karger, pp. 273–280.

Jeffreys, A.J., Wilson, V. and Thein, S.L. (1985). Hypervariable 'minisatellite' regions in human DNA. *Nature*, 314, 67–73.

Jensen-Seaman, M.I. and Li, W.H. (2003). Evolution of the hominoid semenogelin genes, the major proteins of ejaculated semen. *Journal of Molecular Evolution*, 57, 261–270.

Jerison, H.J. (1973). *Evolution of the Brain and Intelligence*. New York: Academic Press.

Ji, Q., Luo, Z.-X., Yuan, C.-X., Wible, J.R., Zhang, J.-P., *et al.* (2002). The earliest known eutherian mammal. *Nature*, 416, 816–822.

Jia, Z.Y., Jiang, Z.G. and Wang, Z.W. (2001). Copulatory behavior in captive masked palm civets, *Paguma larvata*. *Folia Zoologica*, 50(4), 271–279.

Jöchle, W.J. (1975). Current research in coitus-induced ovulation: a review. *Journal of Reproduction and Fertility, Supplement*, 22, 165–207.

Johnson, C.M. and Norris, K.S. (1994). Social behavior. In *The Hawaiian Spinner Dolphin*, eds. K.S. Norris, B. Würsig, R.S. Wells and M. Würsig. Berkeley, CA: University of California Press, pp. 243–286.

Johnson, L.M. and Gay, V.L. (1981). Luteinizing hormone in the cat. 11. Mating-induced secretion. *Endocrinology*, 109, 247–252.

Johnson, R.D. and Halata, Z. (1991). Topography and ultrastructure of sensory nerve endings in the glans penis of the rat. *Journal of Comparative Neurology*, 312, 299–310.

Johnson, R.D., Kitchell, R.I. and Gilanpour, H. (1986). Rapidly and slowly adapting mechano-receptors in the glans penis of the cat. *Physiology and Behavior*, 37, 69–78.

Johnston, S.D., O'Callaghan, P., McGowan, M.R. and Phillips, N.J. (1997). Characteristics of koala (*Phascolarctos cinereus adustus*) semen collected by artificial vagina. *Journal of Reproduction and Fertility*, 109, 319–323.

Johnston, S.D., McGowan, M.R., O'Callahan, P., Cox, R. and Nicolson, V. (2000a). Studies of the oestrous cycle, oestrus and pregnancy in the koala (*Phascolarctos cinereus*). *Journal of Reproduction and Fertility*, 120, 49–57.

Johnston, S.D., McGowan, M.R., O'Callahan, P., Cox, R. and Nicolson, V. (2000b). Natural and artificial methods for inducing the luteal phase in the koala (*Phascolarctos cinereus*). *Journal of Reproduction and Fertility*, 120, 59–64.

Johnston, S.D., O'Callaghan, P., Nilsson, K., Tzipori, G. and Curlewis, J.D. (2004). Semen-induced luteal phase and identification of a LH surge in the koala (*Phascolarctos cinereus*). *Reproduction*, 128, 629–634.

Johnston, S.D., Smith, B., Pyne, M., Stenzel, D. and Holt, W.V. (2007). One-sided ejaculation of echidna sperm bundles. *American Naturalist*, 170, E162.

Jones, E.F., Bain, J.B. and Odell, W.D. (1976). Postcoital luteinizing hormone release in male and female rabbits as determined by radioimmunoassay. *Fertility and Sterility*, 27, 848–852.

Jones, G. and Barratt, E.M. (1999). *Vespertilio pipistrellus* Schreber, 1774 and *V. pygmaeus* Leach, 1825 (currently *Pipistrellus pipistrellus* and *P. pygmaeus*; Mammalia, Chiroptera): proposed designation of neotypes. *Bulletin of Zoological Nomenclature*, 56, 182–186.

Jones, M. (1995). Tasmanian devil, *Sarcophilus harissii*. In *Mammals of Australia*, ed. R. Strahan. Washington, DC: Smithsonian Institution Press, pp. 82–84.

Jones, R.C., Djakiew, D. and Dacheux, J. (2004). Adaptations of the short-beaked echidna *Tachyglossus aculateus* for sperm production, particularly in an arid environment. *Australian Mammalogy*, 26, 199–204.

Joshi, A.R., Smith, J.L.D. and Garshelis, D.L. (1999). Sociobiology of the myrmecophagous sloth bear in Nepal. *Canadian Journal of Zoology*, 77, 1690–1704.

Joubert, S.C.J. (1975). The mating behaviour of the tsessebe (*Damaliscus lunatus lunatus*) in the Kruger National Park. *Zeitschrift für Tierpsychologie*, 37, 182–191.

Kano, T. (1992). *The Last Ape: Pygmy Chimpanzee Behavior and Ecology*. Stanford, CA: Stanford University Press.

Kappeler, P.M. (1997). Intrasexual selection and testis size in strepsirhine primates. *Behavioral Ecology*, 8, 10–19.

Katila, T. (2012). Post-mating inflammatory responses of the uterus. *Reproduction in Domestic Animals*, 47(Supplement 5), 31–41.

Katz, D.F., Slade, D.A. and Nakajima, S.T. (1997). Analysis of preovulatory changes in cervical mucus hydration and sperm penetrability. *Advances in Contraception*, 13, 143–151.

Kauffman, A.S. and Rissman, E.F. (2006). Neuroendocrine control of mating-induced ovulation. In *Knobil and Neill's Physiology of Reproduction, Vol. 2*. Second edn, ed. J.D. Neill. New York: Elsevier: Academic Press, pp. 2283–2326.

Kaufman, J.H. (1965). Studies on the behavior of captive treeshrews (*Tupaia glis*). *Folia Primatologica*, 3, 50–74.

Kays, R.W. and Gittleman, J.L. (2001). The social organization of the kinkajou *Potos flavus* (Procyonidae). *Journal of Zoology, London*, 253, 491–504.

Keeley, A.T.H. and Keeley, B.W. (2004). The mating season of *Tadarida brasiliensis* (Chiroptera: Molossidae) in a large highway bridge colony. *Journal of Mammalogy*, 85(1), 113–119.

Keener, W., Webber, M.A., Szczepaniak, I.D., Markowitz, T.M. and Orbach, D.N. (2018). The sex life of harbor porpoises (*Phocoena phocoena*): lateralized and aerial behavior. *Aquatic Mammals*, 44(6), 620–632.

Kelly, D.A. (2000). Anatomy of the baculum-corpus cavernosum interface in the Norway rat (*Rattus norvegicus*) and implications for force transfer during copulation. *Journal of Morphology*, 244, 69–77.

Kemp, T.S. (2005). *The Origin and Evolution of Mammals*. Oxford: Oxford University Press.

Kenagy, G.J. and Trombulak, S.C. (1986). Size and function of mammalian testes in relation to body size. *Journal of Mammalogy*, 67, 1–22.

Kenney, A.M., Hartung, T.G. and Dewsbury, D.A. (1979). Copulatory behavior and the initiation of pregnancy in California voles (*Microtus californicus*). *Brain Behavior and Evolution*, 16, 176–191.

Kenyon, K.W. (1969). The sea otter in the eastern Pacific Ocean. *North American Fauna*, 68, 1–352.

Kershaw-Young, C.M., Druart, X., Vaughan, J. and Maxwell, W.M.C. (2012). β-Nerve growth factor is a major component of alpaca seminal plasma and induces ovulation in female alpacas. *Reproduction, Fertility and Development*, http://dx.doi.org/10.1071/RD12039.

Kierdorf, U.V. (1996). Verheilte baculum-fraktur bei einem Iltis (*Mustela putorius*). *Zeitschrift für Jagdwissenschaft*, 42, 308–310.

Kihara, K., Sato, K., Ando, M., Azuma, H. and Oshima, H. (1995). Antegrade and retrograde fluid transport through the vas deferens. *American Journal of Physiology*, 38, R1197–R1203.

Kiley-Worthington, M. (1978). The causation, evolution and function of the visual displays of the eland. *Behaviour*, 66, 179–222.

Kim, E., Yamashita, M., Kimura, M., Honda, A., Kashiwabara, S.-I. (2008). Sperm penetration through the cumulus mass and zona pellucida. *International Journal of Developmental Biology*, 52, 677–682.

King, C. (1989). *The Natural History of Weasels and Stoats*. London: Christopher Helm.

Kingdon, J. and Hoffmann, M., eds. (2013a). *Mammals of Africa, Vol. VI. Pigs, Hippopotamuses, Chevrotain, Giraffes, Deer and Bovids*. London: Bloomsbury Press.

Kingdon, J. and Hoffmann, M., eds. (2013b). *Mammals of Africa, Vol. V. Carnivores, Pangolins, Equids, and Rhinoceroses*. London: Bloomsbury Press.

Kinsey, A.C., Pomeroy, W.B. and Martin, C.E. (1948). *Sexual Behavior in the Human Male*. Philadelphia, PA: W.B. Saunders.

Kitchen, D.W. (1974). Social behavior and ecology of the pronghorn. *Wildlife Monographs*, No. 38, 3–96.

Kleiman, D.G. (1968). Reproduction in the Canidae. *International Zoo Yearbook*, 8, 1–8.

Kleiman, D.G. (1971). The courtship and copulatory behaviour of the green acouchi, *Myoprocta pratti*. *Zeitschrift für Tierpsychologie*, 29, 259–278.

Kleiman, D.G. (1974). Patterns of behaviour in hystricomorph rodents. In *The Biology of Hystricomorph Rodents*, eds. I.W. Rowlands and B.J. Weir. Symposia of the Zoological Society of London, 34, 171–209.

Kleiman, D.G. (1977). Monogamy in mammals. *The Quarterly Review of Biology*, 52(1), 39–69.

Kleiman, D.G. and Racey, P.A. (1969). Observations on noctule bats (*Nyctalus noctula*) breeding in captivity. *Lynx*, 10, 65–77.

Kleisener, K., Ivell, R. and Flegr, J. (2010). The evolutionary history of testicular external-ization and the origin of the scrotum. *Journal of Biosciences*, 35(1), 27–37.

Knight, T.W., Gherardi, S. and Lindsay, D.R. (1987). Effects of sexual stimulation on testicular size in the ram. *Animal Reproduction Science*, 13, 105–115.

Knörnschild, M., Feifel, M. and Kalko, E.K.V. (2014). Male courtship displays and vocal communication in the polygynous bat *Carollia perspicillata*. *Behaviour*, 151, 781–798.

Koehler, C.E. and Richardson, P.R.K. (1990). *Proteles cristatus*. *Mammalian Species*, No. 363, 1–6.

Köhler, D. (2012). On reproductive and breeding behaviour of the European water shrew *Neomys fodiens* (Soricidae). *Der Zoologische Garten*, 81, 113–125.

Koilraj, J.A., Agoramoothy, G. and Marimuthu, G. (2001). Copulatory behavior of the Indian flying fox *Pteropus giganteus*. *Current Science*, 80, 15–16.

Komisaruk, B.R. (2016). Commentary on 'The evolutionary origin of female orgasm' by M. Pavlicev and G. Wagner. *Journal of Experimental Zoology Part B: Molecular and Developmental Evolution*, 326, 504–506.

Komisaruk, B.R. and Sansone, G. (2003). Neural pathways mediating vaginal friction: the vagus nerves and spinal cord oxytocin. *Scandinavian Journal of Psychology*, 44, 241–250.

Koretsky, I.A., Barnes, L.G. and Rahmat, S.J. (2016). Re-evaluation of morphological characters questions current views of pinniped origins. *Vestnik Zoologii*, 50(4), 327–354.

Koyama, N. (1988). Mating behavior of ring-tailed lemurs (*Lemur catta*) at Berenty, Madagascar. *Primates*, 29, 163–175.

Kozlowski, J. and Stearns, S.C. (1989). Hypotheses for the production of excess zygotes: models of bet-hedging and selective abortion. *Evolution*, 43(7), 1369–1377.

Kraaijeveld-Smit, F.J.L., Ward, S.J. and Temple-Smith, P.D. (2002). Multiple paternity in a field population of a small carnivorous marsupial, the agile antechinus, *Antechinus agilis*. *Behavioral Ecology and Sociobiology*, 52, 84–91.

Kraus, S.D., Pace, R.M. and Fraser, T.R. (2007). High investment, low return: The strange case of reproduction in *Eubalaena glacialis*. In *The Urban Whale: North Atlantic Right Whales at the Crossroads*, eds. S.D. Kraus and R.M. Rolland. Cambridge, MA: Harvard University Press.

Kruuk, H. (1972). *The Spotted Hyena: A study of Predation and Social Behavior*. Chicago: University of Chicago Press.

Kuchling, G. (2015). Ultrasound scanning as an effective tool in the conservation of chelonians. *International Zoo Yearbook*, 49, 22–30.

Kummer, H. (1984). From laboratory to desert and back: a social system of hamadryas baboons. *Animal Behaviour*, 32, 965–971.

Kummer, H. (1990). The social system of hamadryas baboons and its presumable evolution. In *Baboons: Behavior and Ecology, Use and Care*, eds. M.T. de Melo, A. Whitten and R.W. Byrne. Brasil: Brasilia, pp. 43–60.

Lagunes-Córdoba, R., Tsutsumi, V. and Muñoz-Matínez, E.J. (2009). Structure, innervation, mechanical properties and reflex activation of a striated sphincter in the vestibule of the cat vagina. *Reproduction*, 137, 371–377.

Laidler, L. (1982). *Otters in Britain*. London: David and Charles.

Langendijk, P., Soede, N.M. and Kemp, B. (2005). Uterine activity, sperm transport, and the role of boar stimuli around insemination in sows. *Theriogenology*, 63, 500–513.

Langtimm, C.A. and Dewsbury, D.A. (1991). Phylogeny and evolution of rodent copulatory behaviour. *Animal Behaviour*, 41, 217–225.

Lanier, D.L. and Dewsbury, D.A. (1976). A quantitative study of copulatory behaviour of large Felidae. *Behavioural Processes*, 1(4), 327–333.

Larivière, S. (1998). *Lontra felina. Mammalian Species*, No. 575, 1–5.

Larivière, S. and Ferguson, S. H. (2002). On the evolution of the mammalian baculum: vaginal friction, prolonged intromission or induced ovulation? *Mammal Review*, 32, 283–294.

Larsson, K. (1956). *Conditioning and Sexual Behavior in the Male Albino Rat*. Stockholm: Almqvist and Wiksell.

Larsson, K. (1979). Features of the neuroendocrine regulation of masculine sexual behavior. In *Endocrine Control of Sexual Behavior*, ed. C. Beyer. New York: Raven Press, pp. 77–163.

Laurie, A. (1982). Behavioural ecology of the greater one-horned rhinoceros (*Rhinoceros unicornis*). *Journal of Zoology, London*, 196, 307–341.

Lawick, H. van and Lawick-Goodall, J. van (1971). *Innocent Killers*. London: Collins.

Lawler, D.F., Johnston, S.D., Hegstad, R.L., Keltner, D.G. and Owens, S.F. (1993). Ovulation without cervical stimulation in domestic cats. *Journal of Reproduction and Fertility, Supplement*, 47, 57–61.

Laws, R.M. (1956). The elephant seal (*Mirounga leonina* Linn.). 111. The physiology of reproduction. Falkland Islands Dependencies Survey. *Scientific Reports*, 15, 1–66.

Layne, J.N. and Caldwell, D.K. (1964). Behavior of the Amazon dolphin, *Inia geoffrensis* (Blainville), in captivity. *Zoologica*, 49(5), 81–107.

Le Boeuf, B.J. (1972). Sexual behavior in the northern elephant seal *Mirounga angustirostris*. *Behaviour*, 41(1–2), 1–26.

Lechleitner, R.R. (1958). Certain aspects of behavior of the black-tailed jackrabbit. *The American Midland Naturalist*, 60(1), 145–155.

Lee, A.K. and Cockburn, A. (1985). *Evolutionary Ecology of Marsupials*. Cambridge: Cambridge University Press.

Lehmann, T., Vignaud, P., Likius, A. and Brunet, M. (2005). A new species of Orycteropodidae (Mammalia, Tubilidentata) in the Mio–Pliocene of northern Chad. *Biological Journal of the Linnean Society*, 143, 109–131.

Leiner, N.O., Setz, E.Z.F. and Silva, W.R. (2008). Semelparity and factors affecting the reproductive activity of the Brazilian slender opossum (*Marmosops paulensis*) in south-eastern Brazil. *Journal of Mammalogy*, 89(1), 153–158.

Lemmon, W.B. and Oakes, E. (1967). Tieing between stumptailed macaques during mating. *Laboratory Primate Newsletter*, 6, 14–15.

Leonard, J.L. (2010). Celebrating and understanding reproductive diversity. In *The Evolution of Primary Sexual Characters in Animals*, eds. J.L. Leonard and A. Córdoba-Aguilar. New York: Oxford University Press, pp. 1–5.

Leone, E. (1954). Ergothioneine in the equine ampullar secretion. *Nature*, 174, 404–405.

Leonhard-Marek, S. (2000). Why do trace elements have an influence on fertility? *Tierarzliche Praxis Ausgabe Grobtiere Nutztiere*, 28, 60–65.

Leslie, D.M. and Schaller, G.B. (2009). *Bos grunniens* and *Bos mutus* (Artiodactyla: Bovidae). *Mammalian Species*, No. 836, 1–17.

Levin, R.J. (2020). The clitoris: an appraisal of its reproductive function during the fertile years. *Clinical Anatomy*, 33(1), 136–145.

Li, B. and Zhao, D. (2007). Copulation behavior within one-male groups of *Rhinopithecus roxellana* in the Qinling mountains of China. *Primates*, 48, 190–196.

Liers, E.E. (1951). Notes on the river otter (*Lutra canadensis*). *Journal of Mammalogy*, 32(1), 1–9.

Lin, T.-T., You, E.-M. and Lin, Y.K. (2009). Social and genetic mating systems of the Asian lesser white-toothed shrew, *Crocidura shantungensis*, in Taiwan. *Journal of Mammalogy*, 90 (6), 1370–1380.

Lindsay, D.R. and Fletcher, I.C. (1972). Ram seeking activity associated with oestrous behaviour in ewes. *Animal Behaviour*, 20, 452–456.

Lippert, W. (1973). On the breeding behavior of the maned wolf *Chrysocyon brachyurus*, Illiger. *Der Zoologische Garten*, 43, 225–247.

Liu, D., Ng, M.L., Zhou, L.P. and Haeberle, E.J. (1997). *Sexual Behavior in Modern China*. New York: Continuum Publishing Company.

Lloyd, E.A. (2005). *The Case of the Female Orgasm: Bias in the Science of Evolution*. Cambridge, MA: Harvard University Press.

Londoño, G.C. and Muñaz, N.T. (2006). Reproduction, behaviour and biology of the giant river otter *Pteronura brasiliensis* at Cali Zoo. *International Zoo Yearbook*, 40, 360–371.

Long, C.A. and Frank, T. (1968). Morphometric variation and function in the baculum, with comments on correlation of parts. *Journal of Mammalogy*, 49, 32–43.

Long, K.I. (2001). Spatio-temporal interactions among male and female long-nosed poteroos, *Potorous tridactylus* (Marsupialia: Macropodoidea); mating system implications. *Australian Journal of Zoology*, 49(1), 17–26.

Loughry, W.J. and McDonough, C.M. (2013). *The Nine-Banded Armadillo: A Natural History*. Norman, OK: University of Oklahoma Press.

Loughry, W.J., Prodöhl, P.A., McDonough, C.M. and Avise, J.C. (1998). Polyembryony in armadillos: an unusual feature of the female nine-banded armadillo's reproductive tract may explain why her litters consist of four genetically identical offspring. *American Scientist*, 86 (3), 274–279.

Lovecky, D.V., Estep, D.Q. and Dewsbury, D.A. (1979). Copulatory behaviour of cotton mice (*Peromyscus gossipinus*) and their reciprocal hybrids with white-footed mice (*P. leucopus*). *Animal Behaviour*, 27, 371–375.

Ludlow, J.C. (1976). Observations on the breeding of captive black bears, *Ursus americanus*. In *Bears: Their Biology and Management, Vol. 3*. IUCN Publications, New Series, 40, 65–69.

Luhrs, M.-L. and Kappeler, P.M. (2014). Polyandrous mating in treetops: how male competition and female choice interact to determine an unusual carnivore mating system. *Behavioral Ecology and Sociobiology*, 68, 879–889.

Lumpkin, S. and Koontz, F.W. (1986). Social and sexual behavior of the rufous elephant-shrew (*Elephantulus rufescens*). *Journal of Mammalogy*, 67(1), 112–119.

Luo, Z.-X., Ji, Q., Wible, J.R. and Yuan, C.-X. (2003). An early Cretaceous tribosphenic mammal and metatherian evolution. *Science*, 302, 1934–1940.

Luo, Z.-X., Yuan, C.X., Meng, Q.J. and Ji, Q. (2011). A Jurassic eutherian mammal and divergence of marsupials and placentals. *Nature*, 476(7361), 442–445.

Lüpold, S. and Fitzpatrick, J.L. (2015). Sperm number trumps sperm size in mammalian ejaculate evolution. *Proceedings of the Royal Society of London, B*, 282, 20152122.

Lüpold, S., Linz, G.M., Rivers, J.W., Westneat, D.F. and Birkhead, T.R. (2009). Sperm competition selects beyond relative testes size in birds. *Evolution*, 63(2), 391–402.

MacFadden, B.J. (2005). Fossil horses – evidence for evolution. *Science*, 307, 1728–1730.

Macleod, C.D. and D'Amico, A. (2006). A review of beaked whale behaviour in relation to assessing and mitigating impacts of anthropogenic noise. *Cetacean Research and Management*, 7(3), 211–221.

Magallanes, I., Parham, J.F., Santos, G-P. and Velez-Juarbe, J. (2018). A new tuskless walrus from the Miocene of Orange County, California, with comments on the diversity and taxonomy of odobenids. *Peer J*, 6, e5708.

Magoun, A.J. and Volkenburg, P. (1983). Breeding behavior of free ranging wolverines (*Gulo gulo*). *Acta Zoologica Fennica*, 174, 175–177.

Mahla, A.S., Vyas, S., Kumar, H., Singh, G., Das, G.K., *et al.* (2015). Studies on sexual behaviour in female dromedary camels (*Camelus dromedarius*). *Journal of Camel Practice and Research*, 22(1), 145–149.

Maliniak, E. and Eisenberg, J.F. (1971). The breeding of *Proechimys semispinosus* in captivity. *International Zoo Yearbook*, 11, 93–98.

Malo, A.F., Gomendio, M., Garde, J., Lang-Lenton, B., Soler, A.J., *et al.* (2006). Sperm design and sperm function. *Biology Letters*, 2, 246–249.

Manire, C.A., Byrd, L., Therrien, C.L. and Martin, K. (2008). Mating-induced ovulation in loggerhead sea turtles, *Caretta caretta*. *Zoo Biology*, 27, 213–225.

Mann, K.H. (1962). *Leeches (Hirudinea): Their Structure, Physiology, Ecology, and Embryology*. New York: Pergamon Press.

Mann, T. and Lutwak-Mann, C. (1951). Secretory function of male accessory organs of reproduction in mammals. *Physiological Reviews*, 31, 27–55.

Mann, T. and Lutwak-Mann, C. (1981). *Male Reproductive Function and Semen: Themes and Trends in Physiology, Biochemistry, and Investigative Andrology*. Berlin: Springer-Verlag.

Manno, T.G., DeBarbieri, L.M. and Davidson, J. (2008). Why do Columbian ground squirrels copulate underground? *Journal of Mammalogy*, 89(4), 828–888.

Manson, J.H. (1992). Measuring female mate choice in Cayo Santiago rhesus macaques. *Animal Behaviour*, 44, 405–416.

Maranesi, M., Zerani, M., Leonardi, L., Pistilli, A., Arruda-Alencar, A.M., *et al.* (2015). Gene expression and localization of NGF and its cognate receptors NTRK1 and NGFR in the sex organs of male rabbits. *Reproduction in Domestic Animals*, 50, 918–925.

Mariappa, D. (1986). *Anatomy and Histology of the Indian Elephant*. Oak Park, MI: Indira Publishing House, pp. 119–125.

Marks, C.A. (1998). Courtship and mating in a pair of free-ranging common wombats, *Vombatus ursinus*. In *Wombats*, eds. R.T. Wells and P.A. Pridmore. Chipping Norton: Surrey Beatty and Sons, pp. 125–128.

Markus, N. (2002). Behaviour of the black flying fox *Pteropus alecto*: 2. Territoriality and courtship. *Acta Chiropterologica*, 4(2), 153–160.

Marlow, B.J. (1961). Reproductive behaviour of the marsupial mouse, *Antechinus flavipes* (Waterhouse) (Marsupialia) and the development of the pouch young. *Australian Journal of Zoology*, 9, 203–217.

Marlow, B.J. (1967). Mating behaviour in the leopard seal, *Hydrurga leptonix* (Mammalia: Phocidae), in captivity. *Australian Journal of Zoology*, 15, 1–5.

Marsh, H. (1980). Age determination of the dugong (*Dugong dugon* (Miller)) and its biological implications. *International Whaling Commission Report* (Special Issue 3), 181–201.

Marsh, H., Heinsohn, G.E. and Marsh, L.M. (1984). Breeding cycle, life history and population dynamics of the dugong, *Dugong dugon* (Sirenia: Dugongidae). *Australian Journal of Zoology*, 32, 767–788.

Marson, J., Gervais, D., Cooper, R.W. and Jouannet, P. (1989). Influence of ejaculation frequency on semen characteristics in chimpanzees (*Pan troglodytes*). *Journal of Reproduction and Fertility*, 85, 43–50.

Martan, J. and Hruban, Z. (1970). Unusual spermatozoa formations in the epididymis of the flying squirrel (*Glaucomys volans*). *Journal of Reproduction and Fertility*, 21, 167–170.

Martan, J. and Shepherd, B.A. (1973). Spermatozoa in rouleaux in the female guinea pig genital tract. *Anatomical Record*, 175, 626–630.

Martan, J. and Shepherd, B.A. (1976). The role of copulatory plugs in reproduction in the guinea pig. *Journal of Experimental Zoology*, 196, 79–83.

Martin, G.B., Oldham, C.M. and Lindsay, D.R. (1980). Increased plasma LH levels in seasonally anovular merino ewes following the introduction of rams. *Animal Reproductive Science*, 3, 125–132.

Martin, R. and Handasyde, K. (1999). *The Koala: Natural History, Conservation and Management*. Second edn. Sydney: University of New South Wales Press.

Martin, R.D. (1990). *Primate Origins and Evolution: A Phylogenetic Reconstruction*. London: Chapman and Hall.

Martin, R.D. (1995). Phylogenetic aspects of primate reproduction: the context of advanced maternal care. In *Motherhood in Human and Non-Human Primates*, eds. C.R. Pryce, R.D. Martin and D. Skuse. Basel: Karger, pp. 16–26.

Martin, R.D. (2013). *How We Do It: The Evolution and Future of Human Reproduction*. New York: Basic Books.

Martinet, L. and Raynaud, F. (1972). Méchanisme possible de la superfetation chez la hase. *Compte Rendus de L'Académie des Sciences Paris*, 274, 2683–2686.

Martinet, L. and Raynaud, F. (1975). Prolonged spermatozoa survival in the female hare uterus: explanation of superfetation. In *The Biology of Spermatozoa: Transport Survival and Fertilizing Capacity*, eds. E.S.E. Hafez and G.G. Thibault. Basel: Karger, pp. 134–144.

Martinez, A.C., Oliveira, F.S., Abreu, C.O., Martins, L.L., Pauloni, A.P., *et al.* (2013). Colheita de sêmen por eletroejaculação em cutia-parda (*Dasyprocta azarae*). *Pesquiza Veterinária Brasileira*, 33(1), 86–88.

Masters, W.H. and Johnson, V.E. (1966). *Human Sexual Response*. London: Churchill Ltd.

Mate, B., Duley, P., Lagerquist, B., Wenzel, F., Stimpert, A., *et al.* (2005). Observations of a female North Atlantic right whale (*Eubalaena glacialis*) in simultaneous copulation with two males: supporting evidence for sperm competition. *Aquatic Mammals*, 31(2), 157–160.

Matlaga, D. (2006). Mating behavior of the northern tamandua (*Tamandua mexicana*) in Costa Rica. *Edentata*, 7, 46–48.

Matsuzaki, O. (2002). The force driving mating behavior in the house musk shrew (*Suncus murinus*). *Zoological Science*, 19(8), 851–869.

Matthews, L.H. (1935). The oestrous cycle and intersexuality in the female mole (*Talpa europaea* Linn.). *Proceedings of the Zoological Society of London, Series 2*, 347–383.

Matthews, L.H. (1939). Reproduction of the spotted hyaena (*Crocuta crocuta* Erxleben). *Philosophical Transactions of the Royal Society of London, B*, 230, 1–78.

Matthews, L.H. (1942). Notes on the genitalia and reproduction of some African bats. *Proceedings of the Zoological Society of London, B*, 111, 289–346.

Matthews, M. and Adler, N.T. (1977). Facilitative and inhibitory influences of reproductive behavior on sperm transport in rats. *Journal of Comparative and Physiological Psychology*, 91(4), 727–741.

Maust-Mohl, M., Soltis, J. and Reiss, D. (2018). Underwater click train production by the hippopotamus (*Hippopotamus amphibius*) suggests an echo-ranging function. *Behaviour*, 155(2–3), 231–251.

Mayr, E. (1963). *Animal Species and Evolution*. Cambridge, MA: Belknap Press.

McCarley, H. (1966). Annual cycle, population dynamics and adaptive behavior of *Citellus tridecemlineatus*. *Journal of Mammalogy*,47, 294–316.

McClintock, M.K. (1984). Group mating in the domestic rat as a context for sexual selection: consequences for the analysis of sexual behavior and neuroendocrine responses. *Advances in the Study of Behavior*, 14, 1–50.

McClintock, M.K. and Adler, N.T. (1978). The role of the female during copulation in wild and domestic Norway rats (*Rattus norvegicus*). *Behaviour*, 67(1–2), 67–96.

McCloskey, R.J. and Shaw, K.C (1977). Copulatory behavior of the fox squirrel. *Journal of Mammalogy*, 58, 663–665.

McComb, K. (1987). Roaring by red deer stags advances the date of oestrus in hinds. *Nature*, 330, 648–649.

McCreight, J.C., DeWoody, J.A. and Waser, P.M. (2011). DNA from copulatory plugs can give insights into sexual selection. *Journal of Zoology, London*, 284, 300–304.

McDonough, C. M. (1997). Pairing behavior of the nine-banded armadillo (*Dasypus novem-cinctus*). *The American Midland Naturalist*, 138, 290–298.

McDonough, C.M. (2000). Social organization of nine-banded armadillos. *The American Midland Naturalist*, 144, 139–151.

McIlroy, J.C. (1995). Common wombat, *Vombatus ursinus*. In *Mammals of Australia*, ed. R. Strahan. Washington, DC: Smithsonian Institution Press, pp. 204–205.

McIlroy, J .C. (1976). Aspects of the ecology of the common wombat, 1. Capture, handling, marking and radio-tracking techniques. *Australian Wildlife Research*, 3, 105–116.

McKenna, A. (2005). Husbandry and breeding of the striped possum, *Dactylopsila trivirgata*, at London ZSL. *International Zoo Yearbook*, 39, 169–176.

McLean, I.G. and Schmitt, N.T. (1999). Copulation and associated behaviour in the quokka, *Setonix brachyurus*. *Australian Mammalogy*, 21, 139–142.

McNeilly, A.S. and Folley, S.J. (1970). Blood levels of milk ejection activity (oxytocin) in the female goat during mating. *Journal of Endocrinology*, 48, ix–x.

McPherson, F.J., Nielsen S.G. and Chenoweth, P.J. (2014). Semen effects on insemination outcomes in sows. *Animal Reproduction Science*, 151, 28–33.

Meek, A. (1918). The reproductive organs of Cetacea. *Journal of Anatomy*, 52, 186–210.

Mellen, J.D. (1993). Comparative analysis of scent-marking, social and reproductive behavior in 20 species of small cats (*Felis*). *American Zoologist*, 33(2), 151–166.

Mendonça, M.T. and Crews, D. (1989). Effect of fall mating on ovarian development in the red-sided garter snake. *American Journal of Physiology*, 237, R1548–1550.

Mendonça, M.T., Chernetsky, S.D., Nester, K.E. and Gardner, G.L. (1996). Effects of gonadal steroids on sexual behavior in the big brown bat, *Eptesicus fuscus*, upon arousal from hibernation. *Hormones and Behavior*, 30, 153–161.

Michener, G.R. (1969). Notes on the breeding and young of the crest-tailed marsupial mouse, *Dasycercus cristicauda*. *Journal of Mammalogy*, 50(3), 633–635.

Miller, E.A., Beasely, D.E., Dunn, R.R. and Archie E.A. (2016). Lactobacilli dominance and vaginal pH: why is the human vaginal biome unique? *Frontiers in Microbiology*, 7, doi: 10.3389/fmicb.2016.01936.

Miller, E.H. (2010). Genitalic traits of mammals. In *The Evolution of Primary Sexual Characters in Animals*, eds. J.L. Leonard and A. Córdoba-Aguilar. New York: Oxford University Press, pp. 471–493.

Miller, E.J., Eldridge, M.D.B. and Herbert, C.A. (2010a). Dominance and paternity in the tammar wallaby. In *Macropods: The Biology of Kangaroos, Wallabies and Rat-*

Kangaroos, eds. G. Coulson and M. Eldridge. Collingwood: CSIRO Publishing, pp. 77–86.

Miller, E.J., Eldridge, M.D.B., Thomas, N., Marlow, N. and Herbert, C.A. (2010b). The genetic mating system, male reproductive success and lack of selection on male traits in the greater bilby. *Australian Journal of Zoology*, 58, 113–120.

Milligan, S.R. (1975). The copulatory behavior of *Microtus agrestis*. *Journal of Mammalogy*, 56, 220–224.

Milligan, S.R. (1979). The copulatory pattern of the bank vole (*Clethrionomys glareolus*) and speculation on the role of penile spines. *Journal of Zoology, London*, 188, 279–300.

Mills, M.G.L. (1983). Mating and denning behaviour of the brown hyaena *Hyaena brunnea* and comparisons with other Hyaenidae. *Zeitschrift für Tierpsychologie*, 63, 331–342.

Milton, K.M. (1985). Mating patterns of woolly spider monkeys, *Brachyteles arachnoides*: implications for female choice. *Behavioral Ecology and Sociobiology*, 17, 53–59.

Minchin, A.K. (1937). Notes on the weaning of a young koala (*Phasclarctos cinereus*). *Records of the South Australian Museum*, 6, 1–3.

Mitchell, K.J., Pratt, R.C., Watson, L.N., Gibb, G.C., Llamas, B., *et al.* (2014). Molecular phylogeny, biogeography, and habitat preference evolution of marsupials. *Molecular Biology and Evolution*, 31, 2322–2330. doi:10.1093/molbev/msu176

Miura, S. (1984). Social behavior and territoriality in sika deer (*Cervus nippon* Temminck 1838) during the rut. *Zeitschrift für Tierpsychologie*, 64, 33–73.

Miura, S., Kaji, K., Otaishi, N., Koizumi, T., Tokida, K., *et al.* (1993). Social organization and mating behavior of white-lipped deer in the Qinghai-Xizang plateau, China. In *Deer of China: Biology and Management*, eds. N. Otaishi and H.L. Sheng. Amsterdam: Elsevier Science Publishers, pp. 220–234.

Mobarak, A.M., El-Wishy, A.B. and Samira, M.F. (1972). The penis and prepuce of the one-humped camel (*Camelus dromedarius*). *Zentralblatt für Veterinärmedzin*, 19, 787–795.

Moehlman, P.D. (1974). Behavior and Ecology of Feral Asses (*Equus asinus*). PhD Thesis, University of Wisconsin, Madison.

Moghissi, K.S. (1984). The function of the cervix in human reproduction. *Current Problems in Obstetrics, Gynecology and Fertility*, 7, 1–57.

Møller, A.P. and Birkhead, T.R. (1989). Copulation behaviour in mammals: evidence that sperm competition is widespread. *Biological Journal of the Linnean Society*, 38, 119–131.

Mollineau, W., Adogwa, A., Jasper, N., Young. K. and Garcia, G. (2005). The gross anatomy of the male reproductive system of a neotropical rodent: the agouti (*Dasyprocta leporina*). *Anatomia, Histologia, Embryologia*, 35, 47–52.

Mollison, B.C. (1955). Copulation in the wild rabbit, *Oryctolagus cuniculus*. *Behaviour*, 8, 81–84.

Montgomerie, R. (2010). Sexual conflict and the intromittent organs of male birds. In *The Evolution of Primary Sexual Characters in Animals*, eds. J.L. Leonard and A. Córdoba-Aguilar. New York: Oxford University Press, pp. 453–470.

Montoto, L.G., Sanchez, M.V., Touremente, M., Martín-Coello, J., Luque-Larina, J.J., *et al.* (2011). Sperm competition differentially effects swimming velocity and size of spermatozoa from closely related muroid rodents: head first. *Reproduction*, 142, 819–830.

Moore, C.R. (1926). The biology of the mammalian testis and scrotum. *The Quarterly Review of Biology*, 1(1), 4–50.

Moore, H.D.M. and Taggart, D.A. (1995). Sperm pairing in the opossum increases the efficiency of sperm movement in a viscous environment. *Biology of Reproduction*, 52, 947–953.

Moore, H.D.M., Dvoráková, K., Jenkins, N. and Breed, W.G. (2002). Exceptional sperm cooperation in the wood mouse. *Nature*, 418, 174–177.

Morales, P., Overstreet, J.W. and Katz, D.F. (1988). Changes in human sperm motion during capacitation *in vitro*. *Journal of Reproduction and Fertility*, 83, 119–128.

Morales-Pineyrua, J.T. and Ungerfeld, R. (2012). Pamoas deer (*Ozotoceros bezoarticus*) courtship and mating behavior. *Acta Veterinaria Scandinavica*, 54, 60–65.

Morali, G. and Beyer, C. (1992). Motor aspects of masculine sexual behavior in rats and rabbits. *Advances in the Study of Behavior*, 21, 201–238.

Moran, S., Turner, P.D. and O'Reilly, C. (2009). Multiple paternity in the European hedgehog. *Journal of Zoology, London*, 278, 349–353.

Moreira, J.R., Clarke, J.R. and MacDonald, D.W. (1997). The testis of capybaras (*Hydrochoerus hydrocaeiris*). *Journal of Mammalogy*, 78(4), 1096–1100.

Mori, T., Oh, Y.K. and Uchida, T.A. (1982). Sperm storage in the oviduct of the Japanese greater horseshoe bat, *Rhinolophus ferrumequinum nippon*. *Journal of the Faculty of Agriculture Kyushu University*, 27, 47–53.

Morimoto, J., McDonald, G., Smith, E., Smith, D.T., Perry, J.C., *et al.* (2019). Sex peptide receptor-regulated polyandry modulates the balance of pre- and post-copulatory sexual selection in *Drosophila. Nature Communications*, 10, 283. https://doi.org/10.1038/s41467-018-08113-w.

Morin, P.A., Baker, C.S., Brewer, R.S., Burdin, A.M., Dalebout, M.L., *et al.* (2017). Genetic structure of the beaked whale genus *Berardius* in the North Pacific, with genetic evidence for a new species. *Marine Mammal Science*, 33, 96–111. DOI: 10.1111/mms.12345

Morris, D.J. and Van Aarde, R.J. (1985). Sexual behavior of the female porcupine *Hystrix africaeaustralis*. *Hormones and Behavior*, 19, 400–412.

Morrow, G. and Nicol, S.C. (2009). Cool sex? Hibernation and reproduction overlap in the echidna. *PLoS ONE*, 4, e6070.

Moss, C.J. (1983). Estrous behaviour and female choice in the African elephant. *Behaviour*, 86, 167–196.

Moss, C.J. (1988). *Elephant Memories: Thirteen Years in the Life of an Elephant Family*. New York: W. Morrow.

Mossman, J., Slate, J., Humphries, S. and Birkhead, T. (2008). Sperm morphology and velocity are genetically codetermined in the zebra finch. *Evolution*, 63(10), 2730–2737.

Muizon, C. de and Cifelli, R.L. (2001). A new basal 'didelphoid' (Marsupialia, Mammalia) from the early Paleocene of Tiupampa (Bolivia). *Journal of Vertebrate Paleontology*, 21(1), 87–97.

Mullins, K.J. and Saacke, R.J. (1989). Study of the functional anatomy of bovine cervical mucosa with special reference to mucus secretion and sperm transport. *The Anatomical Record*, 225, 106–117.

Mundy, K.R.D. and Flook, D.R. (1964). Notes on the mating activity of grizzly and black bears. *Journal of Mammalogy*, 45(4), 637–638.

Munoz-Romo, M. and Kunz, T.H. (2009). Dorsal patch and chemical signalling of males of the long-nosed bat, *Leptonycteris curasoae* (Chiroptera: Phyllostomidae). *Journal of Mammalogy*, 90, 1139–1147.

Munshi-South, J. (2007). Extra-pair paternity and evolution of testis size in a behaviorally monogamous tropical mammal, the large treeshrew (*Tupaia tana*). *Behavioral Ecology and Sociobiology*, 62(2), 201–212.

Murali, K.C., Ramachandran, S. and Mutthulingam, P. (2012). An observation of Indian grey mongoose *Herpestes edwardsii* mating. *Small Carnivore Conservation*, 47, 75–76.

Murie, J.O. (1995). Mating behavior of Columbian ground squirrels. 1. Multiple mating by females and multiple paternity. *Canadian Journal of Zoology*, 73, 1819–1826.

Murphy, W.J., Elzirik, E., Johnson, W.E., Zhang, Y.P. Ryder, O.A., *et al.* (2001). Molecular phylogenetics and the origins of placental mammals. *Nature*, 409, 614–618.

Myers, K. and Poole, W.E. (1962). A study of the biology of the wild rabbit, *Oryctolagus cuniculus* (L.), in confined populations. III. Reproduction. *Australian Journal of Zoology*, 10, 225–267.

Myslenkov, A.I. and Voloshina, I.V. (1998). Sexual behaviour of the Amur goral. In *Proceedings of the Second World Conference on Mountain Ungulates*, pp. 75–80.

Nadler, R.D. (1988). Sexual and reproductive behavior. In *Orang-Utan Biology*, ed. J.H. Schwartz. New York: Oxford University Press, pp. 105–116.

Nakamura, F., Suzuki, Y. and Yoshimura, F. (1986). A quantitative immunohistochemical study on the pituitary LH gonadotrophs in the female Afghan pika after copulation. *Endocrinologia Japonica*, 33(1), 1–9.

Napier, J.R. and Napier, P.H. (1967). *A Handbook of Living Primates: Morphology, Ecology and Behaviour of Nonhuman Primates*. London: Academic Press.

Nater, A., Mattle-Greminger, M., Nurcahyo, A., Nowak, M.G., de Manuel, M., *et al.* (2017). Morphometric, behavioral, and genomic evidence for a new orangutan species. *Current Biology*, 27, 3487–3498.

Neal, E. (1986). *The Natural History of Badgers*. London: Croom Helm.

Nekaris, K.A.I. (2003). Observations on mating, birthing and parental care in three subspecies of slender loris in India and Sri Lanka (*Loris tardigradus* and *Loris lydekkerianus*). *Folia Primatologica*, 74(supplement), 312–336.

Nevo, E. (1969). Mole rats *Spalax ehrenbergi*: mating behaviour and its evolutionary significance. *Science*, 163, 484–486.

Nickel, R., Schummer, A., Seiferle, E. and Sack, W.O., eds. (1979). *The Viscera of Domestic Animals*. Berlin: Verlag Paul Parey, pp. 282–392.

Nicoll, M.E. and Racey, P.A. (1985). Follicular development, ovulation, fertilization and fetal development in tenrecs (*Tenrec ecaudatus*). *Journal of Reproduction and Fertility*, 74, 47–55.

Nielsen, C.L.R. and Nielsen, C.K. (2007). Multiple paternity and relatedness in southern Illinois raccoons (*Procyon lotor*). *Journal of Mammalogy*, 88(2), 441–447.

Nikaido, M., Rooney, A.P. and Okada, N. (1999). Phylogenetic relationships among cetartiodactyls based on insertions of short and long interspersed elements: hippopotamuses are the closest extant relatives of whales. *Proceedings of the National Academy of Sciences USA*, 96, 10261–10266.

Nogueira, J.C., Martinelli, P.M., Costa, S.F., Carvalho, G.A. and Câmara, B.G.O. (1999). The penis morphology of *Didelphis*, *Lutreolina*, *Metachirus* and *Caluromys* (Marsupialia, Didelphidae). *Mammalia*, 63(1), 79–92.

Nogueira, J.C., Castro, A.C.S., Cámara, E.V.C. and Cámara, B.G.O. (2004). Morphology of the male genital system of *Chironectes minimus* and comparison to other didelphid marsupials. *Journal of Mammalogy*, 85(5), 834–841.

Notides, A.C. and Williams-Ashman, H.C. (1967). The basic protein responsible for the clotting of guinea-pig semen. *Proceedings of the National Academy of Sciences USA*, 58, 199.

Noureen, S., Nadeem, M.S., Beg, M.A. and Anwar, M. (2014). Seasonal variation in the reproductive tract of the Indian flying fox, *Pteropus giganteus* (Brünnich, 1782). *Animal Biology*, 64, 343–364.

Novacek, M.J., Brown, T.M. and Schankler, D. (1985). On the classification of the early Tertiary Erinaceomorpha (Insectivora, Mammalia). *American Museum Novitates*, 2813, 1–22.

Nowak, R.M. (1999). *Walker's Mammals of the World*. Sixth edn. Baltimore, MD: Johns Hopkins University Press.

Nunn, C.L. (1999). The evolution of exaggerated sexual swellings in female primates and the graded-signal hypothesis. *Animal Behaviour*, 58, 229–246.

Nunn, C.L., Gittleman, J.L. and Anthonovics, J. (2000). Promiscuity and the primate immune system. *Science*, 290, 1168–1170.

O'Shea, T.J., Ackerman, B.B. and Percival, H.F., eds. (1995). *Population Biology of the Florida Manatee*. U.S. Department of the Interior, National Biological Service, Information and Technology Report 1.

Ohsawa, H., Inoue, M. and Takenata, O. (1993). Mating strategy and reproductive success of male patas monkeys (*Erythrocebus patas*). *Primates*, 34, 533–544.

Ojala-Barbour, R., Pinto, C., Britto, J., Albuja, L., Lee, T., *et al.* (2013). A new species of shrew-opossum (Paucituberculata: Caenolestidae) with a phylogeny of extant caenolestids. *Journal of Mammalogy*, 94(5), 967–982.

Olds, N. and Shoshani, J. (1982). *Procavia capensis. Mammalian Species*, 171, 1–7.

Olsen, S.J. (1959). The baculum of the miocene carnivore *Amphicyon. Journal of Paleontology*, 33(3), 449–450.

Orbach, D.N., Packard, J.M. and Würsig, B. (2014). Mating group size in dusky dolphins (*Lagenorhynchus obscurus*): costs and benefits of scramble competition. *Ethology*, 120, 804–815.

Orbach, D.N., Marshall, C.D., Mesnick, S.L. and Würsig, B. (2017a). Patterns of cetacean vaginal folds yield insights into functionality. *PLoS ONE*, 12(3), e0175037.

Orbach, D.N., Kelly, D.A., Solano, M. and Brennan, P.L.R. (2017b). Genital interactions during simulated copulation among marine mammals. *Proceedings of the Royal Society, B*, 284, 20171265.

Orbach, D.N., Brennan, P.L.R., Hedrick, B.P., Keener, W., Webber, M.A., *et al.* (2020). Asymmetric and spiraled genitalia coevolve with unique lateralized mating behavior. *Nature: Scientific Reports*, 10, 3257.

Orgebin-Crist, M.C. and Olson, G.E. (1984). Epididymal sperm transport. In *The Male in Farm Animal Reproduction*, ed. M. Courot. Boston, MA: Matinus Nijhoff Publishers, pp. 80–102.

Orr, T.J. and Brennan, P.L.R. (2016). All features great and small – the potential roles of the baculum and penile spines in mammals. *Integrative and Comparative Biology*, 56(4), 635–643.

Ortiz-Jaureguizar, E. and Pascual, R. (2011). The tectonic setting of the Caribbean region and the K/T turnover of the South American land-mammal fauna. *Boletin Geologico y Minero*, 122(3), 333–344.

Ottow, B. (1955). *Biologische Anatomie der Genitalorgane und der Fortpflanzung der Säugetiere*. Jena: G. Fischer.

Overstreet, J.W. (1983). Transport of gametes in the reproductive tract of the female mammal. In *Mechanism and Control of Animal Fertilization*, ed. J.R. Hartmann. New York: Academic Press, pp. 499–543.

Owen-Smith, N. (1975). The social ethology of the white rhinoceros *Ceratotherium simum* (Burchell, 1817). *Zeitschrift für Tierpsychologie*, 38, 337–384.

Paduschka, W. (1974). Das paarungsverhalten des groben igel-tenrek (*Setifer setosus*, Froriep, 1806) und die frage des phylogenetischen alters einiger paarungseinzelheiten. *Zeitschrift für Tierpsychologie*, 34, 345–358.

Paplinska, J.Z., Bencini, R., Fisher, D.O., Newell, G.R., Goldizen, A.W., *et al.* (2010). Sperm competition in the Macropodoidea: a review of the evidence. In *Macropods: The Biology of Kangaroos, Wallabies and Rat-Kangaroos*, eds. G. Coulson and M. Eldridge. Collingwood: CSIRO Publishing, pp. 66–76.

Parag, A., Bennett, N.C., Faulkes, C.G. and Bateman, P.W. (2006). Penile morphology of African mole-rats (Bathyergidae): structural modification in relation to mode of ovulation and degree of sociality. *Journal of Zoology, London*, 270: 323–329.

Parga, J.A. (2003). Copulatory plug displacement evidences sperm competition in *Lemur catta*. *International Journal of Primatology*, 24, 889–899.

Parga, J.A., Maga, M. and Overdorff, J. (2006). High-resolution X-ray computed tomography scanning of primate copulatory plugs. *American Journal of Physical Anthropology*, 129, 567–576.

Parga, J.A., Sauther, M.L., Cuozzo, F.P., Jacky, I.A.U., Lawler, R.R., *et al.* (2016). Paternity in wild ring-tailed lemurs (*Lemur catta*): implications for male mating strategies. *American Journal of Primatology*, 78, 1316–1325.

Parker, G.A. (1970). Sperm competition and its evolutionary consequences in the insects. *Biological Reviews*, 45, 525–567.

Parker, G.A. (2016). The evolution of expenditure on testes. *Journal of Zoology, London*, 298, 3–19.

Parkes, A.S. (1966). The testes of certain Choeromorpha. In *Comparative Biology of Reproduction in Mammals*, ed. I.W. Rowlands. *Symposia of the Zoological Society of London*, 15, 141–154.

Parrott, M.L., Ward, S.J. and Taggart, D.A. (2005). Multiple paternity and communal maternal care in the feathertail glider (*Acrobates pygmaeus*). *Australian Journal of Zoology*, 53, 79–85.

Parvathy, S., Rao, M., Kumer, V. and Umapathy, G. (2014). Observations on reproductive performance of Indian mouse deer (*Moschiola indica*) in captivity. *Current Science*, 106(3), 439–441.

Pascual, R., Archer, M., Ortiz-Jaureguizar, E., Prado, J.L., Godthelp, H., *et al.* (1992). First discovery of monotremes in South America. *Nature*, 356, 704–705.

Patterson, B. D. and Thaeler, C. S. (1982). The mammalian baculum: hypotheses on the nature of bacular variability. *Journal of Mammalogy*, 63(1), 1–15.

Pauli, J.N. and Peery, M.Z. (2012). Strong polygyny in the brown-throated three-toed sloth. *PLoS ONE*, 7, e51389.

Paulraj, S., Sundrarajan, N., Manimozhi, A. and Walker, S. (1992). Reproduction of the Indian wild dog (*Cuon alpinus*) in captivity. *Zoo Biology*, 11, 235–241.

Pavlicev, M. and Wagner, G.P. (2016). The evolutionary origin of female orgasm. *Journal of Experimental Zoology Part B: Molecular and Developmental Evolution*, 326(6), 326–337.

Pavlicev, M., Zupan, A.M., Barry, A., Walters, S., Milan, K.M., *et al.* (2019). An experimental test of the ovulatory homolog model of female orgasm. *Proceedings of the National Academy of Sciences USA*, 116(41), 20267–20273.

Payne, K. (1998). *Silent Thunder: The Hidden Voice of Elephants*. London: Weidenfeld and Nicolson.

Pearson, O.P. (1944). Reproduction in the shrew (*Blarina brevicauda* Say). *American Journal of Anatomy*, 75, 39–93.

Pearson, O.P. and Bassett, C.F. (1946). Certain aspects of reproduction in a herd of silver foxes. *The American Naturalist*, 80, 45–67.

Peery, M.Z. and Pauli, J.N. (2012). The mating system of a 'lazy' mammal, Hoffmann's two-toed sloth. *Animal Behaviour*, 84, 555–562.

Penfold, M.J., Solely, J.T. and Hartman, M.J. (2019). Morphology of the uterotubal junction of the cheetah (*Acinomyx jubatus*). *The Anatomical Record*, 302, 1855–1864.

Pepin, J. (2011). *The Origins of AIDS*. Cambridge: Cambridge University Press.

Pereira, M.E. and Weiss, M.L. (1991). Female mate choice, male migration and the threat of infanticide in ring-tailed lemurs. *Behavior Ecology and Sociobiology*, 18, 141–152.

Peretti, A.V. and Aisenberg, A., eds. (2015). *Cryptic Female Choice in Arthropods: Patterns, Mechanisms and Prospects*. New York: Springer.

Perry, J.M., Izard, M.K. and Fail, P.A. (1992). Observations on reproduction, hormones, copulatory behavior, and neonatal mortality in captive *Lemur mongoz* (mongoose lemur). *Zoo Biology*, 11, 81–97.

Persson, E. and Rodriguez-Martinez, H. (1990). The ligamentum infundibulo-cornuale in the pig: morphological and physiological studies of the smooth muscle component. *Acta Anatomica*, 138, 111–120.

Petter, F. (1957). La reproduction du fennec. *Mammalia*, 21, 307–309.

Pettigrew, J.D. (1999). Electroreception in monotremes. *Journal of Experimental Biology*, 202, 1447–1454.

Pfaff, D.W. (1980). *Estrogens and Brain Function*. New York: Springer-Verlag.

Pfaff, D.W., Lewis, C., Diakow, C. and Keiner, M. (1972). Neurophysiological analysis of mating behavior responses as hormone-sensitive reflexes. In *Progress in Physiological Psychology, Vol. 5*, eds. E. Stellar and J.M. Sprague. New York: Academic Press, pp. 253–297.

Pfaff, D.W., Diakow, C., Montgomery, M. and Jenkins, F.A. (1978). X-ray cinematographic analysis of lordosis in female rats. *Journal of Comparative and Physiological Psychology*, 92, 937–941.

Philbrick, N. (2000). *In the Heart of the Sea: The Tragedy of the Whaleship Essex*. New York: Penguin Books.

Phillips, D.M. (1970). Development of spermatozoa in the woolly opossum with special reference to the shaping of the sperm head. *Journal of Ultrastructural Research*, 33, 369–380.

Phillips, D.M. and Bedford, J.M. (1987). Sperm–sperm associations in the loris epididymis. *Gamete Research*, 18, 17–25.

Phillips, M.J., Bennett, T.H. and Lee, M.S.Y. (2009). Molecules, morphology, and ecology indicate a recent, amphibious ancestry for echidnas. *Proceedings of the National Academy of Sciences USA*, 106, 17089–17094.

Phoenix, C.H., Copenhaver, K.H. and Brenner, R.M. (1976). Scanning electron microscopy of penile papillae in intact and castrated rats. *Hormones and Behavior*, 7, 217–227.

Pitlay, N. (1997). Copulatory behaviour of the vlei rat *Otomys irroratus*. *South African Journal of Zoology*, 32(3), 95–98.

Pitnik, S., Hosken, D. and Birkhead, T.R. (2010). Sperm morphological diversity. In *Sperm Biology: an Evolutionary Perspective*, eds. T.R. Birkhead, D.J. Hosken and S. Pitnick. Burlington, MA: Elsevier/Academic Press, pp. 69–149.

Pizzari, T. and Parker, G.A. (2010). Sperm competition and sperm phenotype. In *Sperm Biology: An Evolutionary Perspective*, eds. T.R. Birkhead, D.J. Hosken and S. Pitnick. Burlington, MA: Elsevier/Academic Press, pp. 207–245.

Plön, S. and Bernard, R.T.F. (2006). A review of spermatozoan morphology in Cetacea with new data for the Genus *Kogia*. *Journal of Zoology, London*, 269, 466–473.

Poole, J.H. and Moss, C.J. (1981). Musth in the African elephant (*Loxodonta africana*). *Nature*, 292, 830–831.

Popp, J.W. (1982). Observations on the behavior of captive sitatunga (*Tragelaphus spekei*). *Zoo Biology*, 1(1), 59–63.

Preston, B.T., Stevenson, I.R., Pemberton, J.M. and Wilson, K. (2001). Dominant rams lose out by sperm depletion. *Nature*, 409, 681–682.

Price, D. and Williams-Ashman, H.G. (1961). The accessory reproductive glands of mammals. In *Sex and Internal Secretions, Vol. 1*. Third edn, ed. W.C. Young. Baltimore, MD: Williams and Wilkins, pp. 366–448.

Prins, G.S. and Zaneveld, L.J.D. (1980). Radiographic study of fluid transport in the rabbit vas deferens during sexual rest and after sexual activity. *Journal of Reproduction and Fertility*, 58, 311–319.

Proske, U., Gregory, J.E. and Iggo, A. (1998). Sensory receptors in monotremes. *Philosophical Transactions of the Royal Society of London, B*, 353, 1187–1198.

Pullen, S.L., Bearder, S.K. and Dixson, A.F. (2000). Preliminary observations on sexual behavior and the mating system in free-ranging lesser galagos (*Galago moholi*). *American Journal of Primatology*, 51, 79–88.

Purohit, R.C. and Beckett, S.D. (1976). Penile pressures and muscle activity associated with erection and ejaculation in the dog. *American Journal of Physiology*, 231(5), 1343–1348.

Quill, T.A., Sugden, S.A., Rossi, K.L., Doolittle, L.K., Hammer, R.E., *et al.* (2003). Hyperactivated sperm motility driven by CatSper2 is required for fertilization. *Proceedings of the National Academy of Sciences USA*, 100(25), 14869–14874.

Racey, P.A. (1974). The reproductive cycle in male noctule bats, *Nyctalus noctula*. *Journal of Reproduction and Fertility*, 41, 169–182.

Racey, P.A. (1979). The prolonged storage and survival of spermatozoa in Chiroptera. *Journal of Reproduction and Fertility*, 56, 391–402.

Racey, P.A. and Kleiman, D.G. (1970). Maintenance and breeding in captivity of some verspertilionid bats, with special reference to the noctule, *Nyctalus noctula*. *International Zoo Year Book*, 10, 65–69.

Raleigh, V.S. (1999). Trends in world population growth: how will the millennium compare with the past? *Human Reproduction Update*, 5(5), 500–505.

Ralls, K., Barasch, C. and Minkowski, K. (1975). Behavior of captive mouse deer, *Tragulus napu*. *Zeitschrift für Tierpsychologie*, 37, 356–378.

Ramirez, V.D. and Soufi, W.L. (1994). The neuroendocrine control of the rabbit ovarian cycle. In *The Physiology of Reproduction, Vol. 2*. Second edn, eds. E. Knobil and J.D. Neill. New York: Raven Press, pp. 585–611.

Ramm, S.A. and Stockley, P. (2010). Sperm competition and sperm length influence the rate of mammalian spermatogenesis. *Biology Letters*, 6, 219–221.

Ramm, S.A., Parker, G.A. and Stockley, P. (2005). Sperm competition and the evolution of male reproductive anatomy in rodents. *Proceedings of the Royal Society of London, B*, 272, 949–955.

Ramm, S.A., Oliver, P.L., Ponting, C.P., Stockley, P. and Emes, R.D. (2008). Sexual selection and the adaptive evolution of mammalian ejaculate proteins. *Molecular Biology and Evolution*, 25, 207–219.

Ramm, S.A., McDonald, L., Hurst, J.L., Beynon, R.J. and Stockley, P. (2009). Comparative proteomics reveals evidence for evolutionary diversification of rodent seminal fluid and its functional significance in sperm competition. *Molecular Biology and Evolution*, 26(1), 189–198.

Ramm, S.A., Edward, D.A., Claydon, A.J., Hammond, D.E., Brownridge, P., *et al.* (2015). Sperm competition risk drives plasticity in seminal fluid composition. *BMC Biology*, DOI 10.1186/s12915-015-0197-2.

Ramondt, J., Verhoeff, A., Garfield, R.E. and Wallenburg, H.C.S. (1994). Effects of estrogen treatment and inhibition of prostanoid synthesis on myometrial activity and gap junction formation in the oophorectomized ewe. *European Journal of Obstetrics, Gynecology, and Reproductive Biology*, 54, 63–69.

Ramos, A.S. Jr. (1979). Morphologic variations along the length of the monkey vas deferens. *Archives of Andrology*, 3, 187–196.

Rasa, O.A.E. (1977). The ethology and sociology of the dwarf mongoose (*Helogale undulata rufula*). *Zeitschrift für Tierpsychologie*, 43, 337–406.

Rathbun, G.B. (1979). The social structure and ecology of elephant-shrews. *Advances in Ethology*, 20, 1–75.

Rathbun, G.B. and Rathbun, C.D. (2006). Social structure of the bushveld sengi (*Elephantulus intufi*) in Namibia and the evolution of monogamy in the Macroscelidea. *Journal of Zoology, London*, 269, 391–399.

Ratto, M.H., Leduc, Y.A., Valderrama, X.P., van Straaten, K.E., Delbaere, L.T.J., *et al.* (2012). The nerve of ovulation-inducing factor in semen. *Proceedings of the National Academy of Sciences, USA*, 109(37), 15042–15047.

Ratto, M.H., Berland, M., Silva, M.E. and Adams, G.P. (2019). New insights of the role of β-NGF in the ovulation mechanism of induced ovulating species. *Reproduction*, 157, R199–R207.

Raynaud, A. (1969). Mammeles. In *Traité de Zoologie: Anatomie, Systématique, Biologie. Tome 16. Fascicule 6, Mammeles. Appareil Génital Gamétogenèse, Fecondation, Gestation*, ed. P.-P. Grassé. Paris: Masson et Cie, pp. 1–853.

Reddi, A.H. and Prasad, M.R.N. (1967). Action of testosterone propionate and growth hormone on the os penis of the Indian palm squirrel, *Funambulus pennanti* (Wroughton). *General and Comparative Endocrinology*, 8, 143–151.

Redford, K.H. and Eisenberg, J.F. (1992). *Mammals of the Neotropics: The Southern Cone.* Chicago, IL: Chicago University Press.

Reid, A. (2009). *Sepioloidea magna* sp. nov.: a new bottletail squid (Cephalopoda: Sepiadariidae) from northern Australia. *The Beagle, Records of the Museums and Art Galleries of the Northern Territory*, 25, 103–109.

Reid, B.L. and Cleland, K.W. (1957). The ultrastructure and function of the epididymis. *Australian Journal of Zoology*, 5, 223–246.

Retief, T.A., Bennett, N.C., Kinahan, A.A. and Bateman P.W. (2013). Sexual selection and genital allometry in the Hottentot golden mole (*Amblysomus hottentotus*). *Mammalian Biology*, 78, 356–360.

Ribble, D.O. and Perrin, M.R. (2005). Social organization of the eastern rock elephant-shrew (*Elephantulus myurus*): the evidence for mate guarding. *Belgian Journal of Zoology, Supplement*, 135, 167–173.

Rich, T.H., Vickers-Rich, P., Trusler, P., Flannery, T.F., Cifelli, R.L., *et al.* (2001). Monotreme nature of the Australian early Cretaceous mammal *Teinolophus trusleri*. *Acta Palaeontologica Polonica*, 46, 113–118.

Richard, A. (1976). Patterns of mating in *Propithecus verreauxi verreauxi*. In *Prosimian Behavior*, eds. R.D. Martin, G.A. Doyle and A.C. Walker. London: Duckworth, pp. 49–74.

Richard-Hansen, C. and Taube, E. (1997). Note on the reproductive behavior of the three-toed sloth, *Bradypus tridactylus*, in French Guiana. *Mammalia*, 61(2), 259–263.

Riedelsheimer, B., Unterberger, P., Künzle, H. and Welsch, U. (2007). Histological study of the cloacal region and associated structures in the hedgehog tenrec *Echinops telfairi*. *Mammalian Biology*, 72(6), 330–341.

Riedman, M.R. (1990). *The Pinnipeds: Seals, Sea lions, and Walruses*. Berkeley, CA: University of California Press.

Rieger, I. (1979). Breeding the striped hyaena, *Hyaena hyaena*, in captivity. *International Zoo Yearbook*, 19, 193–198.

Riffell, J.A., Krug, P.J. and Zimmer, R.K. (2004). The ecological and evolutionary consequences of sperm chemo-attraction. *Proceedings of the National Academy of Sciences USA*, 101, 4501–4506.

Rioja, T., Lorenzo, C., Naranjo, E., Scott, L. and Carrillo-Reyes, A. (2008). Polygynous mating behavior in the endangered Tehuantepec jackrabbit (*Lepus flavigularis*). *Western North American Naturalist*, 68(3), 343–349.

Rioux-Paquette, E., Garant, D., Martin, A.M., Coulson, G. and Festa-Bianchet, M. (2015). Paternity in eastern grey kangaroos: moderate skew despite strong sexual dimorphism. *Behavioral Ecology*, 26(4), 1147–1155.

Rismiller, P. (1999). *The Echidna: Australia's Enigma*. Hong Kong: Hugh Lauter Levin Associates.

Rissmiller, P.D. and McKelvey, M.W. (2000). Frequency of breeding and recruitment in the short-beaked echidna, *Tachyglossus aculeatus*. *Journal of Mammalogy*, 81(1), 1–17.

Robeck, T.R., Curry, B.E., McBain, J.F. and Kraemer, D.C. (1994). Reproductive biology of the bottlenose dolphin (*Tursiops truncatus*) and the potential application of advanced reproductive technologies. *Journal of Zoo and Wildlife Medicine*, 25(3), 321–336.

Roberts, M.S. and Kessler, D.S. (1979). Reproduction in red pandas (*Ailurus fulgens*) (Carnivora: Ailuropodidae). *Journal of Zoology, London*, 188, 235–249.

Robinson, P.T., Flacke, G.L. and Hentschel, K.M., eds. (2017). *The Pygmy Hippo Story: West Africa's Enigma of the Rainforest*. New York: Oxford University Press.

Rodger, J.C. (1982). The testis and its excurrent ducts in American caenolestid and didelphid marsupials. *The American Journal of Anatomy*, 163, 269–282.

Rodger, J.C. and Bedford, J.M. (1982). Induction of oestrus, recovery of gametes, and the timing of fertilization events in the opossum, *Didelphis virginiana*. *Journal of Reproduction and Fertility*, 64, 159–169.

Rodger, J.C. and White, I.G. (1975). Electro-ejaculation of Australian marsupials and analyses of the sugars in the seminal plasma from three macropod species. *Journal of Reproduction and Fertility*, 43, 233–239.

Rodgers, C.H. (1971). Influence of copulation on ovulation in the cycling rat. *Endocrinology*, 88, 433–436.

Rodgers, C.H. and Schwartz, N.B. (1973). Serum LH and FSH levels in mated and unmated proestrus female rats. *Endocrinology*, 92, 1475–1479.

Rodriguez, E., Weiss, D.A., Yang, J.H., Menshenina, J., Ferretti, M., *et al.* (2011). New insights on the morphology of adult mouse penis. *Biology of Reproduction*, 85, 1216–1221.

Rodriquez-Sierra, J.F., Crowley, W.R. and Komisaruk, B.R. (1975). Vaginal stimulation in rats induces prolonged lordosis responsiveness and sexual receptivity. *Journal of Comparative and Physiological Psychology*, 89, 79–85.

Roeder, J.J. (1979). La reproduction de la genette (*Genetta genetta* L.) en captivité. *Mammalia*, 43, 531–542.

Roellig, K., Goeritz, F., Fickel, J., Hermes, R., Hofer, H., *et al.* (2010). Superconception in mammalian pregnancy can be detected and increases reproductive output per breeding season. *Nature Communications*, 1(6), 78. DOI: 10.1038/ncomms1079.

Roemer, G.W., Smith, D.A., Garcelon, D.K. and Wayne, R.K. (2001). The behavioural ecology of the island fox (*Urocyon littoralis*). *Journal of Zoology, London*, 255, 1–14.

Roer, H. and Egsbaek, W. (1969). Uber die Balz der Wasserfledermaus (*Myotis daubentonii*) (Chiroptera) im Winterquartier. *Lynx* (N.S.), 10, 85–91.

Roger, J.C. and Hughes, R.L. (1973). Studies of the accessory glands of male marsupials. *Australian Journal of Zoology*, 21, 303–320.

Roldan, E.R.S. (2019). Sperm competition and the evolution of sperm form and function in mammals. *Reproduction in Domestic Animals*, 54, 14–21.

Romer, A.S. (1962). *Vertebrate Paleontology*. Chicago, IL: Chicago University Press.

Rood, J.P. (1958). Habits of the short-tailed shrew in captivity. *Journal of Mammalogy*, 39(4), 499–507.

Rood, J.P. (1972). Ecological and behavioural comparisons of three genera of Argentine cavies. *Animal Behaviour Monographs*, 5(1), 1–83.

Rose, K.D. and Archibald, J.D., eds. (2005). *The Rise of Placental Mammals: Origins and Relationships of the Major Extant Clades*. Baltimore, MD: Johns Hopkins University Press.

Rose, R.W. (1985). The Reproductive Biology of the Tasmanian Bettong, *Bettongia gaimardi*. PhD Dissertation, University of Tasmania.

Rose, R.W., Nevison, C.M. and Dixson, A.F. (1997). Testis weight, body weight and mating systems in marsupials and monotremes. *Journal of Zoology, London*, 243, 523–531.

Roseweir, A.K. and Millar, R.P. (2009). The role of kisspeptin in the control of gonadotrophin secretion. *Human Reproduction Update*, 15, 206–212.

Roth, T.L., O'Brien, J.K., McRae, M.A., Bellem, A.C., Romo, S.J., *et al.* (2001). Ultrasound and endocrine evaluation of ovarian cyclicity and early pregnancy in the Sumatran rhinoceros (*Dicerorhinus sumatrensis*). *Reproduction*, 121, 139–149.

Roth, T.L., Stoops, M.A., Atkinson, M.W., Blumer, E.S., Campbell, M.K., *et al.* (2005). Semen collection in rhinoceroses (*Rhinoceros unicornis, Diceros bicornis, Ceratotherium simum*) by electroejaculation with a uniquely designed probe. *Journal of Zoo and Wildlife Medicine*, 36(4), 617–627.

Rowe, M., Albrecht, T., Cramer, E.R.A., Johnsen, A., Laskemoen, T., *et al.* (2015). Postcopulatory sexual selection is associated with accelerated evolution of sperm morphology. *Evolution*, 69(4), 1044–1052.

Rowell, T.E. and Dixson, A.F. (1975). Changes in social organization during the breeding season of wild talapoin monkeys. *Journal of Reproduction and Fertility*, 43, 419–434.

Rudd, C.D. (1994). Sexual behaviour of male and female tammar wallabies (*Macropus eugenii*) at post-partum oestrus. *Journal of Zoology, London*, 232, 151–162.

Ruggiero, L.F. and Henry, S.E. (1993). Courtship and copulatory behavior of *Martes americana*. *Northwestern Naturalist*, 74(1), 18–22.

Ryan, R.M. (1966). Observations on the broad-nosed bat, *Scoteinus balstoni*, in Victoria. *Journal of Zoology, London*, 148, 162–166.

Ryser, J. (1992). The mating system and male mating success of the Virginia opossum (*Didelphis virginiana*) in Florida. *Journal of Zoology, London*, 228, 127–139.

Sachs, B.D. (1982). Role of the rat's striated penile muscles in penile reflexes, copulation and induction of pregnancy. *Journal of Reproduction and Fertility*, 66, 433–443.

Sachs, B.D. (1983). Potency and fertility: hormonal and mechanical causes and effects of penile actions in rats. In *Hormones and Behaviour in Higher Vertebrates*, eds. J. Balthazart, E. Prove and R. Gilles. Berlin: Springer, pp. 86–110.

Sachs, B.D. and Meisel, R. (1988). The physiology of male sexual behavior. In *The Physiology of Reproduction, Vol. 2*, eds. E. Knobil and J.D. Neill. New York: Raven Press, pp. 1393–1485.

Safaris, V., Lambert, R.W. and Breed, W.G. (1981). Sperm head morphology of the plains mouse *Pseudomys australis*. *Journal of Reproduction and Fertility*, 61, 399–401.

Sale, M.G., Kraaijeveld-Smit, F.J.L. and Arnould, J.P.Y. (2013). Multiple paternity in the swamp antechinus (*Antechinus minimus*). *Australian Mammalogy*, 35, 227–230.

Samsudewa, D., Capitan, S.S., Sevilla, C.C., Vega, R.S.A. and Ocampo, P.P. (2013). Comparative reproductive behavior of α-male, β-male and subordinate male timor deer (*Cervus timorensis* Blainville) raised in captivity. *International Journal of Environmental and Rural Development*, 4(2), 98–103.

Sandera, M., Albrecht, T. and Stopka, P. (2013). Variation in apical hook length reflects the intensity of sperm competition in murine rodents. *PLoS ONE*, 8(7), e68427.

Sanger, T.J., Gredler, M.L. and Cohn, M.J. (2015). Resurrecting embryos of the tuatara, *Sphenodon punctatus*, to resolve vertebrate phallus evolution. *Biology Letters*, 11, 20150694.na

Sarsaifi, K., Rosnina, Y., Ariff, M.O., Wahid, H., Hani, H., *et al.* (2013). Effect of semen collection methods on the quality of pre- and post-thawed Bali cattle (*Bos javanicus*) spermatozoa. *Reproduction in Domestic Animals*, 48, 1006–1012.

Satake, N., Elliott, R.M.A., Watson, P.F. and Holt, W.V. (2006). Sperm selection and competition in pigs may be mediated by differential motility activation and suppression of sperm subpopulations within the oviduct. *Journal of Experimental Biology*, 209, 1560–1572.

Scarlata, C.D., Elias, B.A., Godwin, J.R., Powell, R.A., Shepherdson, D., et al. (2012). Relationship between fecal hormone concentrations and reproductive success in captive pigmy rabbits (*Brachylagus idahoensis*). *Journal of Mammalogy*, 93(3), 759–770.

Schaller, G.B. (1998). *Wildlife of the Tibetan Steppe*. Chicago, IL: University of Chicago Press.

Schipper, J., Chanson, J.S., Chiozza, F., Cox, N.A., Hoffmann, M., *et al.* (2008). The status of the world's land and marine mammals: diversity, threat, and knowledge. *Science*, 322(5899), 225–230.

Schmidt, F. (1934). Ober die Fortpflanzungsbiologie von sibirischen Zobel (*Martes zibellina*) und europaischem Baummarder (*Martes martes* L.). *Zeitschrift für Saugetierkunde*, 9, 392–403.

Schmidt, F. (1943). Naturgeschichte des baum und des steinmarders. *Monographien der Wildsäugetiere*, 10, 1–258.

Schramm, P. (1961). Copulation and gestation in the pocket gopher. *Journal of Mammalogy*, 42, 167–170.

Schramm, R.D., Briggs, M.B. and Reeves, J.J. (1994). Simultaneous and induced ovulation in the lion (*Panthera leo*). *Zoo Biology*, 13, 301–307.

Schubert, M., Pillay, N., Ribble, D.O. and Schradin, C. (2009). The round-eared sengi and the evolution of social monogamy: factors that constrain males to live with a single female. *Ethology*, 15, 972–984.

Schülke, O., Kappeler, P.M. and Zischler, H. (2004). Small testes size despite extra-pair paternity in the pair-living nocturnal primate *Phaner furciver*. *Behavioral Ecology and Sociobiology*, 55, 293–301.

Schulte, T. L. (1937). The genito-urinary system of the *Elephas indicus* male. *American Journal of Anatomy*, 61(1), 131–157.

Schultz, A.H. (1938). The relative weights of the testes in primates. *Anatomical Record*, 72, 387–394.

Schultz, N.G., Lough-Stevens, M., Abreu, E., Orr, T. and Dean, M.D. (2016). The baculum was gained and lost multiple times during mammalian evolution. *Integrative Comparative Biology*, 56, 635–643.

Schulze, H. and Meier, B. (1995). Behavior of captive *Loris tardigradus nordicus*: a qualitative description, including some information about morphological bases of behavior. In *Creatures of the Dark, the Nocturnal Prosimians*, eds. L. Alterman, G.A. Doyle and M.K. Izard. New York: Plenum, pp. 221–249.

Schurmann, C. (1982). Mating behaviour of wild orangutans. In *The Orangutan: Its Ecology and Conservation*, ed. L.E.M. de Boer. The Hague: Dr. W. Junk, pp. 269–284.

Schusterman, R.J. (1968). Steller sea lion *Eumetopias jubatus* (Schreber 1776). In *Handbook of Marine Mammals, Vol. 1*, eds. S.H. Ridgeway and R.J. Harrison. New York: Academic Press, pp. 119–141.

Schwartz, J.H. (1987). *The Red Ape: Orang-utans and Human Origins*. London: Elm Tree Books.

Scott, C.S. (2006). A new erinaceid (Mammalia, Insectivora) from the late Paleocene of western Canada. *Canadian Journal of Earth Sciences*, 43(11), 1695–1709.

Seidel, G.E. and Foote, R.H. (1969). Motion picture analysis of ejaculation in the bull. *Journal of Reproduction and Fertility*, 20, 313–317.

Seifert, E. (2007). A new estimate of afrotherian phylogeny based on simultaneous analysis of genomic, morphological, and fossil evidence. *BMC Evolutionary Biology*, 7, 13.

Setchell, B.P. and Carrick, F.N. (1973). Spermatogenesis in some Australian marsupials. *Australian Journal of Zoology*, 21, 491–499.

Setchell, B.P., Maddocks, S. and Brooks, D.E. (1994). Anatomy, vasculature, innervation and fluids of the male reproductive tract. In *The Physiology of Reproduction, Vol. 1*, eds. E. Knobil and J.D. Neill. New York: Raven Press, pp. 1063–1175.

Settlage, D.S.F., Motoshima, M. and Tredway, D.R. (1973). Sperm transport from the external cervical os to the fallopian tubes in women: a time and quantitation study. *Fertility and Sterility*, 24(9), 655–661.

Seuánez, H.N. (1980). Chromosomes and spermatozoa of the African great apes. *Journal of Reproduction and Fertility, Supplement*, 28, 96–104.

Shadle, A.R. (1946). Copulation in the porcupine. *The Journal of Wildlife Management*, 10(2), 159–162.

Shadle, A.R., Smelzer, M. and Metz, M. (1946). The sex reactions of porcupines (*Erethizon d. dorsatum*) before and after copulation. *Journal of Mammalogy*, 27(2), 116–121.

Shafik, A. (1993). Vagino-cavernosus reflex. Clinical significance and role in [the] sexual act. *Gynecologic and Obstetric Investigation*, 35, 114.

Shafik, A. (1995). Vagino-levator reflex: description of a reflex and its role in sexual performance. *European Journal of Obstetrics and Gynecology*, 60, 161–164.

Shafik, A. (1996). Study of the intramural oviduct response to tubal and uterine distension: identification of tubo-uterine sphincter and reflex. *Human Reproduction*, 11, 2527–2530.

Sharma, V., Lehmann, T., Stuckas, H., Funke, L. and Hiller, M. (2018). Loss of *RXFP2* and *INSL3* genes in Afrotheria shows that testicular descent is the ancestral condition in placental mammals. *PLoS Biology*, 16(6), e2005293. https://doi.org/10.1371/journal.pbio.2005293

Sharman, G.B. (1976). Evolution of viviparity in mammals. In *Reproduction in Mammals, Vol. 6, The Evolution of Reproduction*, eds. C.R. Austin and R.V. Short. Cambridge: Cambridge University Press, pp. 32–70.

Sharman, G.B., Calaby, J.H. and Poole, W.E. (1966). Patterns of reproduction in female diprotodont marsupials. In *Comparative Biology of Reproduction in Mammals*, ed. I.W. Rowlands. *Symposia of the Zoological Society of London*, 15, 205–232.

Sharpe, R.M. (1994) Regulation of spermatogenesis. In *The Physiology of Reproduction, Vol. 1*. Second ed., eds. E. Knobil, and J.D. Neill. New York: Raven Press, pp. 1363–1434.

Sherman, P.W. and Morton, M.L. (1979). Four months of the ground squirrel. *Natural History*, 88, 50–57.

Sherman, P.W., Jarvis, J.U.M. and Alexander, R.D., eds. (1991). *The Biology of the Naked Mole-Rat*. Princeton, NJ: Princeton University Press.

Shimmin, G.A., Jones, M., Taggart, D.A. and Temple-Smith, P.D. (1999). Sperm transport and storage in the agile antechinus (*Antechinus agilis*). *Biology of Reproduction*, 60, 1353–1359.

Shimmin, G.A., Taggart, D.A. and Temple-Smith, P.D. (2002). Mating behaviour in the agile antechinus *Antechinus agilis* (Marsupialia: Dasyuridae). *Journal of Zoology, London*, 258, 39–48.

Short, J., Richards, J.D. and Turner, B. (1998). Ecology of the western barred bandicoot *Perameles bougainville* (Marsupialia: Peramelidae) on Dorre and Bernier Islands, Western Australia. *Wildlife Research*, 25(6), 567–586.

Short, R.V. (1984). Oestrous and menstrual cycles. In *Reproduction in Mammals, Vol. 3*. Second edn, eds. C.R Austin and R.V. Short. Cambridge: Cambridge University Press, pp. 115–152.

Short, R.V., Mann, T. and Hay, M.F. (1967). Male reproductive organs of the African elephant, *Loxodonta africana. Journal of Reproduction and Fertility*, 13, 517–536.

Shoshani, J. and Tassy, P. (1996). *The Proboscidea: Evolution and Palaeoecology of Elephants and Their Relatives*. Oxford: Oxford University Press.

Shultz, S. and Roberts, D. (2013). *Dendrohyrax dorsalis* western tree hyrax. In *Mammals of Africa. Volume I: Introductory Chapters and Afrotheria*, eds. J. Kingdon, D. Happold, M. Hoffman, T. Butynski, M. Happold and J. Kalina. London: Bloomsbury Publishing, pp. 155–157.

Signoret, J.P. (1970). Reproductive behaviour in pigs. *Journal of Reproduction and Fertility (Supplement)*, 11, 105–117.

Signoret, J.P., Cognie, Y. and Martin, G.B. (1984). The effect of males on female reproductive physiology. In *The Male in Farm Animal Reproduction*, ed. M. Courot. Netherlands: Martinus Nijhoff Publishers, pp. 290–304.

Silberberg, A. and Adler, N. (1974). Modulation of the copulatory sequence of the male rat by a schedule of reinforcement. *Science*, 185(No. 4148), 374–376.

Sillero-Zuberi, C., Gottelli, D. and MacDonald, D. W. (1996). Male philopatry, extra-pack copulations and inbreeding avoidance in Ethiopian wolves (*Canis simensis*). *Behavioral Ecology and Sociobiology*, 38, 331–340.

Silva, M., Nino, A., Guerra, M., Letelier, C., Valderrama, X.P., *et al.* (2011). Is an ovulation-inducing factor (OIF) present in the seminal plasma of rabbits? *Animal Reproduction Science*, 127, 213–221.

Simmons, L.W. and Firman, R.C. (2014). Experimental evidence for the evolution of the mammalian baculum by sexual selection. *Evolution*, 68, 276–283.

Simmons, N.B., Seymour, K.L., Habersetzer, J. and Gunnell, G.F. (2008). Primitive early Eocene bat from Wyoming and the evolution of flight and echolocation. *Nature*, 451, 818–821.

Simpson, G.G. (1945). The principles of classification and a classification of mammals. *Bulletin of the American Museum of Natural History*, 85, 1–350.

Simpson, G.G. (1980). *Splendid Isolation: The Curious History of South American Mammals*. New Haven, CT: Yale University Press.

Sinha, A., Datta, A., Madhusudan, M.D. and Mishra, C. (2005). The Arunachal macaque: a new species from Western Arunachal Pradesh, north eastern India. *International Journal of Primatology*, 26, 977–989.

Skarén, U. (1979). Mating behaviour of *Sorex isodon* Turov. *Annales Zoologici Fennici*, 16, 291–293.

Slijper, E.J. (1962). *Whales*. New York: Basic Books.

Slijper, E.J. (1976). *Whales and Dolphins*. Ann Arbor, MI: University of Michigan Press.

Slob, A.K., Groeneveld, W.H. and Van der Werff Ten Bosch, J.J. (1986). Physiological changes during copulation in male and female stumptail macaques (*Macaca arctoides*). *Physiology and Behavior*, 38, 891–895.

Smith, C.C. (1968). The adaptive nature of social organization in the genus of tree squirrels *Tamiasciurus*. *Ecological Monographs*, 38, 31–63.

Smith, D.A. and Smith, L.C. (1975). Oestrus, copulation, and related aspects of reproduction in eastern chipmunks, *Tamias striatus* (Rodentia: Sciuridae). *Canadian Journal of Zoology*, 53, 756–767.

Smith, M. (1980). Behaviour of the koala, *Phascolarctos cinereus* (Goldfuss), in captivity. V. Sexual behaviour. *Australian Wildlife Research*, 7, 41–51.

Smith, M.S. and Neill, J.D. (1976). Termination at midpregnancy of the two daily surges of plasma prolactin initiated by mating in the rat. *Endocrinology*, 98(3), 696–701.

Smith, R.L. (1984). Human sperm competition. In *Sperm Competition and the Evolution of Animal Mating Systems*, ed. R. L. Smith. New York: Academic Press, pp. 601–659.

Smith, S.J. and Leslie, D.M. (2006). *Pteropus livingstonii*. *Mammalian Species*, No. 792, 1–5.

Smith, T. and Yanagimachi, R. (1990). The viability of hamster spermatozoa stored in the isthmus of the oviduct: the importance of sperm–epithelium contact for sperm survival. *Biology of Reproduction*, 42, 450–457.

Smith, T.G. and Aars, J. (2015). Polar bears (*Ursus maritimus*) mating during late June on the pack ice of northern Svalbard, Norway. *Polar Research*, 34(1), 25786. https://doi.org/10.3402/polar.v34.25786

Smith, T.T., Koyanagi F. and Yanagimachi, R. (1988). Quantitative comparison of the passage of homologous and heterologous spermatozoa through the uterotubal junction of the golden hamster. *Gamete Research*, 19, 227–234.

Smithwick, E.B. and Young, L.G. (1997). Sequential histology of the adult chimpanzee epididymis. *Tissue and Cell*, 29(4), 383–412.

Smithwick, E.B., Gould, K.G. and Young, L.G. (1996). Estimate of epididymal transit time in the chimpanzee. *Tissue and Cell*, 28, 485–493.

Soede, N.M. (1993). Boar stimuli around insemination affect reproductive process in pigs: a review. *Animal Reproduction Science*, 32, 107–125.

Solomon, N.G. and Keane, B. (2007). Reproductive strategies in female rodents. In *Rodent Societies: an Ecological and Evolutionary Perspective*, eds. J.O. Wolff and P.W. Sherman. Chicago, IL: Chicago University Press, pp. 42–56.

Sorenson, M.W. (1970). Observations on the behavior of *Dasycercus cristicauda* and *Dasyuroides byrnei* in captivity. *Journal of Mammalogy*, 51(1), 123–130.

Soulsbury, C.D. (2010). Ovulation mode modifies paternity monopolization in mammals. *Biology Letters*, 6, 39–41.

Spencer, P.B.S., Lapidge, S., Hampton, J. and Pluske, J. (2005). The sociogenetic structure of a controlled feral pig population. *Wildlife Research*, 32(4), 297–304.

Spinage, C.A. (1969). Reproduction in the Uganda defassa waterbuck, *Kobus defassa ugandae* Neumann. *Journal of Reproduction and Fertility*, 18, 445–457.

Stallmann, R.R. and Harcourt, A.H. (2006). Size matters: the (negative) allometry of copulatory duration in mammals. *Biological Journal of the Linnean Society*, 87, 185–193.

Stansfield, F.J. (2015). A novel objective method of estimating the age of mandibles from African elephants (*Loxodonta africana africana*). *PLoS ONE*, 10(5), e0124980.

Stephenson, P.J. (1993). Reproductive biology of the large-eared tenrec, *Geogale aurita* (Insectivora: Tenrecidae). *Mammalia*, 57, 553–564.

Sterling, E.J. (1993). Patterns of range use and social organization in aye-ayes (*Daubentonia madagascariensis*) on Nosy Mangabé. In *Lemur Social Systems and Their Ecological Basis*, eds. P. Kappeler and J.U. Ganzhorn. New York: Plenum, pp. 1–10.

Stirling, I. (1971). Studies on the behaviour of the South Australian fur seal, *Arctocephalus forsteri* (Lesson). I. Annual cycle, postures and calls, and adult males during the breeding season. *Australian Journal of Zoology*, 19, 243–266.

Stockley, P. (2002). Sperm competition risk and male genital anatomy: comparative evidence for reduced duration of female sexual receptivity in primates with penile spines. *Evolutionary Ecology*, 16, 123–137.

Stockley, P., Ramm S.A., Sherborne, A.L., Thom, M.D.F., Paterson, S., *et al.* (2013). Baculum morphology predicts reproductive success of male house mice under sexual selection. *BMC Biology*, 11, 66.

Stodart, E. (1966). Management and behaviour of breeding groups of the marsupial *Perameles nasuta* Geoffroy in captivity. *Australian Journal of Zooloogy*, 14, 611–623.

Strahan, R. (1995). *Mammals of Australia*. Second edn. Washington, DC: Smithsoniam Institution Press.

Strahan, R. and Thomas, D.E. (1975). Courtship of the platypus *Ornithorhynchus anatinus*. *Australian Zoologist*, 18(3), 165–178.

Stringer, C. and Andrews, P. (2005). *The Complete World of Human Evolution*. London: Thames and Hudson.

Stuart, C.C., Vaughan, J.L., Kershaw-Young, C.M., Wilkinson, J., Bathgate, R., *et al.* (2015). Effects of varying doses of β-nerve growth factor on the timing of ovulation, plasma progesterone concentration and corpus luteum size in female alpacas (*Vicuna pacos*). *Reproduction Fertility and Development*, 27, 1181–1186. http://dx.doi.org/10.1071/RD14037.

Suarez, S.S. (1987). Sperm transport and motility in the mouse oviduct: observations *in situ*. *Biology of Reproduction*, 36, 203–210.

Suarez, S.S. (2007). Interactions of spermatozoa with the female reproductive tract: inspiration for assisted reproduction. *Reproduction Fertility and Development*, 19, 103–110.

Suarez, S.S. (2008a). Control of hyperactivation in sperm. *Human Reproduction Update*, 14(6), 647–657.

Suarez, S.S. (2008b). Regulation of sperm storage and movement in the mammalian oviduct. *International Journal of Developmental Biology*, 52, 455–462.

Suarez, S.S. (2010). How do sperm get to the egg? Bioengineering expertise needed! *Experimental Mechanics*, 50, 1267–1274.

Suarez, S.S. and Pacey, A.A. (2006). Sperm transport in the female reproductive tract. *Human Reproduction Update*, 12(1), 23–37.

Suarez, S.S., Marquez, B., Harris, T.P. and Schimenti, J.C. (2007). Different regulatory systems operate in the midpiece and principal piece of the mammalian sperm flagellum. *Society for Reproduction and Fertility, Supplement*, 65, 331–334.

Suchentrunk, F. and Hackländer, K. (2005). Maternal and fetal microsatellite genotypes reveal multiple paternity in a brown hare (*Lepus europaeus*) population. *Mammalian Biology, Supplement*, 70, 39.

Suckling, G.C. (1995). Sugar glider, *Petaurus breviceps*. In *Mammals of Australia*, ed. R. Strahan. Washington, DC: Smithsonian Institution Press, pp. 229–231.

Sumbera, R., Burda, H. and Chitaukali, W.N. (1988). Reproductive biology of a solitary subterranean bathyergid rodent, the silvery mole-rat (*Heliophobius argentocinereus*). *Journal of Mammalogy*, 84, 278–287.

Sun, F., Giojalas, L.C., Rovasio, R.A., Tur-Kaspa, I., Sanchez, R., *et al.* (2003). Lack of species specificity in mammalian sperm chemotaxis. *Developmental Biology*, 255(2), 423–427.

Sun, L. and Dai, N. (1995). Male and female association and mating system in the Chinese water deer (*Hydropotes inermis*). *Mammalia*, 59, 171–178.

Superina, M. (2007). Natural History of the Pichi (*Zaedyus pichiy*) in Mendoza Province, Argentina. PhD Dissertation, University of New Orleans.

Suzuki, F. and Racey, P.A. (1984). Light and electron microscopical observations on the male excurrent duct system of the common shrew (*Sorex araneus*). *Journal of Reproduction and Fertility*, 70, 419–428.

Suzuki, Y. (1984). Comparative aspect of eutherian estrous cycle. In *Endocrine Correlates of Reproduction*, eds. K. Ochiai, Y. Arai, T. Shioda and M. Takahashi. Tokyo: Japan Scientific Societies Press, pp. 287–305.

Symons, D. (1979). *The Evolution of Human Sexuality*. New York: Oxford University Press.

Synott, A.L., Fulkerson, W.J. and Lindsay, D.R. (1981). Sperm output by rams and distribution amongst ewes under conditions of continual mating. *Journal of Reproduction and Fertility*, 65, 355–361.

Szalay, F.S. (1982). A new appraisal of marsupial phylogeny and classification. In *Carnivorous Marsupials*, ed. M. Archer. Mosman, New South Wales: Royal Zoological Society of New South Wales, pp. 621–640.

Szykman, M., Van Horn, R.C., Engh, A.L., Boydston, E.E. and Holekamp, K.E. (2007). Courtship and mating in free-living spotted hyenas. *Behaviour*, 141(7), 815–846.

Tabuce, R., Asher, R. and Lehmann, T. (2008). Afrotherian mammals: a review of current data. *Mammalia*, 72, 2–14.

Taggart, D.A., Johnson, J.L., O'Brien, H.P. and Moore, H.D.M. (1993). Why do spermatozoa of American marsupials form pairs? A clue from the analysis of sperm-pairing in the epididymis of the grey short-tailed opossum, *Monodelphis domestica*. *Anatomical Record*, 236, 465–478.

Taggart, D.A., Breed, W.G., Temple-Smith, P.D., Purvis, A. and Shimmin, G. (1998). Reproduction, mating strategies and sperm competition in marsupials and monotremes. In *Sperm Competition and Sexual Selection*, eds. T.R. Birkhead and A. P. Møller. San Diego, CA: Academic Press, pp. 623–666.

Tamura, N. (1993). Role of sound communication in mating of Malaysian *Callosciurus* (Sciuridae). *Journal of Mammalogy*, 74(2), 468–476.

Tan, M., Jones, G., Zhu, G., Ye, J., Hong, T., *et al.* (2009). Fellatio by fruit bats prolongs copulation time. *PLoS ONE*, 4(10), e7595.

Tanco, V.M., Van Steelandt, M.D., Ratto, M.H. and Adams, G.P. (2012). Effect of purified llama ovulation-inducing factor (IOF) on ovarian function in cattle. *Theriogenology*, 78, 1030–1039.

Tattersall, I. (1982). *The Primates of Madagascar*. New York: Columbia University Press.

Taylor, A.C., Cowan, P.E., Fricke, B.L. and Cooper, D.W. (2000). Genetic analysis of the mating system of the common brushtail possum (*Trichosurus vulpecula*) in New Zealand farmland. *Molecular Ecology*, 9, 869–880.

Taylor, J.M. and Horner, B.E. (1970). Observations on reproduction in *Leggadinia* (Rodentia, Muridae). *Journal of Mammalogy*, 51(1), 10–17.

Taylor, W.A. and Skinner, J.D. (2003). Activity patterns, home ranges and burrow use of aardvarks (*Orycteropus afer*) in the Karoo. *Journal of Zoology, London*, 261, 291–297.

Teeling, E.C., Springer, M.S., Madsen, O., Bates, P., O'Brien, J., *et al.* (2005). A molecular phylogeny for bats illuminates biogeography and the fossil record. *Science*, 307, 580–584.

Temple-Smith, P.D. (1973). Seasonal Breeding Biology of the Platypus, *Ornithorhynchus anatinus* (Shaw, 1799), with Special Reference to the Male. PhD Thesis, Australian National University, Canberra.

Temple-Smith, P.D. and Grant, T.R. (1986). Sperm structure and marsupial phylogeny. In *Possums and Opossums: Studies in Evolution*, ed. M. Archer. Sydney: Australian Mammal Society.

Temple-Smith, P. and Grant, T. (2001). Uncertain breeding: a short history of reproduction in monotremes. *Reproduction, Fertility and Development*, 13, 487–497.

Terkel, J. and Sawyer, C.H. (1978). Male copulatory behavior triggers nightly prolactin surges resulting in successful pregnancy in rats. *Hormones and Behavior*, 11, 304–309.

Teska, W.R., Rybak, E.N. and Baker, R.H. (1981). Reproduction and development of the pygmy spotted skunk (*Spilogale pygmaea*). *The American Midland Naturalist*, 105(2), 390–392.

Thewissen, J.G.M., Cooper, L.N., Clementz, M.T., Bajpai, S. and Tiwari, B.N. (2007). Whales originated from aquatic artiodactyls in the Eocene epoch of India. *Nature*, 450, 1190–1194.

Thomas, B.B. and Oommen, M.M. (1998). Reproductive behaviour of the South Indian gerbil *Tatera indica cuvieri* with a note on the role of postejaculatory copulations. *Acta Theriologica*, 43(3), 263–270.

Thompson, V.D. (1987). Parturition and development in the Queensland koala. *International Zoo Yearbook*, 26, 217–222.

Thornhill, R. (1983). Cryptic female choice and its implications in the scorpionfly *Harpobittacus nigriceps*. *American Naturalist*, 122, 765–788.

Tipkantha, W., Pukazhenthi, B., Siriaroonrat, B., Thongphakdee, A., Maikaew, U., *et al.* (2011). Ejaculate characteristics of captive Malayan tapirs (*Tapirus indicus*). *Thai Journal of Veterinary Medicine*, 41(4), 499–508.

Tohmé, G. and Tohmé, H. (1980). Contribution a l'etude du porc-epic *Hystrix indica indica* Kerr, 1792 (Rodentia). *Mammalia*, 44, 523–529.

Tomas, W.M., Campos, Z., Desbiez, A.L.J., Kluyber, D., Borges, P.A.L., *et al.* (2013). Mating behavior of the six-banded armadillo *Euphractus sexcinctus* in the Pantanal wetland, Brazil. *Edentata*, 14, 87–89.

Touremente, M., Zarka-Trigo, D. and Roldan, E.R.S. (2016). Is the hook of muroid rodent's sperm related to sperm train formation? *Journal of Evolutionary Biology*, 29, 1168–1177. doi: 10.1111/jeb.12857.

Touremente, M., Varea-Sánchez, M. and Roldan, E.R.S. (2019). Faster and more efficient swimming: energy consumption of murine spermatozoa under sperm competition. *Biology of Reproduction*, 100, 420–428. doi:10.1093/biolre/ioy197.

Travis, S.E., Slobodchikoff, C.N. and Keim, P. (1996). Social assemblages and mating relationships in prairie dogs: a DNA fingerprint analysis. *Behavioral Ecology*, 7(1), 95–100.

Trivers, R. (1985). *Social Evolution*. Menlo Park, CA: Benjamin Cummings.

Trivers, R. and Willard, D.E. (1973). Natural selection of parental ability to vary the sex ratio of offspring. *Science*, 179, 90–92.

Trupin, G.L. and Fadem, B.H. (1982). Sexual behaviour of the grey short-tailed opossum *Monodelphis domestica*. *Journal of Mammalogy*, 63, 409–414.

Tsagkogeorga, G., Parker, J., Stupka, E., Cotton, J.A. and Rossiter, S.J. (2013). Phylogenetic analyses elucidate the evolutionary relationships of bats. *Current Biology*, 23, 2262–2267.

Turek, F.W. and Van Cauter, E. (1994). Rhythms in reproduction. In *The Physiology of Reproduction, Vol. 2*. Second edn, eds. E. Knobil and J.D. Neill. New York: Raven Press, pp. 487–540.

Türk, G., Gür, S., Kandemir, F.M. and Sönmez, M. (2011). Relationship between seminal plasma arginase activity and semen quality in Saanen bucks. *Small Ruminant Research*, 97, 83–87.

Tutin, C.E.G. (1979). Mating patterns and reproductive strategies in a community of wild chimpanzees (*Pan troglodytes schweinfurthii*). *Behavioral Ecology and Sociobiology*, 6, 29–38.

Tyndale-Biscoe, C.H. and Rodger, J.C. (1978). Differential transport of spermatozoa into the two sides of the genital tract of a monovular marsupial, the tammar wallaby (*Macropus eugenii*). *Journal of Reproduction and Fertility*, 52, 37–43.

Tyndale-Biscoe, H. (2005). *Life of Marsupials*. Collingwood: CSIRO Publishing.

Tyndale-Biscoe, H. and Renfree, M. (1987). *Reproductive Physiology of Marsupials*. Cambridge: Cambridge University Press.

Ulloa-Leal, C., Bogle, O.A., Adams, G.P. and Ratto, M.H. (2014). Luteotrophic effect of ovulation-inducing factor/nerve growth factor present in seminal plasma of llamas. *Theriogenology*, 81, 1101–1107.

Ursing, B.M. and Arnason, U. (1998). Analyses of mitochondrial genomes strongly support a hippopotamous–whale clade. *Proceedings of the Royal Society of London, B*, 265, 2251–2255.

Utami Atmoko, S. and Van Hooff, J.A.R.A.M. (2004). Alternative male reproductive tactics: male bimaturism in orang-utans. In *Sexual Selection in Primates: New and Comparative Perspectives*, eds. P. Kappeler and C. Van Schaik. Cambridge: Cambridge University Press, pp. 196–207.

Valdespino, C., Asa, C.S. and Bauman, J.E. (2002). Estrous cycles, copulation, and pregnancy in the fennec fox (*Vulpes zerda*). *Journal of Mammalogy*, 83(1), 99–109.

Valenciano, A., Baskin, J.A., Abella, J., Pérez-Ramos, A., Álvarez-Sierra, M.A., *et al.* (2016). *Megalictis*, the bone-crushing giant mustelid (Carnivora, Mustelidae, Oligobuninae) from the early Miocene of North America. *PLoS ONE*, 11(4), e0152430.

Valomy, M., Hayes, L.D. and Schradin, C. (2015). Social organization in Eulipotyphla: evidence for a social shrew. *Biology Letters*, 11, 20150825.

Van Der Horst, C.J. and Gillman, J. (1940). Mechanism of ovulation and corpus luteum formation in *Elephantulus*. *Nature*, 145, 974.

Van Der Horst, G., Medger, K., Steckler, D., Luther, I. and Bartels, P. (2018). Bottlenose dolphin (*Tursiops truncatus*) sperm revisited: motility, morphology and ultrastructure of fresh sperm of consecutive ejaculates. *Animal Reproduction Science*, 195, 309–320.

Van Horn, R.N. and Resko, J.A. (1977). The reproductive cycle of the ring-tailed lemur (*Lemur catta*): sex steroid levels and sexual receptivity under controlled photoperiods. *Endocrinology*, 101, 1579–1586.

Vanpé, C., Kjellander, P., Gaillard, J.M., Cosson, J.S., Galan, M., *et al.* (2009). Multiple paternity occurs at low frequency in the territorial roe deer, *Capreolus capreolus*. *Biological Journal of the Linnean Society*, 97, 128–139.

Van Wagenen, G. (1936). The coagulating function of the cranial lobe of the prostate gland in the monkey. *Anatomical Record*, 118, 231–251.

Vaughan, J.L., Galloway, D. and Hopkins, D. (2003). The development of artificial insemination technology in alpacas (*Llama pacos*). A report of the Rural Industries Research and Development Corporation. RIRDC Publication No. 03/104.

Vaughan, T.A., Ryan, J.M. and Czaplewski, N.J. (2015). *Mammalogy*. Sixth edn. Burlington, MA: Jones and Bartlett Learning.

Venables, V.M. and Venables, L.S.V. (1957). Mating behaviour of the seal *Phoca vitulina* in Shetland. *Proceedings of the Zoological Society of London*, 128, 387–396.

Venables, V.M. and Venables, L.S.V. (1959). Vernal coition of the seal *Phoca vitulina* in Shetland. *Proceedings of the Zoological Society of London*, 132, 665–669.

Vidyadaran, M.K., Sharma, R.S.K., Sumita, S., Zulkifli, I. and Razeen-Mazlan, A. (1999). Male genital organs and accessory glands of the lesser mouse deer, *Tragulus javanicus*. *Journal of Mammalogy*, 80(1), 199–204.

Viring, S., Einarsson, S., Nicander, L. and Larsson, K. (1980). Localization of the sperm 'reservoir' at the uterotubal junction of the pig. *Proceedings of the 9th International Congress on Animal Reproduction and Artificial Insemination*, Madrid, 5, 224–227.

Von Koenigswald, W.F. (1979). Ein lemurenrest aus dem oezanen Olschiefer der grube messel bei Darmstadt. *Palaeontologische Zeitschift*, 53, 63–76.

Vorhies, C.T. and Taylor, W.P. (1933). The Life Histories and Ecology of Jack Rabbits, *Lepus alleni* and *Lepus californicus*, in Relation to Grazing in Arizona. University of Arizona, College of Agriculture, Technical Bulletin No. 49, 1-587.

Vyas, S., Sharma, N., Sheikh, F.D., Sena, D.S. and Bissa, U.K. (2015). Reproductive status of *Camelus bactrianus* during early breeding season in India. *Asian Pacific Journal of Reproduction*, 4(1), 61–64.

Wallach, S.J.R. and Hart, B.L. (1983). The role of the striated penile muscles of the male rat in seminal plug dislodgement and deposition. *Physiology and Behavior*, 31, 815–821.

Wallage, A., Clarke, L., Thomas, L., Pyne, M., Beard, L., *et al.* (2015). Advances in captive breeding and reproductive biology of the short-beaked echidna (*Tachyglossus aculeatus*). *Australian Journal of Zoology*, 63, 181–191.

Walther, F.R. (1984). *Communication and Expression in Hoofed Animals*. Bloomington, IN: Indiana University Press.

Walton, A. (1960). Copulation and natural insemination. In *Marshall's Physiology of Reproduction, Vol. 1, Part 2*. Third edn, ed. A.S. Parkes. London: Longman, pp. 130–160.

Warburton, N.M., Bateman, P.W. and Fleming, P.A. (2019). Anatomy of the cavernosus muscles of the kangaroo penis highlights marsupial–placental dichotomy. *Journal of Anatomy*, 234, 306–315.

Warren, R.J., Vogelsang, R.W., Kirkpatrick, R.L. and Scanlon, P.F. (1978). Reproductive behaviour of captive white-tailed deer. *Animal Behaviour*, 26, 179–183.

Waser, P.M. and Waser, M.S. (1985). *Ichneumia albicauda* and the evolution of viverrid gregariousness. *Zeitschrift für Tierpsychologie*, 68, 137–151.

Waterman, J.M. (1998). Mating tactics of male Cape ground squirrels, *Xerus inauris*: consequences of year-round breeding. *Animal Behaviour*, 56, 459 466.

Waterman, J. (2007). Male mating strategies in rodents. In *Rodent Societies: an Ecological and Evolutionary Perspective*, eds. J.O. Wolff and P.W. Sherman. Chicago, IL: Chicago University Press, pp. 27–41.

Watkins, J.F. (1990). Observations of an aquatic grey seal (*Halichoerus grypus*) mating. *Journal of Zoology, London*, 222, 677–680.

Watson, J.W. (1964). Mechanism of erection and ejaculation in the bull and ram. *Nature*, 204, 95–96.

Watson, M. (1872). Contributions to the anatomy of the Indian elephant (*Elephas indicus*), Part II. Urinary and generative organs. *Journal of Anatomy and Physiology, London*, 7, 60–70.

Weimann, B., Edwards, M.A. and Jass, C.N. (2014). Identification of the baculum in American pika (*Ochotona princeps*: Lagomorpha) from southwestern Alberta, Canada. *Journal of Mammalogy*, 95(2), 284–289.

Weir, B.J. (1971). The reproductive organs of the female plains viscacha (*Lagostomus maximus*). *Journal of Reproduction and Fertility*, 25, 365–373.

Weir, B.J. (1974). Reproductive characteristics of hystrichomorph rodents. In *The Biology of Hystrichomorph Rodents*, eds. I.W. Rowlands and B.J. Weir. *Symposia of the Zoological Society of London*, 34, 265–301.

Weir, B.J. and Rowlands, I.W. (1973). Reproductive strategies of mammals. *Annual Review of Ecology and Systematics*, 4, 139–163.

Weisbecker, V. and Beck, R.M.D. (2015). Marsupial and monotreme evolution and biogeography. In *Marsupials and Monotremes*, eds. A. Klieve, L. Hogan, S. Johnston and P. Murray. New York: Nova Science Publishers, pp. 1–31.

Wellings, K., Field, J., Johnson, A.M. and Wadsworth, J. (1994). *Sexual Behaviour in Britain*. London: Penguin Books.

Wells, K., Hamede, R.K., Kerlin, D.H., Storfer, A., Hohenlohe, P.A., *et al.* (2017). Infection of the fittest: devil facial tumour disease has greatest effect on individuals with highest reproductive output. *Ecology Letters*, 20, 770–778.

Wemmer, C. and Murtaugh, J. (1981). Behavior and reproduction in the binturong, *Arctis binturong*. *Journal of Mammalogy*, 62(2), 342–352.

Werdelin, L. and Nilsonne, A. (1999). The evolution of the scrotum and testicular descent in mammals. *Journal of Theoretical Biology*, 196(1), 61–72.

Wharton, C.H. (1950). Notes on the life history of the flying lemur. *Journal of Mammalogy*, 31(3), 269–273.

White, L.M., Hosack, D.A., Warren, R.J. and Fayrer-Hosken, R.A. (1995). Influence of mating on duration of estrus in captive white-tailed deer. *Journal of Mammalogy*, 76, 1159–1163.

Whitehead, H. (2003). *Sperm Whales: Social Evolution in the Ocean.* Chicago, IL: The University of Chicago Press.

Whitford, D., Fanning, F.D. and White, A.W. (1982). Some information on reproduction, growth and development in *Planigale gilesi* (Dasyuridae, Marsupialia). In *Carnivorous Marsupials, Vol. 1,* ed. M. Archer. Sydney: Royal Society of New South Wales, pp. 77–81.

Whitsett, J.M., Ayer, M.L. and Muse, K.E. (1980). Androgenic control of phallic papillae in hamsters: a quantitative analysis using the scanning electron microscope. *Biology of Reproduction*, 23, 669–676.

Wible, J.R., Rougier, G.W., Novacek, M.J. and Asher, R.J. (2007). Cretaceous eutherians and Laurasian origin for placental mammals near the K/T boundary. *Nature*, 447, 1003–1006.

Widdig, A., Bercovitch, F.B., Streich, W.J., Sauermann, U., Nürnberg, P., *et al.* (2004). Longitudinal analysis of reproductive skew in male rhesus monkeys. *Proceedings of the Royal Society of London, B*, 271, 819–826.

Wight, H.M. (1931). Reproduction in the eastern skunk (*Mephitis mephitis nigra*). *Journal of Mammalogy*, 12, 42–47.

Wildt, D.E., Seager, S.W.J. and Chakraborty, P.K. (1980). Effect of copulatory stimuli on incidence of ovulation and serum luteinizing hormone in the cat. *Endocrinology*, 107, 1212–1217.

Wildt, L., Kissler, S., Licht, P. and Becker, W. (1998). Sperm transport in the human female genital tract and its modulation by oxytocin as assessed by hysterosalpingoscintigraphy, hysterotonography, electrohysterography and Doppler sonography. *Human Reproduction Update*, 4, 655–666.

Wilkinson, G.S. and McCracken, G.F. (2003). Bats and balls: sexual selection and sperm competition in the Chiroptera. In *Bat Ecology*, eds. T.H. Kunz and M.B. Fenton. Chicago, IL: University of Chicago Press, pp. 128–155.

Williams, E.S., Thorne, E.T., Kwiatkowski, D.R., Anderson, S.L. and Lutz, K. (1991). Reproductive biology and management of black-footed ferrets (*Mustela nigripes*). *Zoo Biology*, 10, 383–398.

Williams, R. and Williams, A. (1982). The life cycle of *Antechinus swainsonii* (Dasyuridae, Marsupialia). In *Carniviorous Marsupials, Vol. 1,* ed. M. Archer. Mosman: The Royal Zoological Society of New South Wales, pp. 89–95.

Williams-Ashman, H.G., Wilson, J., Beil, R.E. and Lorand, L. (1977). Transglutaminase reactions associated with rat semen clotting system: modulation by macromolecular polyanions. *Biochemical and Biophysical Research Communications*, 79, 1192.

Williamson, T.E., Brusatte, S.L. and Wilson, G.P. (2014). The origins and early evolution of metatherian mammals: the Cretaceous record. *Zookeys*, 465, 1–76.

Wilson, D.E. (1971). Ecology of *Myotis nigricans* (Mammalia: Chiroptera) on Barro Colorado Island, Panama Canal Zone. *Journal of Zoology, London*, 163, 1–13.

Wilson, D.E. and Reeder, D.M (2005). *Mammal Species of the World: A Taxonomic and Geographic Reference.* Third edn. Baltimore, MD: Johns Hopkins University Press/ Bucknell University.

Wilson, J.R., Adler, N. and Le Boeuf, B. (1965). The effects of intromission frequency on successful pregnancy in the rat. *Proceedings of the National Academy of Sciences USA*, 53, 1392–1395.

Wimsatt, W.A. (1942). Survival of spermatozoa in the female reproductive tract of the bat. *Anatomical Record*, 83, 299–305.

Wimsatt, W.A. (1944). Further studies on the survival of spermatozoa in the female reproductive tract of the bat. *Anatomical Record*, 88, 193–204.

Wimsatt, W.A. (1945). Notes on breeding behavior, pregnancy, and parturition in some vespertilionid bats of the Eastern United States. *Journal of Mammalogy*, 26, 23–33.

Wimsatt, W.A. and Kallen, F.C. (1952). Anatomy and histophysiology of the penis of a vespertilionid bat, *Myotis lucifugus lucifugus*, with particular reference to its vascular organization. *Journal of Morphology*, 90, 415–466.

Wingfield, J.C., Whaling, C.S. and Marler, P. (1994). Communication in vertebrate aggression and reproduction: the role of hormones. In *The Physiology of Reproduction,Vol. 2*. Second edn, eds. E. Knobil and J.D. Neill. New York: Raven Press, pp. 303–342.

Winter, J.W. (1976). The Behaviour and Social Organization of the Brush-Tail Possum (*Trichosurus vulpecula*: Kerr). PhD Thesis, University of Queensland.

Wislocki, G.B. (1933). The reproductive systems. In *The Anatomy of the Rhesus Monkey*, eds. C.G. Hartman and W.L. Straus. London: Baillière, Tindall, and Cox, pp. 231–247.

Wislocki, G.B. (1936). The external genitalia of the simian primates. *Human Biology*, 8(3), 309–347.

Wistrand, H. (1974). Individual, social, and seasonal behavior of the thirteen-lined ground squirrel (*Spermophilus tridecemlineatus*). *Journal of Mammalogy*, 55, 329–347.

Wlasiuk, G. and Nachman, M.W. (2010). Promiscuity and the rate of molecular evolution of primate immunity genes. *Evolution*, 64(8), 2204–2220.

Wolfe, K.M., Robertson, H. and Bencini, H. (2000). The mating behaviour of the dibbler, *Parantechinus apicalis*, in captivity. *Australian Journal of Zoology*, 48, 541–550.

Woodall, P.F. (1995). The male reproductive system and the phylogeny of elephant shrews (Macroscelidea). *Mammal Review*, 25(1–2), 87–93.

Woodburne, M.O. and Case, J.A. (1996). Dispersal, vicariance, and the late Cretaceous to early Tertiary land mammal biogeography from South America to Australia. *Journal of Mammalian Evolution*, 3, 121–161.

Woodburne, M.O. and Zinsmeister, W.J. (1982). Fossil land mammals from Antarctica. *Science*, 218, 284–286.

Woodburne, M.O., Goin, F.J., Raigemborn, M.S., Heizler, M.G., Gelfo, J.N., *et al.* (2014). Revised timing of the South American Paleogene land mammal ages. *Journal of South American Earth Sciences*, 54, 109–119.

Wooller, R.D., Richardson, K.C., Garavanta, C.A.M., Saffer, V.M. and Bryant, K.A. (2000). Opportunistic breeding in the polyandrous honey possum, *Tarsipes rostratus. Australian Journal of Zoology*, 48, 669–680.

Woolley, P.A. (1966). Reproduction in *Antechinus* spp. and other dasyurid marsupials. In *Comparative Biology of Reproduction in Mammals*, ed. I.W. Rowlands. *Symposia of the Zoological Society of London*, 15, 281–294.

Woolley, P.A. (1982). Phallic morphology of the Australian species of *Antechinus* (Dasyuridae, Marsupialia): a new taxonomic tool? In *Carnivorous Marsupials, Vol. 2*, ed. M. Archer. Sydney: Royal Society of New South Wales, pp. 767–781.

Wright, H.M. (1931). Reproduction in the eastern skunk (*Mephitis mephitis nigra*). *Journal of Mammalogy*, 12(1), 42–47.

Wright, P.L. (1948). Breeding habits of captive long-tailed weasels (*Mustela frenata*). *The American Midland Naturalist*, 39(2), 338–344.

Wrobel, K.-H., Kujat, R. and Fehle, G. (1993). The bovine uterotubal junction: general organization and surface morphology. *Cell and Tissue Research*, 271, 227–239.

Wroblewski, E.E., Murray, C.M., Keele, B.F., Schumacher-Stankey, J.C., Hann, B.H., *et al.* (2009). Male dominance rank and reproductive success in chimpanzees, *Pan troglodytes schweinfurthii. Animal Behaviour*, 77, 873–885.

Wyss, A.R. and Flynn, J.J. (1993). A phylogenetic analysis and definition of the Carnivora. In *Mammal Phylogeny, Placentals, Vol 2*, eds. F.S. Szalay, M.J. Novacek and M.C. McKenna. New York: Springer, pp. 32–53.

Yahner, R.H. (1979). Temporal patterns in male mating behavior of captive Reeve's muntjac (*Muntiacus reevesi*). *Journal of Mammalogy*, 60(3), 560–567.

Yamaguchi, R., Muro, Y., Isotani, A., Tokuhiro, K., Takumi, K., *et al.* (2009). Disruption of ADAM3 impairs the migration of sperm into oviduct in mouse. *Biology of Reproduction*, 81, 142–146.

Yanagimachi, R. (1970). The movement of golden hamster spermatozoa before and after capacitation. *Journal of Reproduction and Fertility*, 23, 193–196.

Yanagimachi, R. (1994). Mammalian fertilization. In *The Physiology of Reproduction, Vol. 1.* Second edn, eds. E. Knobil and J.D. Neill. New York: Raven Press, pp. 189–317.

Young, W.C. and Grunt, J.A. (1951). Pattern and measurement of sexual behavior in the male guinea pig. *Journal of Comparative and Physiological Psychology*, 44, 492–500.

Yudin, A.I., Hanson, F.W. and Katz, D.F. (1989). Human cervical mucus and its interaction with sperm: a fine-structural view. *Biology of Reproduction*, 40, 661–671.

Yunes, R.M. and Castro-Vazquez, A. (1990). An unusual pattern of copulatory behavior in a South American cricetid: *Akodon molinae. Journal of Comparative Psychology*, 104(3), 263–267.

Zahn, A. and Dippel, B. (1997). Male roosting habits and mating behaviour of *Myotis myotis. Journal of Zoology, London*, 243, 659–674.

Zarrow, M.X. and Clark, J.H. (1968). Ovulation following vaginal stimulation in a spontaneous ovulator and its implications. *Journal of Endocrinology*, 40, 343–352.

Zeng, Z., Song. Y.-L. and Zhang, Q. (2011). Copulatory pattern and behavior in a semi-captive population of Eld's deer. *Current Zoology*, 57(3), 284–292.

Zhang, F., Yu, Y., Yu, J., Wu, S., Li, S., *et al.* (2020). Reproductive behavior of the captive Sunda pangolin (*Manis javanica* Desmarest,1822). *Zoo Biology*, 39(2), 65–72. doi:10.1002/zoo.21526

Zhou, T., Wang, G., Chen, M., Zhang, M., Guo, Y., *et al.* (2015). Comparative analysis of macaque and human sperm proteomes: insights into sperm competition. *Proteomics*, 15, 1564–1573.

Index

Printed in the United States
by Baker & Taylor Publisher Services